CUSTODY, CARE & CRIMINALITY

CUSTODY, CARE & CRIMINALITY

FORENSIC PSYCHIATRY AND LAW IN 19TH CENTURY IRELAND

BRENDAN KELLY

The
History
Press
Ireland

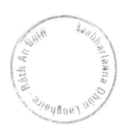
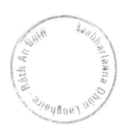

This book is dedicated to my parents, sisters and niece

First published 2014

The History Press Ireland
50 City Quay
Dublin 2
Ireland
www.thehistorypress.ie

© Brendan Kelly 2014

British Library Cataloguing in Publication Data.
A catalogue record for this book is available from the British Library.

ISBN 978 1 84588 829 9

Typesetting and origination by The History Press

Contents

Foreword

It is a pleasure to welcome the reader to this treasure trove of material assembled and analysed by Professor Brendan Kelly from primary sources in Irish hospital archives. Professor Kelly has gone beyond the nineteenth century, delving back into the 1700s and forwards into the twentieth century. Professor Kelly has drawn together the archives of the Irish asylums, case notes and committee minutes, to allow the reader to understand how this extraordinary mass confinement grew and declined. This is an important book for anyone interested in the real history of asylums, the management of mental health services and the care of the severely mentally ill and incapacitated. Those preparing syllabuses at undergraduate or postgraduate level will find this book valuable as a starting point for seminars on care, culture and compassion in mental health services, on mental health law and human rights.

What can the non-historian learn from this review? Professor Kelly raises a number of questions that are familiar, and some that are not.

WERE THE CALCULATIONS WRONG?

Was there a real increase in the number of new cases of severe mental illness in Ireland between the beginning of the eighteenth and end of the nineteenth centuries? Professor Kelly identifies distinguished writers such as Tuke (1894) and Conolly Norman, the forerunners of modern psychiatric epidemiology, who carefully calculated the increasing number of persons detained on the grounds of (legal) insanity in Ireland and concluded that there was a real increase in such disorders in Ireland over the course of the eighteenth and nineteenth centuries. They can be forgiven for confusing legal categories with clinical reality. The means of making such calculations were still being developed. National census data had been compiled from about 1821 onwards and Durkheim in France began calculating population-based suicide rates and the related confounding factors only from the 1890s. Hacking has reviewed the emergence of our modern understanding of probability and risk at about that time.[1]

THE FAMINE 1845–1852

Did the asylums increase in size so dramatically in Ireland because of the famine? They also increased in England, though not to the same extent. Was the growth of asylum care due to urbanisation and the loss of family cohesion and supports? Not in Ballinasloe or the other west of Ireland asylums.[2] Was it due to emigration, leaving the mentally incapacitated behind? This at least is a possible explanation for some of the growth in the numbers dependent on asylums, but as Professor Kelly shows in this excellent book, there are many other factors that may be relevant also.

How would a modern epidemiologist think about the famine and its consequences? The famine in Ireland might have created a dispossessed generation of physically impaired and mentally traumatised survivors.

Biological factors may have contributed to a real increase in severe mental illness. Starvation in utero would produce a generation reaching adulthood in the decades after the famine with impaired intellectual function and vulnerabilities to schizophrenia and other mental illnesses. Pelvic disproportion due to childhood malnutrition might have caused a second generation burdened with birth injury presenting four or five decades after the famine. Even in modern times, birth injury has been described as part of the diathesis for schizophrenia.[3] However, these are only speculations.

CULTURE AND WELFARE

It would be no surprise that the famine and the evictions around the same time should lead to transgenerational welfare dependence. In Ireland two factors may have limited this – the ease of emigration for those who were capable, and the lack of any welfare system on which the incapable could depend, other than the work houses and asylums. This was acknowledged in what may have been a satirical sketch by John Millington Synge who recounts a conversation with a woman in Wicklow, sometime around the end of the nineteenth century –

In Wicklow, as in the rest of Ireland, the union, though it is a home of refuge for the tramps and tinkers, is looked on with supreme horror by the peasants. The madhouse, which they know better, is less dreaded …

'My brother Michael has come back to his own place after being seven years in the Richmond Asylum; but what can you ask of him, and he with a long family of his own? And, indeed, it's a wonder he ever came back when it was a fine time he had in the asylum.'

She saw my movement of surprise and went on:

'There was a son of my own, as fine a lad as you'd see in the county – though I'm his mother that says it, and you'd never think it to look at me. Well, he was a keeper in a kind of private asylum, I think they call it, and when Michael was taken bad, he went to see him, and didn't he know the keepers that were in charge of him, and they promised to take the best of care of him, and, indeed, he was always a quiet man that would give no trouble. After the first three years he was free in the place, and he walking about like a gentleman, doing any light work he'd find agreeable. Then my son went to see him a second time, and 'You'll never see Michael again,' says he when he comes back, 'for he's too well off where he is.' And, indeed, it was well for him, but now he's come home.[4]

RURAL DEPOPULATION, URBAN DRIFT

The subdivision of small holdings by the law of inheritance up to the time of the famine and the evictions that followed it forced the numerous offspring of Irish families to leave the land. Elsewhere in Europe a drift from rural areas to cities was actively facilitated by urban growth and the need for labour in industrial centres. Since there was no industrialisation and little urban growth in Ireland, the young and fit went to industrial centres abroad. Those not fit for emigration gravitated towards the workhouses and asylums. In industrialised countries such as England the urbanised poor had subsistence work and access to a market in rented or social accommodation of a decent standard – they did not have the same expectation of inheritance, of property rights and of a living. The urban disabled could share in what was available without threatening any right of succession, where none was expected. Emigration, for the Irish brought up on a small holding, was a liberation. In Ireland, the only market in rented accommodation was the crowded tenements of Dublin.[5] Paradoxically, family cohesion may have been easier in urban centres abroad than in rural Ireland.

CYCLES OF ASYLUM REFORM AND REGRESSION

The asylums described by Professor Kelly appear to veer cyclically from enlightened and humane 'moral' regimes to custodial and impoverished, and were often inherently lacking in relational care. Asylums were at times designed as places of utopian idealism.[6] The early asylum doctors regarded the design and management of their hospitals as a scientific project,[7,8] as science was understood in their day. The careful description of the roles and duties of all those working in an asylum accords with modern interests in the distinction between care and custody.[9] Relational care is that therapeutic alliance between clinicians and patients that is now recognised as central to recovery. It is the antithesis of custodial control. Why are asylums characterised by cycles of idealism and enlightenment, followed by custodial repression, followed by further cycles of reform and regression? Professor Kelly records the 'moral' humanitarian hospital regime of Dr William Saunders Hallaran in the early years of the nineteenth century in Cork, where he was medical superintendent from 1789 to 1825, as was prevalent also in England, the USA and elsewhere. This was followed by unrestrained growth and regressive, custodial care in the aftermath of the famine. By the 1930s the Inspector's reports on conditions in the Cork asylum described oppressive, unhygienic and impoverished facilities and custodial practices. Dr Robert MacCarthy[10] was medical superintendent at Our Ladies Hospital, Cork from 1961 where he had to reform the 'existing regime of institutional care ... abolishing padded cells and straitjackets ... injected a dose of humanity into what was a harsh environment inherited from Victorian times.'

In Dublin, reform took hold again around the turn of the nineteenth and twentieth centuries with Conolly Norman in Dublin (medical superintendent of the Richmond Asylum Grangegorman 1886–1908), followed by Dunne's reforms (1937–1966) at the same hospital after a further period of regression during the Second World War or 'emergency'. To these reformers could be added Blake in Carlow.[11] Yet by the late 1970s when I first visited Grangegorman as a medical student it was in such a state of decay that closure seemed the only possible course. Closure eventually occurred – in 2013.

Clearly Hallaran's work in Cork had not taken hold, any more than the work of Conolly Norman or Dunne had in Grangegorman. The prolonged recession of the 1970s and '80s led to further set-backs. Why did the asylums grow, and even more to the point, why did they regress from the idealistic havens of moral therapy and humanitarian care, to custodial and neglected places in what appear to have been regular cycles? Simple economic strictures, cycles of public expenditure and austerity, are probably the most obvious explanation.

Table 1 in chapter 2 shows the very low ratio of doctors to patients across all asylums in 1906, and the ratio of ward-based staff was likely to be as low in modern terms. The asylums therefore had to rely on security procedures and physical structures – walls, locked doors and the like, to maintain a safe environment for the patients and for the staff. This has been the downfall of hospital care in all eras. When well-resourced, it is easy to provide a caring and therapeutic service. In times of austerity it is easy to cut staff numbers while increasing bed numbers – doing more for less – though the quality of what is done falls to the point of toxicity. It is a recurrent feature of the history of asylums that in every generation the culture of custody re-emerged and smothered the culture of care. Lack of resources and lack of public esteem will inevitably lead to this regression.

The failure to distinguish between three types of performance moni-toring for psychiatric hospitals may have permitted this cycle of regression and regeneration. First, inspectors charged with the enforcement of absolute compliance with legal rules (and the power to punish non-compliance) have not been in a position to encourage quality initiatives and standards. This second type of performance monitoring to improve quality and minimise risk requires cycles of audit and improvement programmes that always require trust and openness, not the fear of censure. Third, the commissioners of public mental health services generally seek cost efficiency over clinical effectiveness, and will generally prefer customer satisfaction over clinical effectiveness.

POLICY DEVELOPMENT, LEGAL REFORM AND UNINTENDED CONSEQUENCES

Ireland after independence did not continue the pattern of frequent parliamentary reports and Royal Commissions that continuously drove the steady evolution of policy in the UK. Professor Kelly documents the many such reports that modernised Irish mental health legislation up to the first years of the twentieth century. Taking the UK as one example, mental health policy continued to progress before and after the Second World War. On the subject of forensic psychiatry alone the London Parliament published the Emery Report (1961)[12] on high secure hospitals, the Glancy Report (1974) and the Butler Report (1975)[13] on the need for local and regional secure hospitals to fill the gap left between the old asylums and the new open units in district general hospitals. The Reid Report (1995)[14] set out the rights of detained patients to high-quality services. All of these led to real change in policy, legislation and service provision.[15] Similar developments in modern forensic psychiatric services could be traced in the Netherlands and other modern European states, in Canada and Australia. These were seen as a necessary counterbalance to the rapid development of community care in the interests of a comprehensive mental health service in order to include those too disturbed or challenging for community treatment. In Ireland, the prison population grew as the asylums shrank[16] and the mentally ill gravitated towards prisons, as happened throughout the developed world, though to a much greater extent[17] because the counterbalances implemented elsewhere in the 1980s and 1990s did not happen in Ireland.

Yet there were government reports and policy papers in the new state too. Professor Kelly summarises a 1927 Report of the Commission on the Relief of the Sick and Destitute Poor including the Insane Poor[18] that recommended the repeal of the many scattered pieces of legislation inherited from the former regime, to be replaced with a single amending and consolidating Act. A 1933 Committee of Investigation added weight to this. The result was the adoption of recommendations from a 1903 Conference of Irish Asylums Committee and the eventual Mental Treatment Act of 1945, which failed to do anything about the various pieces of legislation regarding insanity or transfers from prisons to hospitals and failed to properly establish the status of 'voluntary' patients. The 1945 Act established an Inspector of Mental Hospitals, but the annual reports of the inspector were not published for several years up to 1987. There followed a Commission of Inquiry on Mental Illness (1966)[19] and an embarrassing sequence of delays (Green Paper on Mental Health 1992, White Paper: A New Mental Health Act 1995) and false starts that came to nothing (Mental Treatment Act 1961, Health (Mental Services) Act 1981 and Disability Act 2005), and policy documents (Planning for the Future 1984[20] and Vision for Change 2006[21]) that have made very slow progress. The introduction of new legislation, the Mental Health Act of 2001 and the Criminal Law (Insanity) Act of 2006 has produced real change, but more is required.

While policy led law reform elsewhere, in Ireland law reform often appeared disconnected from or even drove policy and practice, though often because of unintended consequences. The Criminal Lunatics (Ireland) Act of 1838 gave the power to justices of the peace to detain 'dangerous lunatics' without any medical certification. This probably drove much of the growth of the asylums from that date until the Mental Treatment Act of 1945 restored medical control over diagnosis and admission.[22] Contrary to modern expectations, this restoration of medical control was associated with a decline in hospitalisation.[17] Yet the Criminal Law (Insanity) Act 2006 attempted to re-introduce judicial detention without medical certification for those unfit to stand trial. This was only partially reformed in 2010, and only because it was so obviously contrary to the case law of the European Court of Human Rights.[23]

MENTAL HEALTH POLICY IN NATIONAL AND INTERNATIONAL CONTEXT

Dr Dermot Walsh, who was a major influence on the policy makers of the Commission of Inquiry on Mental Illness in 1966, Planning for the Future in 1984 and Vision for Change in 2006, drew attention in 1989 to the misuse of mental health services as local employment schemes.[24] This situation persists. Rural services, with less psychiatric morbidity, have disproportionate resources, while the 'new' urban centres are under-provided and rely disproportionately on the prisons and forensic hospital beds.[25] This political use of one public service to achieve the ends of an unrelated policy, usually regionalism, can be seen as part of a broader pattern in Irish policy and public services, with rejected attempts at regional development policies[26] and inefficient decentralisation of public services.[27]

Ireland was not only slow to modernise mental health services. The British Government published and quickly acted on the Wolfenden Report on Homosexual Offences (1957) as did most other western democracies while in Ireland, only action in the courts and eventually the European Court of Human Rights (1988)[28] produced change in Irish legislation (in 1993).[29] In a more general sense, the governance of the new republic after independence was often inward-looking, reluctant to embrace change and slow to adapt to modernity.[30]

In mental health legislation and service development, it could be argued that it was the European Convention on Human Rights, the European Court of Human Rights[31] and its enforcement agency, the Council of Europe Committee for the Prevention of Torture and Inhumane or Degrading Treatment or Punishment (The Committee for the Prevention of Torture)[32] that has driven the passage of the Mental Health Act 2001, the Criminal Law (Insanity) Act 2006 and 2010, and the still awaited Mental Capacity and Assisted Decision Making Bill. The Criminal Law (Insanity) Acts still fall far short of the reform and consolidation recommended in the 1927 Report,[33] or the 1959 Mental Health Act for England and Wales. The European Union's increasing interest in medical services including mental health[34] may eventually become a further impetus for common standards across the European Union, a development that could not come soon enough if further cycles of reform, stagnation and regression are to be avoided.

THE END OF HISTORY?

Many of the most enlightened reformers of mental health services in recent decades have come to the view that hospital care for any but the shortest periods of time leads inevitably to custodial and harmful care. The only long-term, certain way of preventing the cyclical deterioration of hospital services would be to close all such hospitals. But there is no denying the natural history of severe mental illnesses and other mental incapacities. Those who, because of their illnesses or developmental disorders, are prone to harming others or themselves will need the professional protection of others and protection for the sake of others including their own families and communities. Such persons continue to accumulate in the prisons[35] and although much can be done with modern enhanced prison mental health services,[36,37] these should be seen only as reactions, not as effective solutions. Prison custody for the severely mentally ill is not an intended consequence or a part of modern community mental health policy. Detention and compulsory treatment under mental health legislation, continuing now at the Central Mental Hospital in Dundrum for over 160 years, can be seen from an ideological point of view as paternalistic, discriminatory and more objectively, vulnerable to regression. But safe, therapeutic and humane hospital care followed by structured community care will always be needed for the most severely disturbed and challenging who are mentally incapacitated and mentally disabled, often for prolonged periods. A well-organised, secure hospital must be well-resourced[38] to remain oriented towards care and recovery. It would be better for the future to recognise the pressures that occur during economic recessions and avoid the pit-falls of a return to custodial care by providing fewer, more intensively staffed hospital and community places rather than more but impoverished places.

Harry Kennedy BSc, MB BCh BAO, MD, FRCPI, FRCPsych
Consultant Forensic Psychiatrist and Executive Clinical Director, National
Forensic Mental Health Service, Central Mental Hospital, Dundrum, Dublin
and Clinical Professor of Forensic Psychiatry, Trinity College Dublin.

Acknowledgements

Much of the research that informs this book was performed in the archives of the Central Mental Hospital (previously Central Criminal Lunatic Asylum), Dundrum, Dublin, Ireland. I am deeply grateful for the support of Professor Harry Kennedy of the National Forensic Psychiatry Service throughout this project. I also greatly appreciate his foreword to this book.

This book is primarily based on sixteen published, peer-reviewed research papers on psychiatric history. These papers, along with a 15,000-word critical appraisal, constituted my PhD in history (by means of published works) at the University of Northampton, England in 2011. I am very grateful for the supervision of Dr Cathy Smith (First Supervisor) and Professor Jon Stobart (Director of Studies) at the School of Social Sciences (History) in the University of Northampton. Their encouragement and supervision were crucial factors in completing my PhD and contextualising my archival and historical research work.

I also wish to acknowledge the educational influences of my colleagues in clinical and academic psychiatry, the doctors, nurses, social workers, occupational therapists, psychologists, lecturers, administrators and students with whom I work. I am very grateful for the assistance and support of Dr Larkin Feeney, Dr John Bruzzi and Mr Gerry Devine of the (HSE). In addition, I have benefitted enormously from my contact with mental health service-users and their families, carers, advocates and legal advisors.

I am very grateful to Professor Sharlene Walbaum, her family, colleagues and students at Quinnipiac University, Connecticut. Shar's wisdom, enthusiasm and hospitality have added greatly to my historical work.

I greatly appreciate the teaching and guidance of my teachers at Scoil Chaitríona (Renmore, Galway) and St Joseph's Patrician College, Galway, especially Mr Ciaran Doyle (my history teacher, now principal) who conveyed a genuine enthusiasm for history to me. I also owe a debt of gratitude to my teachers and supervisors at the School of Medicine in the National University of Ireland, Galway.

Most of all, I appreciate deeply the support of my wife (Regina), children (Eoin and Isabel), parents (Mary and Desmond), sisters (Sinéad and Niamh) and niece (Aoife) throughout all of my academic and publishing endeavours.

PUBLICATION ACKNOWLEDGEMENTS AND PERMISSIONS

All reasonable efforts have been made to contact the copyright holders for text used in this book. If any omissions are brought to my attention, appropriate acknowledgement will be included in any future editions of this work.

Quotations from 'Modern Psycho-therapy and out Asylums' by E. Boyd Barrett (*Studies* 1924: 8: 29-43) are reproduced by kind permission of the editor of *Studies: An Irish Quarterly Review*.

Quotations from the Official Report of Dáil Éireann and Official Report of Seanad Éireann are Copyright Houses of Oireachtas.

Quotations from *The Irish Times* are used by kind permission of *The Irish Times*. Quotations from the *Journal of Mental Science* are used by kind permission of the Royal College of Psychiatrists.

Introduction material was drawn from:

Kelly, B.D., 'Poverty, Crime and Mental Illness: Female Forensic Psychiatric Committal in Ireland, 1910-1948', *Social History of Medicine* (2008; 21 (2): 311-28), used with kind permission of Oxford University Press who publish *Social History of Medicine* on behalf of The Society for the Social History of Medicine

Kelly, B.D., 'Criminal Insanity in Nineteenth-Century Ireland, Europe and the United States: Cases, Contexts and Controversies', *International Journal of Law and Psychiatry*, (2009; 32: 362–8), used with kind

permission of Elsevier. www.sciencedirect.com/science/article/pii/
S0160252709001046

Kelly, B.D., 'Intellectual Disability, Mental Illness and Offending Behaviour:
Forensic Cases from Early Twentieth-Century Ireland', *Irish Journal
of Medical Science* (2010; 179: 409–16), used with kind permission
from Springer Science+Business Media: *Irish Journal of Medical Science*,
Intellectual disability, mental illness and offending behaviour: forensic
cases from early twentieth-century Ireland, Volume 79, Year of publication:
2010, Pages: 409–16, Author: Brendan D. Kelly

Material for Chapter 1 was drawn from:

Kelly, B.D., 'Dr William Saunders Hallaran and Psychiatric Practice in
Nineteenth-Century Ireland', *Irish Journal of Medical Science* (2008; 177:
79–84), used with kind permission from Springer Science+Business
Media: *Irish Journal of Medical Science*, Dr William Saunders Hallaran and
Psychiatric Practice in Nineteenth-Century Ireland, Volume: 177, Year of
publication: 2008, Pages: 79–84, Author: Brendan D. Kelly

Kelly, B.D., 'Mental Illness in Nineteenth Century Ireland: A Qualitative
Study of Workhouse Records', *Irish Journal of Medical Science* (2004; 173:
53–5), used with kind permission from Springer Science+Business Media:
Irish Journal of Medical Science, Mental Illness in Nineteenth Century
Ireland: A Qualitative Study of Workhouse Records, Volume 173, Year of
publication: 2004, Pages 53–5, Author: Brendan D. Kelly

Material for Chapter 2 was drawn from:

Kelly, B.D., 'Mental Health Law in Ireland, 1821–1902: Building the Asylums',
Medico-Legal Journal (2008; 76: 19–25), used with kind permission of
SAGE Publications Ltd. http://mlj.sagepub.com/content/76/1/19.full.
pdf+html

Kelly, B.D., 'Mental Health Law in Ireland, 1821–1902: Dealing with the
"Increase of Insanity in Ireland"', *Medico-Legal Journal* (2008; 76: 26–33),
used with kind permission of SAGE Publications Ltd. http://mlj.sagepub.
com/content/76/1/26.full.pdf+html

Kelly, B.D., 'One Hundred Years Ago: The Richmond Asylum, Dublin
in 1907', *Irish Journal of Psychological Medicine* (2008; 24: 108–14), used
with kind permission of MedMedia Group and with the agreement
of Cambridge University Press, current publisher of the *Irish Journal of
Psychological Medicine* on behalf of the College of Psychiatrists of Ireland.

Kelly, B.D., 'Criminal Insanity in Nineteenth-Century Ireland, Europe and
the United States: Cases, Contexts and Controversies', *International Journal*

of Law and Psychiatry (2009; 32: 362–8) used with kind permission of Elsevier. www.sciencedirect.com/science/article/pii/S0160252709001046

Material for Chapter 3 was drawn from:

Kelly, B.D., 'Clinical and Social Characteristics of Women Committed to Inpatient Forensic Psychiatric Care in Ireland, 1868–1908', *Journal of Forensic Psychiatry and Psychology* (2008; 19: 261–73), reprinted by permission of the publisher, Taylor & Francis Ltd, http://www.tandf.co.uk/journals/

Kelly, B.D., 'Poverty, Crime and Mental Illness: Female Forensic Psychiatric Committal in Ireland, 1910–1948', *Social History of Medicine* (2008; 21(2): 311–28), used with kind permission of Oxford University Press who publish *Social History of Medicine* on behalf of The Society for the Social History of Medicine

Kelly, B.D., 'Murder, Mercury, Mental Illness: Infanticide in Nineteenth Century Ireland', *Irish Journal of Medical Science* (2007; 176: 149–52), used with kind permission from Springer Science+Business Media: *Irish Journal of Medical Science*, Murder, Mercury, Mental Illness: Infanticide in Nineteenth Century Ireland, Volume: 176, Year of publication: 2007, Pages: 149–52, Author: Brendan D. Kelly

Material for Chapter 4 was drawn from:

Kelly, B.D., 'Folie à Plusieurs: Forensic Cases from Nineteenth-Century Ireland', *History of Psychiatry* (2009; 20: 47–60), used with kind permission of SAGE Publications Ltd. http://hpy.sagepub.com/content/20/1/47. abstract. I am also very grateful for the suggestions of Professor GE Berrios of the Department of Psychiatry, University of Cambridge, United Kingdom in relation to this paper. Quotations are reproduced by kind permission of the Royal College of Psychiatrists

Kelly, B.D., 'Learning Disability and Forensic Mental Healthcare in Nineteenth-Century Ireland', *Irish Journal of Psychological Medicine* (2008; 25: 116–8), used with kind permission of MedMedia Group and with the agreement of Cambridge University Press, current publisher of the *Irish Journal of Psychological Medicine*, on behalf of the College of Psychiatrists of Ireland

Kelly, B.D., 'Intellectual Disability, Mental Illness and Offending Behaviour: Forensic Cases from Early Twentieth-Century Ireland', *Irish Journal of Medical Science* (2010; 179: 409–16), used with kind permission from Springer Science+Business Media: *Irish Journal of Medical Science*, Intellectual disability, mental illness and offending behaviour: forensic cases from early twentieth-century Ireland, Volume 79, Year of publication 2010, Pages: 409–16, Author: Brendan D. Kelly

Kelly, B.D., 'Syphilis, Psychiatry and Offending Behaviour: Clinical Cases from Nineteenth-Century Ireland', *Irish Journal of Medical Science* (2009; 178: 73–7), used with kind permission from Springer Science+Business Media: *Irish Journal of Medical Science*, Syphilis, Psychiatry and Offending Behaviour: Clinical Cases from Nineteenth-Century Ireland, Volume: 178, Year of publication: 2009, Pages: 73–7

Material for Chapter 5 was drawn from:

Kelly, B.D., 'The Mental Treatment Act 1945 in Ireland: An Historical Enquiry', *History of Psychiatry* (2008; 19: 47–67), used with kind permission of SAGE Publications Ltd. http://hpy.sagepub.com/content/19/1/47.abstract

Kelly, B.D., 'Physical Sciences and Psychological Medicine: The Legacy of Prof John Dunne', *Irish Journal of Psychological Medicine* (2005; 22: 67–72), used with kind permission of MedMedia Group and with the agreement of Cambridge University Press, current publisher of the *Irish Journal of Psychological Medicine*, on behalf of the College of Psychiatrists of Ireland. Professor John Dunne's Presidential Address was delivered to annual meeting of the Royal Medico-Psychological Association (RMPA), the forerunner of the Royal College of Psychiatrists, on 13 July 1955 and was reprinted in the *Journal of Mental Science* in the following year (Dunne, J., 'The Contribution of the Physical Sciences to Psychological Medicine', *Journal of Mental Science* (1956; 102: 209–20)). Quotations from that paper are reprinted with the kind permission of the Royal College of Psychiatrists, and with the consent of Dr David Dunne. The author is grateful for the co-operation of the Royal College of Psychiatrists and Dr David Dunne.

Kelly, B.D., 'Mental Health Law in Ireland, 1945 to 2001: Reformation and Renewal', *Medico-Legal Journal* (2008; 76: 65–72), used with kind permission of SAGE Publications Ltd. http://mlj.sagepub.com/content/76/2/65.full.pdf+html

Introduction

In the early 1890s, Henry, a 77-year-old farmer, was charged with murder, declared insane, and detained 'at the Lord Lieutenant's pleasure' (i.e. indefinitely) in the Central Criminal Lunatic Asylum in Dundrum, Dublin, Ireland's only inpatient forensic psychiatry hospital, designed for individuals with mental disorder who engaged in offending behaviour.[1]

On admission, Henry was diagnosed with 'chronic mania' and described as 'intemperate' (as opposed to 'sober'). The medical officer noted that Henry 'vomits frequently after his meals' and had 'some chronic intestinal trouble but I am unable to discover the exact nature thereof'.

Seven years after admission, 'this impulsive old man' was 'delicate and losing strength' , 'very weakly' and 'confined to bed'. He was diagnosed with 'pleurisy of the left side' (i.e. chest pain) and prescribed 'whiskey, 4 ounces', but 'got rapidly worse'. A couple of days later, Henry died of a chest infection, at the age of 84 years, having spent over fifty years in various psychiatric institutions, including the Central Criminal Lunatic Asylum.

Some years later, in the early 1900s, Patricia, a 45-year-old woman from the south of Ireland was charged with the murder of a child. Owing to her mental state, she was, like Henry, detained indefinitely at the Central Criminal Lunatic Asylum.[2]

Admission notes record that Patricia 'formerly lived with her brother who is a farmer … She threw his child aged nine months into a pond and drowned it'. There was, however, little evidence that Patricia was suffering from mental disorder on admission and considerable evidence that her chief problem was intellectual disability. Clinical notes recorded that Patricia 'lacks intelligence and has evidently been weak-minded from birth. She is practically devoid of reason, speaks with difficulty and is incapable of conversing intelligently'. Seven months later, Patricia had 'given no trouble since admission' but 'seems oblivious to everything'. After five years in the Central Criminal Lunatic Asylum, Patricia was 'incapable of coherent conversation or concentrated effort'.

Occasionally, Patricia became more disturbed for periods of time. Medical notes recorded that 'she hammers on the door and shutters of her cell, whistles and in general creates as much noise as she can. Her reason for this tirade is that she is dead and wishes to get out of her coffin ... She requires large doses of paraldehyde [a medication for epilepsy, sedative or 'hypnotic'] ... ordinary hypnotics are useless ...' Despite these disturbances, Patricia continued 'to work daily in the laundry and is in good bodily health'.

Some twenty-five years after admission to the Central Criminal Lunatic Asylum, Patricia was still firmly behind the asylum walls, now suffering from epilepsy, bronchitis and influenza, as well as her ongoing features of intellectual disability and episodic mental disorder. Her future at that point was not bright: once an individual had been detained in an Irish asylum for more than five years, she or he was virtually certain to die there.[3]

This book is about people like Henry and Patricia, whose histories have been forgotten or misunderstood, and whose fates were determined by the vast, complicated asylum system that developed in Ireland over the nineteenth and early twentieth centuries. This was a time of dramatic change in Irish mental health services, with a rapid increase in asylum populations and multiple changes in legislation, including Ireland's unique criminal insanity legislation of the mid-1800s. In this book, I am concerned with the fate of the mentally ill and intellectually disabled during this period, with a particular focus on women charged with crimes, declared insane, and committed to the Central Criminal Lunatic Asylum, a remarkable institution which was later renamed the Central Mental Hospital and remains part of Ireland's forensic psychiatric services today.[4]

Forensic psychiatric services provide mental health care to individuals with mental disorder who engage in offending behaviour.[5] In most societies, both mental disorder and offending behaviour are associated with socio-economic status; mental ill-health is more common in lower socio-economic groups and individuals in lower socio-economic groups are more likely to be incarcerated for offending behaviour.[6] In addition, individuals with mental disorder are more likely to be taken into custody following an offence, compared to individuals without mental disorder.[7] As a result, rates of mental disorder in prison today are remarkably high: almost 4 per cent of prisoners have a psychotic mental disorder, while over 10 per cent have major depression.[8] Some of these individuals are today transferred from prison to modernised forensic psychiatric facilities, such as the Central Mental Hospital, for specialist care, with the result that admission profiles to forensic facilities also show a strong socio-economic gradient. In Ireland, the majority of forensic psychiatric admissions are from deprived inner-city areas with limited provision of social and health-care resources.[9]

These phenomena are not new. Incarceration has been a constant feature of the experience of mental disorder over many centuries and individuals with enduring disorders have consistently experienced social prejudice, downward 'social drift' and systematic exclusion from the social, political and economic lives of societies in which they have lived.[10] The roots of these problems are complex and likely relate to myriad factors, including the effects of mental disorder itself, specific social, political and economic circumstances, and the legal context in which prosecution, committal and incarceration occur.

In order to tell the complicated stories of people like Henry and Patricia as fully and accurately as possible, I explore their medical case histories from the archives of the Central Criminal Lunatic Asylum in a number of ways throughout this book. First, I outline the general historical background to the network of institutions in which these stories unfolded, through analysis of workhouse records, asylum committee minutes, inspectors' reports, mental health legislation, nineteenth-century textbooks and other published materials. Secondly, as both an historian and practicing psychiatrist, I integrate the material from these historical sources with careful clinical consideration of individual case records from the archives of the Central Criminal Lunatic Asylum, dating from the late 1800s to the early 1900s. In this way, historical analysis is combined with 'the clinical gaze' to integrate clinical dimension of patients' experiences with their institutional and legislative experiences of Ireland's courts and asylum system.[11]

The heart of this book lies in these case histories which explore the stories of women who killed their children, individuals who developed shared mental disorders (e.g. an entire family that developed a belief that one child was a changeling and together killed that child), individuals with intellectual disability (charged with crimes they poorly understood), individuals with syphilis (rightly or wrongly diagnosed), and many other vividly drawn cases of mental disorder, physical illness, social deprivation and crime.

For the most part, these are piercing stories of poverty, illness, crime and tragedy. However, these histories also demonstrate much that is positive, especially in the efforts of certain doctors to reform Ireland's system of institutional care and develop more humane treatments for the mentally ill and intellectually disabled. The history of this period is also much more complex than a cursory examination at first suggests, especially as the case histories presented in this book commonly demonstrate real physical and mental health need among those detained. While the asylums commonly failed to meet these needs in a comprehensive or humane way, the alternatives for these individuals included committal to workhouses or prison, or lives of vagrancy and early death. As a result, these are complicated, nuanced histories which need to be explored in context in order to determine their true lessons for reformers today.

Chapter 1 is concerned with 'Mental Health Care in Nineteenth-Century Ireland'. This chapter outlines the background to mental health care in early nineteenth-century Ireland, when many individuals with mental disorder or intellectual disability were either homeless or placed in workhouses or one of the few asylums that existed at that time. While there may have been few asylums, however, there was already great enthusiasm for new treatments for 'lunacy' within those asylums and Chapter 1 explores some of the treatments used in a particular Cork asylum, including bleeding, purging, a broad range of medications (e.g. digitalis, opium, camphor, mercury), 'moral treatment' and the infamous 'Dr Cox's Circulating Swing'. Chapter 1 also examines the fate of the large number of individuals with physical or mental disorders who entered the Irish workhouse system during the nineteenth century. This exploration is based on examination of original workhouse records and minutes from the Ballinrobe Poor Law Union, County Mayo which was located in an area especially badly affected by the Great Irish Famine (1845–52).

Against this background, Chapter 2, titled 'Creating the Asylums and the Insanity Defence', examines the emergence of Ireland's cavernous asylum system, an extraordinary creation which grew at an unprecedented rate throughout the 1800s: in 1851 there were 3,234 individuals in Irish asylums and by 1891 this had more than tripled, to 11,265.[12] While there were similar problems with high committal rates in other countries, including Britain, France, and the United States, Ireland's admission rates were especially high at their peak, and especially slow to decline.[13] Chapter 2 examines the legal underpinnings of this system, the widespread belief that insanity was increasing uniquely quickly in Ireland, and the kind of asylums that emerged from these concerns in the nineteenth and early twentieth centuries. This chapter also examines the emergence of the idea of criminal insanity in Ireland, Europe and the United States, with particular emphasis on the insanity defence, using case histories from the archives of the Central Criminal Lunatic Asylum to demonstrate specific clinical and legal issues in the Irish context.

Chapter 3 focuses on one specific group within Ireland's asylum system: 'Women in the Central Criminal Lunatic Asylum, Dublin' between 1868 and 1948. Most of the women admitted to the hospital during this period had been charged with crimes, deemed insane by the courts, and sent to the Central Criminal Lunatic Asylum for indefinite periods of custody and care. Chapter 3 uses original archival case records to examine the clinical and social characteristics of these women, and presents histories of mental disorder, social deprivation and infanticide (the killing of infants). In these discussions, I place particular emphasis on the clinical dimensions of these cases, unearthing and decoding, as best as possible at this remove, signs and symptoms of mental disorder in these women.

Chapter 4 examines, in greater depth, specific 'Clinical Aspects of Criminal Insanity in Eighteenth and Nineteenth-Century Ireland' and presents further case histories of men and women committed to the Central Criminal Lunatic Asylum in the late 1800s and early 1900s, examining both clinical and social aspects of their cases. This chapter includes cases of syphilis, intellectual disability and folie à plusieurs, an unusual disorder in which one or more delusions (fixed, false beliefs, not amenable to reason) are shared by several individuals, often within a close-knit group or family. Forensic complications of these physical and mental conditions are explored in the broader context of the clinical and social challenges these individuals and families faced.

Chapter 5 is titled 'Reformation and Renewal: Into the Twentieth Century' and concludes the book by examining the process of reform of Ireland's mental health laws and institutions in the early to mid-twentieth century. This movement found its clearest expression in the Mental Treatment Act 1945 which coincided with new enthusiasm for increasingly scientific approaches to treatment. This chapter completes the story by drawing conclusions for reformers of today, based on the case histories explored throughout the book.

A NOTE ON TERMINOLOGY

In order to maintain confidentiality, patients' names in the case histories drawn from the archives of the Central Criminal Lunatic Asylum have all been changed so as to render them unidentifiable. In all other respects, original language and terminology from the nineteenth-century records have been maintained. This represents an attempt to optimise fidelity to historical sources and does not represent an endorsement of the broader use of such terminology in contemporary settings.

1

Mental Health Care in Nineteenth-Century Ireland

INTRODUCTION

The nineteenth century was a time of significant change in mental health care in Ireland. At the start of the century, the majority of individuals with mental disorder or intellectual disability were either living with their families, homeless or placed in workhouses or one of the few asylums that existed at that time.[1]

While there may have been few asylums, there was already substantial enthusiasm for new treatments for 'lunacy' within those asylums. The first part of this chapter explores some of the treatments used in a particular Cork asylum in the early 1800s, including bleeding, purging, 'moral treatment', a broad range of medications (e.g. digitalis, opium, camphor and mercury) and the infamous 'Dr Cox's Circulating Swing'.[2]

Asylum care was, however, the exception rather than the rule at the start of the 1800s, and the second part of this chapter examines the fate of the much greater number of individuals with physical or mental disorders who entered the Irish workhouse system during the nineteenth century. This exploration is based on examination of original workhouse records and minutes from the Ballinrobe Poor Law Union, County Mayo, which was located in an area especially badly affected by the Great Famine (1845–1852).[3]

The therapeutic enthusiasm within the asylums (as demonstrated in the Cork asylum) and the difficult conditions facing the physically and mentally ill outside the asylums (as demonstrated in the Ballinrobe Workhouse) formed the background to the great asylum-building era of the 1800s, which is examined in the next chapter.

DR WILLIAM SAUNDERS HALLARAN AND PSYCHIATRIC PRACTICE IN THE EARLY 1800s

In Ireland, there was scant provision for individuals with mental disorders throughout the seventeenth and eighteenth centuries.[4] In 1817, the House of Commons (of Great Britain, then including Ireland) established a committee to investigate the plight of the mentally ill in Ireland. The committee reported a disturbing picture:

> When a strong man or woman gets the complaint [mental disorder], the only way they have to manage is by making a hole in the floor of the cabin, not high enough for the person to stand up in, with a crib over it to prevent his getting up. This hole is about five feet deep, and they give this wretched being his food there, and there he generally dies.[5]

The situation in nineteenth-century Ireland was not unique, as the majority of individuals with mental disorder in Ireland, England and many other countries lived lives of vagrancy, destitution, illness and early death.[6] Toward the end of the 1700s there were, however, signs of reform, most notably in Paris where Dr Phillipe Pinel (1745–1862) pioneered less custodial approaches to asylum care,[7] and York where William Tuke (1732–1822), an English Quaker businessman, founded the York Retreat in 1796, based on policies of care and gentleness, combined with benevolent medical supervision.[8]

These reforms were accompanied by a clear commitment to the 'moral management' paradigm of treatment.[9] This approach was based on the idea that 'insanity' found its roots in disorders of the emotions and thoughts, and that traditional medical treatment and physical restraints might not always be appropriate. The principles of moral management included the idea that the doctor should speak with the patient in a rational fashion, and the patient should have a healthy diet, exercise frequently and, where possible, engage in gainful occupation.

Jean-Étienne Dominique Esquirol (1772–1840), a French psychiatrist, described moral treatment as 'the application of the faculty of intelligence and of emotions in the treatment of mental alienation'.[10] This approach represented a significant break from the past which had emphasised custodial care rather than engagement with the patient as an individual. Today, such an approach would likely be described as 'milieu therapy' involving the establishment of therapeutic communities and a group-based approach to recovery.[11]

MENTAL HEALTH REFORM IN IRELAND

In Ireland, the leading proponent of these kinds of reforms was Dr William Saunders Hallaran, the most prominent and prolific Irish psychiatrist of the nineteenth century.[12] Born in 1765, Hallaran studied medicine at Edinburgh and spent much of his working life as Senior Physician to the South Infirmary and Physician to the House of Industry and Lunatic Asylum of Cork. Throughout his career, Hallaran was not only an industrious and progressive clinician and teacher, but also a tireless advocate for a more scientific and systematic approach to mental disorder and its treatment.

In 1810, Hallaran published the first Irish textbook of psychiatry, impressively titled *An Enquiry into the Causes Producing the Extraordinary Addition to the Number of Insane together with Extended Observations on the Cure of Insanity with Hints as to the Better Management of Public Asylums for Insane Persons.*[13] This book outlined many of the central themes that defined Hallaran's approach to the treatment of mental disorder, including:

- Recognition of physical or bodily factors (e.g. syphilis) as important causes of mental disorder
- Deep concern about the apparent increase in mental disorder in nineteenth-century Ireland, a concern which Hallaran shared with many others at that time
- Engagement with the causes, courses and outcomes of mental disorder in a more systematic fashion than was customary
- Careful reconsideration of traditional treatments, such as blood-letting, vomiting and purgatives, which were widely used during this period
- Detailed exploration of novel treatment modalities, such as 'Dr Cox's Circulating Swing'
- Careful re-evaluation of traditional medicinal remedies, such as digitalis (foxglove), opium, camphor and mercury
- Critical re-consideration of other contemporary, non-medicinal, physical treatments for insanity, such as shower baths, diet and exercise
- The role of physical factors in causing mental disorder

In the opening section of his 1810 textbook, Hallaran clearly outlined the importance of physical or bodily factors (such as infections) in causing mental disorder in many people:

A principal object of this essay is to point out what heretofore seems to have escaped the observation of authors on the subject, namely, the practical distinction between that species of insanity which can evidently be referred to mental causes, and may therefore be denominated mental insanity, and that species of nervous excitement, which, though partaking of like effects, so far as the sensorium may be engaged, still might appear to owe its origin merely to organic [i.e. physical or bodily] injury, either idiopathically [i.e. inexplicably] affecting the brain itself, or arising from a specific action of the liver, lungs or mesentry; inducing an inflammatory disposition in either, and thereby exciting in certain habits those peculiar aberrations, which commonly denote an unsound mind. That this distinction is material in the treatment of insane persons, cannot well be denied, any more than that the due observance of the causes connected with the origin of this malady, is the first step towards establishing a basis upon which a hope of recovery may be founded.[14]

This distinction between causes 'of the mind' and physical or bodily causes of mental disorder was clearly important when planning treatment:

In the mode of cure, however, I would argue the necessity of the most cautious attention to this important distinction, lest as I have often known to be the case, that the malady of the mind which is for the most part to be treated on moral principles, should be subjected to the operation of agents altogether more foreign to the purpose; and that the other of the body, arising from direct injury to one or more of the vital organs, may escape the advantages of approved remedies … this discrimination has been found to be of the highest importance where a curative indication was to be looked for, nor need there be much difficulty in forming a prognosis, where either from candid report, or from careful examination, the precise nature of the excitement shall be ascertained.

Hallaran paid particular attention to his belief in the role of the liver in causing mental disorder, recommending that 'the actual state of the liver in almost every case of mental derangement should be a primary consideration;

even though the sensorium should be largely engaged'. Hallaran concluded his textbook's opening discussion by re-emphasising both the distinction and the links between the 'sensorium' (or mind) and the body:

> Here we have sufficient evidence of the existence of insanity on the principle of mere organic [i.e. physical or bodily] lesion; holding a connection as it would appear, with the entire glandular system. Hence we may be led to suppose than an imperfect or a specific action in certain portions of this important department tends to lay the foundation of that affection, which I would under such circumstances, denominate the 'mania corporea' of Cullen; including at the same time within this species, the different varieties of the complaint as described by authors, depending upon the various causes, whether mechanical or otherwise, as affecting the sensorium, and the other important organs of the animal economy.

This opening discussion clearly outlines one of Hallaran's greatest contributions to psychiatric thinking: a clear recognition of the importance of physical or bodily factors in causing certain cases of mental disorder.[15] As he concluded this discussion, Hallaran made reference to Dr William Cullen (1710–1790), a prominent Edinburgh physician who had a substantial influence on a generation of leading asylum-doctors including Hallaran, John Ferriar, Benjamin Rush and Thomas Trotter, author of *A View of the Nervous Temperament*.[16] Cullen was the first to use the term 'neurosis' to describe various mental disorders that occurred in the absence of any physical or bodily illness. Consistent with this, Hallaran's distinction between mental factors and physical or bodily factors in causing mental disorder laid the foundation for much subsequent progress in determining the causes of insanity throughout the nineteenth and twentieth centuries.

Syphilis, for example, was a major cause of admission to psychiatric institutions throughout nineteenth-century Europe, with syphilitic 'general paralysis' accounting for over 30 per cent of voluntary admissions of men to Sainte Anne asylum in Paris between 1876 and 1914 (Chapter 3).[17] 'Syphilis-related disorders' would later be one of the three main focuses of the Würzburger Schlüssel classification of psychological disorders in Germany.[18] Hallaran gathered the first systematic data on the apparent causes of psychiatric admissions in Ireland and also found that a significant proportion of psychiatric disorders in Cork were attributable to venereal disease, including syphilis.[19] Combined with observations from Paris and elsewhere, these findings further supported the emphasis that Hallaran laid on the relevance of physical or bodily factors (such as syphilis) in causing many cases of mental disorder.

'THE EXTRAORDINARY INCREASE OF INSANITY IN IRELAND'

The next topic to concern Hallaran in his 1810 textbook was the 'cause of the extraordinary increase of insanity in Ireland':

> It has been for some few years back a subject of deep regret, as well as of speculative research, with several humane and intelligent persons of this vicinity, who have had frequent occasions to remark the progressive increase of insane persons, as returned at each Assizes to the Grand Juries, and claiming support from the public purse. To me it has been at times a source of extreme difficulty to contrive the means of accommodation for this hurried weight of human calamity!

Characteristically, Hallaran believed that the reasons for this apparent increase in insanity related to both 'corporeal' (physical or bodily) and 'mental excitement' (in the mind):

> To account therefore correctly for this unlooked for pressure of a public and private calamity, it appears to be indispensably requisite to take into account the high degree of corporeal as well as of mental excitement, which may be supposed a consequence of continued warfare in the general sense … In some it was evident that terror merely had its sole influence, producing in most instances an incurable melancholia. In others where disappointed ambition had been prevalent, the patients were of an opposite cast, and were in general cheerful, gay and fanciful; but extremely treacherous and vindictive.

In addition to the effects of social unrest and conflict in increasing rates of illness, Hallaran was also concerned about 'the unrestrained use and abuse of ardent spirits' (i.e. alcohol):

> So frequently do instances of furious madness present themselves to me, and arising from long continued inebriety, that I seldom have occasion to enquire the cause, from the habit which repeated opportunities have given me at first sight, of detecting its well-known ravages.

Once an individual had developed 'the habit of daily intoxication', Hallaran noted that 'the countenance now bespeaks a dreary waste of mind and body; all is confusion and wild extravagance. The temper which previously partook of the grateful endearments of social intercourse, becomes dark, irritable and suspicious.' The challenges of treatment were only too apparent, 'Perhaps there is not in nature a greater difficulty than that of restoring a professed drunkard to a permanent abhorrence of such a habit'. At population level, the solution to the problems presented by alcohol lay in reforming revenue laws, limiting availability and optimising the quality of alcohol consumed:

> As I have every reason to suppose that the revenue laws, so far at least as they relate to this part of the Empire, give ample opportunity of regulating and inspecting the quantum of this valuable commodity, at its first shot, I would also consider of the possibility of officers in this department laying such restraint upon it, as must effectually prevent its making further progress in society … I would therefore, at the fountain head, commence the measures of reform, by enforcing the necessary limitations to its unreserved dispensation … If then we must admit the expediency of indulging the lower orders with a free admission to the bewitching charms of our native whiskey, let it be, in the name of pity, in the name of decency and good order, under such stipulations, as that it may at least be dealt out to them in its purity, free from those vicious frauds which not only constitute the immediate cause of the most inveterate maladies in the general sense, but also render them particularly liable to the horrors of continued insanity.

Hallaran also identified 'terror from religious enthusiasm' as a cause for increasing rates of 'mental derangement':

> On the whole, I am much inclined to indulge the hope, that however well-disposed my fellow countrymen may be, to cherish and hold fast the full impression of a pure and rational religion, still, that possessing a strong and lively discriminating faculty, they will continue to resist all charlatanical efforts to dissuade them from the substantial blessings which they now enjoy: either by submitting themselves to the distorted doctrines of the libertine, any more than to the circumscribed dogmas of our modern declaimers.

Hallaran was by no means alone in his efforts to explain the apparent rise in mental disorder in Ireland. This issue was a recurring concern for psychiatrists, policy-makers and governments in Ireland throughout the nineteenth and twentieth centuries. Even in the early 1700s there was a clear recognition that the needs of increasing numbers of mentally ill individuals were not being met by existing provisions in workhouses, prisons or hospitals.[20]

Concern about this problem grew steadily throughout the 1700s and 1800s, despite efforts to increase provision for the mentally ill through the opening of St Patrick's Hospital, Dublin in 1757[21] and various developments and initiatives at workhouses, such as that in Cork, aimed at assisting the mentally ill.[22] Despite these measures, Dr D. Hack Tuke,[23] toward the end of the nineteenth century, warned that the number of 'certified lunatics' in Irish workhouses was still increasing rapidly, which was particularly worrying given the poor care available to the mentally ill in these settings.[24] Similarly, the Irish Inspectors of Lunatics were increasingly concerned about overcrowding in general asylums[25] and by this time there was compelling evidence of similar overcrowding in the Central Criminal Lunatic Asylum in Dundrum, Dublin, too.[26]

Hallaran's 1810 textbook, combined with evidence of apparently increasing rates of insanity, played a critical role in prompting the authorities to instigate the building of the Richmond Asylum in Dublin, Ireland's largest asylum, which opened in 1814.[27] Later known as Grangegorman Mental Hospital and St Brendan's Hospital, this institution was quickly filled with individuals transferred from workhouses, and came under sustained pressure to take admissions well beyond its original capacity.[28] These events prompted the building of further asylums at multiple locations including Dublin, Derry, Belfast, Limerick, Armagh, Killarney, Kilkenny, Omagh, Mullingar and Sligo.[29] All of these developments were informed, in no small part, by the observations of Hallaran in his 1810 textbook and his personal efforts to ensure adequate provision of care and accommodation for the mentally ill, within the conceptual and therapeutic frameworks of the times.

CAUSES, COURSES AND OUTCOMES OF MENTAL DISORDER DURING THE 1800s

In terms of the causes of mental disorder, Hallaran recognised not only the effects of socio-political context and excessive alcohol consumption, but also the role of inherited predisposition:

> The lamentable and undeniable proofs of the existence of this complaint by inheritance, cannot be considered by the serious and intelligent, without feelings of the strongest emotion ... I can at this instant produce several young persons of from six to fourteen years old, who are now insane, and who have been reported to me as being mischievous since their infancy, and who since then, have continued to evince strong evidence of insanity. In the generality of those, I have been able to trace the cause by inheritance even to two generations, and almost invariably taking its course in the male and female line, without deviation from its original inclination.

Hallaran also noted that the mentally ill tended to die relatively young:

> It does not often happen that insane persons will arrive at what may be termed old age. I have seen some who have arrived at the sixtieth year, but those were for the most part such as had enjoyed long intervals between each paroxysm, or who had only continued in a state of relative quiescence from the commencement.

In terms of recovery, Hallaran noted that:

> The appearances which chiefly denote a prospect of recovery, are not at all times easily to be defined: though they are in themselves, evident proofs of the approaching event. It has been universally allowed in those cases, where the violence of the symptoms has been most remarkable, that the expectation of a favourable issue may be the more confidently entertained.

Hallaran further wrote:

> The interval between any two paroxysms is in duration regulated by the continuance of that which had preceded, and that as the complaint assumes a more benign aspect, the length of the paroxysm, as well as the interval, will increase in mutual proportion: till at length, by taking advantage of the opportunity, the disease ceases to attract observation. [Moreover] as the paroxysms begin to assume a more protracted form, the intervals will be less distinct, though of longer duration, and as the disease advances, they will run into the continued form, with occasional remissions only.

Hallaran felt the period toward the end of recovery from an acute illness was a time that presented particular risks:

> Insane persons at this period will require the strictest watching … Under such circumstances, and having attained a thorough knowledge of the state that had so recently overwhelmed them, they are ever disposed to become alarmed for the supposed consequences: they will frequently assume a sullen silence, bordering on despondency, suspicious to a great degree, of every measure, however obviously intended for their advantage. This, as it may be termed, the secondary state of the complaint, has been too often neglected … Too much attention cannot be paid at this important period.

Almost two centuries of clinical observation have confirmed the importance of this observation. The 'sullen silence, bordering on despondency' described by Hallaran is consistent with today's diagnosis of 'post-schizophrenic depression', characterised by persistent low mood, loss of enjoyment and disturbances of appetite, energy and sleep, following an episode of schizophrenia.[30] Hallaran's observation that the recovery phase following such illness 'has been too often neglected' is also apt in light of evidence that risk of suicide is particularly high in the period immediately following discharge from hospital.[31] On this basis, Hallaran was clearly correct in saying that 'too much attention cannot be paid at this important period' following an episode of illness.

'METHOD OF CURE' – BLOODLETTING, VOMITING AND PURGATIVES

Hallaran issued a clear warning against reliance on force in managing the mentally ill, consistent with the relatively enlightened principles of moral management:

> Maniacs, when in a state to be influenced by moral agents, are not to be subdued ex efficio, by measures of mere force, and he who will attempt to impose upon their credulity by aiming it at too great a refinement in address or intellect, will often find himself detected, and treated by them with marked contempt … I have in consequence made it a special point on my review days, to converse for a few minutes with each patient,

on the subject which appeared to be most welcome to his humour. By a
regular attention to the duties of this parade, I am generally received
with as much politeness and decorum as if every individual attached to it,
had a share of expectancy from the manner in which he may happen to
acquit himself on the occasion. The mental exertion employed amongst
the convalescents by this species of address is very remarkable, and the
advantages flowing from it are almost incredible.

In terms of specific treatments for insanity, Hallaran

refrained as much as possible from directing venesection [bloodletting] …
I have not been able to note its good effects in any instance, or to observe
those appearances in the blood drawn, which might be supposed to
correspond with the general character of the disease … Bleeding to any
great extent does not often seem to be desirable, and except in recent
cases, does not even appear to be admissible.

Bloodletting had been a common treatment for mental disorder for many
centuries[32] and was widely practiced in ancient Greece and the early
Roman period, although some thinkers, such as Asclepiades, objected to
the practice and called for more humane treatments for the mentally ill.[33]
Nonetheless, bloodletting was still commonly performed in psychiatric
settings throughout the 1700s[34] and often involved the use of leeches.[35]
As Hallaran's comments suggest, certain physicians gradually became
disenchanted with indiscriminate bloodletting during the course of the
nineteenth century,[36] with prominent psychiatrists such as Philippe Pinel
at the Salpêtrière in Paris explicitly rejecting the practice.[37] Nonetheless,
the use of bloodletting persisted in certain areas and would later enjoy a
revival towards the end of the nineteenth century, largely due to the work
of Benjamin Rush in America and Broussais in France.[38]

   The administration of emetics (substances to make the patient vomit)
was another treatment that was commonly used and widely discussed by
physicians during the nineteenth century. While acknowledging 'the use of
emetics in all febrile affections', Hallaran was cautious about the indiscriminate use of emetics for mental disorder:

Were it possible for a practitioner at all times to meet the incipient form
of insanity, as he not unfrequently does the first approaches of fever,
and other acute diseases, he might with effect, interrupt its progress, or at

least deprive it of its severity, by the timely interposition of an emetic. But unless he may happen to be so fortunate, or should he only meet the complaint at its maturity, he had better argue with himself, previous to his complying with a too generally received opinion as to their indiscriminate utility ... I have been a witness to very disagreeable consequences arising from the want of necessary precaution on this head, which have deterred me from directing full emetics in any case.

In some cases, particularly large doses of emetic medication were required, on occasion amounting to 'four times the usual quantity'. One particular patient required some

sixteen grains of the tartarised antimony, before the action of the stomach had been excited. In this case, nothing beyond the common appearances of insanity had presented themselves, and although the lady had been of the most delicate form, still the effect of such an immoderate portion of the medicine was far from being excessive or troublesome.

The usual dose of 'tartarised antimony' (a metalloid now used in lead batteries) was 'four grains of it with four ounces of vitriolated magnesia in eight ounces of hot water. Of this solution one ounce is given every hour, till some vomiting or purging be produced'.

Hallaran had little doubt about the effectiveness of this technique in certain cases:

I can safely undertake to say, that in recent cases of insanity, by persisting in this mode of treatment, I have frequently without any other remedy, completely effected a reduction of the maniacal hallucinations, within ten or fourteen days from the commencement; so as to be able to follow up the plan of cure in a most satisfactory manner.

The use of emetics and purgatives has a long history in both medicine and psychiatry. In 1615, Curtius Marinello published an Italian textbook of psychiatry and neurology that endorsed the use of both bloodletting and purging on the basis that such disorders represented an excess of black humour in the body.[39] Throughout the nineteenth century the use of bloodletting, purgatives and emetics persisted in the majority of psychiatric settings, despite substantial changes in physicians' views about the causes of mental disorder.[40] In effect, there were few alternative therapeutic strategies available to psychiatrists and physicians at that time, so these treatments persisted despite growing disenchantment with them.

In Ireland, emetics and purgatives were commonly used for a range of physical and mental disorders. In 1810, the same year that Hallaran published his textbook of psychiatry, Dr Martin Tuomy, a Fellow of the Royal College of Physicians of Ireland, published his *Treatise on the Principal Diseases of Dublin* in which he explicitly endorsed the use of purgatives and emetics, which might be administered daily for up to twenty-one days.[41] As was the case with bloodletting, however, there was a growing disenchantment with the indiscriminate use of emetics and purgatives, with prescriptions for more violent emetic and purgative agents declining as the nineteenth century progressed. During this period, various other novel forms of treatment emerged, providing possible alternatives. These included 'Dr Cox's Circulating Swing', which Hallaran discussed in considerable detail in his 1810 textbook.

DR COX'S CIRCULATING SWING

In his consideration of emetics and purgatives, Hallaran noted that patients occasionally exhibited 'excessive obstinacy' in complying with treatment, with very worrying results:

> Such a degree of constipation, as well as an obduracy in refraining from every kind of remedy or sustenance, becomes so alarming that all hope of even prolonging the life of the patient seems at an end, and death has in several cases on record, quickly ensued from this sole cause. Fortunately for practitioners in this department of the medical profession, a safe and effectual remedy for the unhappy disposition of maniacs here referred to, has been made known to the public through the practical work of Doctor Cox, who, though he generously gives the credit of the invention to the late Doctor Darwin, was the first who had the courage to apply to practice the use of the circulating swing, and which is now become of so much consequence in the cure of maniacs of almost every description.

The circulating swing was developed by Dr Joseph Mason Cox (1763–1818), a Scottish physician,[42] and was described as 'both a moral and a medical mean in the treatment of maniacs'.[43] Building on the work of Dr Erasmus Darwin (1731–1802), who described a 'rotative couch' aimed at inducing sleep,[44] Cox suggested suspending a chair from the ceiling by means of ropes; seating a patient securely in the chair; and instructing an asylum attendant to rotate the chair at a given speed, thus spinning the patient around a vertical axis for a given period of time.[45] This technique was employed at many asylums throughout nineteenth-century Europe, especially in German-speaking countries, following the translation of Cox's work into German and French.[46]

In Ireland, Hallaran pointed out that he 'was not slow in taking advantage of Dr Cox's observations on this subject and accordingly set about erecting machinery for this purpose'. The apparatus that Hallaran assembled was 'so contrived, that four persons can if necessary, be secured in it at once, by dividing the platform attached to the perpendicular shaft into four equal compartments, which may, by removing the partitions, be occasionally adapted to the horizontal position'.

Hallaran was extremely pleased with the results of this work:

> Having completed it to my satisfaction, I have been enabled in a most ample manner, to put fairly to the test, the extent of credit due to this invention … I also feel the most particular satisfaction, in having it fully in my power to acknowledge the debt owing to Doctor Cox, by the public at large, for the value of his labours, and especially for his excellent application of the circulating swing, as 'a moral and medical mean' in the cure of insanity.

Hallaran used this 'Herculean remedy' for selected patients only, including:

> those who have been recently attacked with maniacal symptoms, and who, previous to its employment had been sufficiently evacuated by purgative medicines. Or those, who after reiterated attacks at short intervals, had been subjected to its operation immediately on the accession of a paroxysm. There are also others for whom it has been found particularly useful, and to whom Doctor Cox has strongly alluded. I mean those already mentioned, where no influence can be exerted sufficient to effect a medical purpose, or even to maintain the common energies of life.

Hallaran also used the swing with patients who had difficulty sleeping; in these cases using the swing 'at a moderate rate' could 'induce the most placid sleep, and so very soundly, as scarcely to be disturbed by the attendants when in the act of removing him to bed'. Dr Cox's Circulating Swing had different effects on patients presenting with different symptoms: in the 'obstinate and furious' it generated 'a sufficiency of alarm to insure obedience' while in the 'melancholic' it generated 'a natural interest in the affairs of life'.

Despite these enthusiastic observations, Hallaran warned against the indiscriminate use of the apparatus, which 'should be held in reserve as long as possible, and should not be repeated unless where the necessity of doing so may be equally imperious as at first'. He advised caution with tall patients and noted that particular patterns of rotation could produce 'sudden action of the bowels, stomach and urinary passages, in quick succession'. While clearly aware of such adverse effects, Hallaran still believed that use of the swing was in the best interests of selected patients as it 'prevents the possibility of injury' in a patient who might otherwise 'strike or beat himself against a wall or bed-post. By this means he can be completely invested, and kept sufficiently warm.'

Hallaran also used the principles of Dr Cox's Circulating Swing outside the hospital, by placing his patients

> in hammocks, slung by two parallel ropes from the ceiling, and supported from the angles by cords with eyes, hooked to the perpendicular supporters; which, after the oscillatory motion had been continued for some time, by twisting the ropes to their full extent, so as to let them return by relaxation to their former position, has been eventually found sufficient to create nausea and vomiting to a considerable degree. This, from its vertiginous quality, having produced surprise, and some share of tranquillity, has been followed by sound sleep, and the attendant continuing a rocking motion of the hammock for some time after in a dark room, has contributed to prolong it for eight or ten hours without interruption.

Finally, Dr Cox's Circulating Swing was also a source of entertainment in the evenings at the asylum:

> The idiots belonging to the establishment have used it sometimes when permitted, as a mode of amusement, without any inconvenience or effect whatever, and others during the intervals, with equal satisfaction; who, on the recurrence of the paroxysm, have not been able to resist its most gentle rotation for five minutes in continuance.

Despite Hallaran's awareness of the adverse effects of the apparatus, his insistence on 'careful superintendence' and his belief that he was acting in patients' best interests, it is clear that Dr Cox's Circulating Swing belonged to an era prior to the development of more humane treatments for the mentally ill and prior to clear enunciation and recognition of the human rights of the mentally ill.[47] On this basis, it is essential that Hallaran's enthusiasm for Dr Cox's Circulating Swing is interpreted in its historical setting and in the context of contemporary societal attitudes to the mentally ill.[48] Some 200 years after both Hallaran's textbook and Dr Cox's Circulating Swing[49] first appeared, it is to be hoped that increased emphasis on the rights of the mentally ill will ensure sustained importance is placed on the dignity of patients during all forms of treatment and enhance the provision of evidence-based therapies that are humane, safe, effective and acceptable to patients and their families.[50]

MEDICINAL REMEDIES: DIGITALIS, OPIUM, CAMPHOR AND MERCURY

The asylums of the nineteenth century were filled with medicinal remedies which had been in use for decades, if not centuries, including digitalis (foxglove), opium, camphor and mercury. Some of these agents were specific to psychiatry but most were used for multiple conditions across many fields of medical practice, with varying degrees of effectiveness. Digitalis was one of the most commonly used of these remedies, especially in the asylums.

While Hallaran could not 'have any pretensions to originality by avowing a confidence in the use of the digitalis, when adapted to the cure of insanity, I yet have the satisfaction to think, that I have contributed to place its merits as an anti-maniacal remedy, on as high a scale as can well belong to any one subject of materia medica, which still holds rank and credit in the cure of diseases'.

Digitalis appeared to act by 'restraining the inordinate action of the heart and arteries' and its clinical effects included a lowering of pulse and the production of 'sound and refreshing sleep', both of which were key indicators of clinical improvement in nineteenth-century asylums. Digitalis was, however, 'not admissible unless where the system has been previously reduced by proper evacuants' (i.e. agents to induce vomiting or purging) and 'although its sedative quality cannot be questioned ... it cannot be usefully exerted under the circumstances of high arterial action'.

For several centuries, digitalis had been commonly used in Ireland for
the management of a range of medical conditions[51] and was widely used for
psychiatric disorders throughout the eighteenth and nineteenth centuries.[52]
The current understanding of the biological action of digitalis at the cellular
level suggests that digitalis may indeed have had an effect on the brain, but it
was not until the work of Dr William Withering (1741–99) that the issues of
standardised preparation and dose-response characteristics were identified
as critical for the effective and safe use of the drug.[53]

Notwithstanding Hallaran's statement of belief in the powers of digitalis,
he again cautioned against excessive therapeutic zeal:

> Having made an assertion of so very positive a nature, I feel myself called
> upon, at least to qualify such an expression, by admitting, what very few
> will doubt, that there are daily to be met with those cases of insanity,
> which no human power can remedy: as depending upon causes connected
> with advanced age; hereditary disposition appearing at a late period of
> life; mechanical pressure arising either from accidents, or malconforma-
> tion; deep mental excitement, producing the excess of melancholia, or its
> alternation, with extravagant gaiety and frivolity.

Hallaran felt that opium, like digitalis, had 'deservedly obtained a principal
character amongst anti-maniacal remedies. To those however, who are
well acquainted with the stimulant and exhilarating powers of opium, few
precautions will be necessary, as to its indiscriminate employment, under the
degree of high arterial excitement which so generally prevails with insane
persons'. Even though the use of opium declined following the introduction of Dr Cox's Circulating Swing, there were still 'certain cases of insanity,
where the use of opium has been found to subdue the first approaches of
the paroxysm in its most violent form, and even to cut it short where it had
already assumed a positive character'.

Opium appeared to work 'by interrupting the quick succession of
morbid ideas, where a long absence of natural sleep had been an aggravation' and thus 'effecting an entire and lasting return of the mental faculty'.
There could, however, be significant adverse effects with opium and 'unless
the exact moment for such determined practice be seized upon, mischief
of a serious nature must ensue, and … at all events, it is a remedy which
cannot be persisted in longer than the first effort, or even hazarded, where
the source of the disorder can bear a reference to, or even a connection
with, the causes which induce an over-distension of the vessels of the head,

and the acute febrile diathesis which is its certain attendant'. Like digitalis, there was a long history of the use of opium in medical settings, especially for disorders attributed to excessive 'stimulation' of tissues[54] and psychiatric conditions such as 'melancholia' and 'mania'.[55]

Camphor was another common treatment for mental disorder throughout the eighteenth and nineteenth centuries[56] and was later used by Ladislas von Meduna (1896–1964) to induce seizures as a 'convulsive' treatment for certain mental disorders (a forerunner of today's electro-convulsive therapy or ECT).[57] Hallaran noted that many authors believed camphor had a particular role in the treatment of mania on the basis 'of its general effects in other febrile disorders [infections] and … its specific influence over the worst symptoms of insanity'. However, despite camphor's 'soporific quality' and ability to assist occasionally in the 'reduction of the febrile diatheses' (reducing high temperature), Hallaran believed that camphor 'frequently failed altogether' in the treatment of mania. Ultimately, he had 'no hesitation in looking upon the plan of treating maniacal patients, on a curative principle, by a continued course of camphor and opium, or of either, as an egregious loss of time, and as most liable to fatal consequences'.

Hallaran also had doubts about the use of mercury in the treatment of insanity and 'from the early opportunity of a few cases, in which mercury had been employed as an agent in the cure of insanity, I was taught to expect more from it even as a specific, than I find myself justified in allowing it, from subsequent efforts to ascertain its value'. He had, however, 'a high opinion of its utility, as a preparative for the commencement of the digitalis'. There was a long history of the use of mercury for the treatment of syphilis in eighteenth-century Ireland[58] and throughout the nineteenth century, mercury was still commonly used in the management of syphilitic disorders of the nervous system.[59]

On occasion, mercury was used in combination with potassium iodide for this purpose, although Hallaran was not the only clinician to express doubts about this practice: in France, Dr Jean-Alfred Fournier (1832–1914) also noted its failures and went on to define 'parasyphilis' as the non-syph-ilitic sequelae of syphilis, which might require an alternative therapeutic approach.[60] Many of these alternative approaches were discussed in some detail in Hallaran's 1810 textbook and included physical treatments such as shower baths, dietary regulation and exercise.

PHYSICAL TREATMENTS:
SHOWER BATHS, DIET AND EXERCISE

Water treatment was a common component of treatment programmes for mental disorder throughout the eighteenth and nineteenth centuries.[61] Specific techniques included washing, bathing and the 'shower bath'. Hallaran wrote:

> The general influence of the shower bath so fully supplies all the purposes of more minute attention, that in the larger hospitals set apart for lunatics, there can seldom occur a case of acute madness, which will not at its commencement meet the most decided relief, by being placed under it two or three times a day, as the case may require.

This therapeutic technique appeared to work 'by immediately tranquilizing the high degree of febrile action, which on the formation of the maniacal paroxysm, rages with such determined violence' (i.e. it calmed the patient down). The shower bath also 'answers an extremely good purpose in enforcing cleanliness at all seasons, and more especially in warm weather'. Hallaran had little doubt about its effectiveness, once certain conditions were met:

> The advantages arising from the use of the shower bath, in the more advanced stage of convalescence from a maniacal paroxysm, when the patient is in a state to use active exercise, are, on the tonic principle, of the first consequence, and superior to any I have ever met with: provided that at this period, the state of the bowels be particularly attended to.

Hallaran recognised the importance of diet in the asylum and described the Cork asylum's 'farinaceous diet' (i.e. consisting of meal or flour) in some detail:

> This is composed of a plentiful meal of oatmeal porridge and new milk in the mornings, and of potatoes, with a sufficiency of the same description of milk in the evenings. There are several who prefer the indulgence of oaten bread in lieu of porridge, and who also have the same for supper; though two meals are the usual allowance of the house. To this may be added, that in many instances amongst the aged and infirm, and particularly those in a state of convalescence, an allowance of animal food is admitted, so long as it may seem to be necessary.

'Animal food' was carefully restricted to 'certain seasons of the year' owing to its tendency to produce a 'disposition to riot' and an 'aggravation of insanity'. Regarding wine, Hallaran felt that 'in the higher classes of society, where it had been an indispensable article of indulgence, and where at the eve of recovery it could not be entirely withheld, I have found it in strict moderation, to answer a good purpose, by adding strength to the patient'. However, 'those who have been prevailed upon to abstain from it entirely have been also the most fortunate in escaping a return of the malady'. Overall, 'in addressing myself to medical practitioners there need not be any pains taken to point out the necessity of a scrupulous observance of temperance, as the only security to persons predisposed to insanity or recently afflicted with an insane paroxysm'.

Regulation of diet was a key element in programmes of moral management which were in place in most Irish asylums throughout the nineteenth century; other elements included regular exercise and gainful employment.[62] This therapeutic approach had a critical influence on the design of many Irish asylums constructed in the nineteenth century.[63]

Consistent with this approach, Hallaran paid considerable attention to exercise and occupation in his 1810 textbook. He wrote that 'exercise, as forming a very material department of regimen, and as intimately connected with the treatment of maniacs in their convalescent state, requires to be conducted with much precaution and address'. He emphasised the benefits of initiating programmes of graded physical activity at an early stage in a patient's admission to an asylum:

> The advantages to be acquired by an early attention to bodily exercise, as connected with regimen in general, cannot exceed those which may particularly be obtained from the union of corporeal action with the regular employment of the mind.

Gainful activity was another key element in programmes of moral management and Hallaran was particularly concerned about asylum patients who, apart from their mental disorder, were in generally 'rude health' but were 'obliged to loiter away the day in listless apathy! The consequences of this neglected and unavoidable sloth, attendant on the present principles of the institution, are deeply to be lamented; as constituting in many instances a pabulum [sustenance] for the disease which it was intended to remove'.

On this basis, 'the earliest attention is paid to the capacity of every individual, in order to ascertain at the period of convalescence, the practicability of employing the mind, by any species of bodily exertion'. Such activity 'seldom fails to confirm and to accelerate the prospect of recovery'. Hallaran recommended:

> adopting on a general principle, a systematic arrangement of daily labour, by which incurable maniacs, capable of corporeal exertion, may still acquire the habit of rendering themselves useful to society, by thus diminishing a portion of the expense allowed for their maintenance, and also, on the very important principle, of affording them the most certain means of enjoying a term of repose from the horrors of a hopeless malady.

Developing this theme further, Hallaran discussed 'removing the convalescent and incurable insane, to convenient distances from large cities and towns, to well enclosed farms, properly adapted to the purposes of employing them with effect, in the different branches of husbandry and horticulture'. Patients in the asylum 'might on convalescence, be conveyed in covered carriages to the farms, each of which, holding an intimate communication with, and depending on the original foundation, should make daily returns of their proceedings to the principal master, for the weekly inspection of the board of trustees, according to the present invariable custom in this city'. This was an early version of occupational therapy, aimed at re-establishing normal patterns of daily activity among the mentally ill.

HALLARAN'S CONTRIBUTION TO THERAPEUTIC ENTHUSIASM WITHIN THE ASYLUMS

Hallaran was an industrious clinician and tireless teacher, and the themes and qualities that defined his life's work were clearly enunciated in his 1810 textbook, the first Irish textbook of psychiatry. As well as a clinician and scientist, Hallaran was a tireless advocate for improved services for individuals with mental disorder. It is, perhaps, this central, over-arching advocacy that best explains Hallaran's long-standing commitment to the study of psychiatric disorders, his extensive efforts to improve services, and the astonishing comprehensiveness and vigour of his ground-breaking textbook:

> I have expressed my opinion somewhat at large on this interesting subject, from a conviction, of no recent date, of its necessity, as well as of the comparative facility with which its meaning may be put in force; if

I have taken these pains in vain, I must impute my disappointment to the visionary suggestion of a mind, perhaps too sanguine in a cause, which has engaged my most serious attention during a very important season of my life. If, in raising my humble voice, I should perchance, be heard, in behalf of those claims, which the most comfortless of the creation may be allowed to have, on the wisdom and on the humanity of this great and enlightened empire, I even would not despair of meeting, in the stream which emanates from such a source, a ray of that benignity, which marks its mighty progress.

Over the course of the two centuries following Hallaran's 1810 textbook, various developments in psychiatry, including the rapid expansion of Ireland's asylum system, were to tilt the balance away from the broad-based approach recommended by Hallaran towards a more custodial model of care. The closing decades of the twentieth century, however, finally saw the emergence of re-energised models of bio-psycho-social psychiatry which emphasise the role of occupational therapies in the process of recovery, consistent with the approach recommended by Hallaran some two centuries earlier.[64]

MENTAL DISORDER IN THE NINETEENTH-CENTURY WORKHOUSE

The asylum care that Hallaran so enthusiastically described was very much the exception rather than the rule during the early nineteenth century. The second part of this chapter examines the fate of the great number of individuals with mental disorder who entered the Irish workhouse system rather than the asylum system. This exploration is based on an examination of original workhouse records and minutes from the Ballinrobe Poor Law Union, County Mayo, which was located in an area especially badly affected by the Great Irish Famine (1845–52) and serves to demonstrate key issues which were relevant to the poverty-stricken and mentally ill throughout Ireland at this time.[65]

The Great Irish Famine was one of the most devastating natural disasters in the history of modern Europe. Over the ten-year period between 1841 and 1851, the population of Ireland fell by more than 20 per cent. Over 1 million Irish people died as a result of the Famine and approximately 1 million more were to emigrate in its immediate aftermath.[66] Ireland's population was decimated for decades to follow.

Though no part of Ireland fully escaped the effects of the Famine, not all counties were affected equally. Counties in the west of Ireland, such as Galway, Mayo and Roscommon, were particularly badly affected. For example, the death rate in County Mayo between 1846 and 1851 was approximately 60 per 1,000, while the death rate in Kildare and Wexford was less than 5 per 1,000.[67] Western counties had a particular reliance on potato crops, so when the crops failed from 1845 to 1849, western subsistence farmers and their families were especially vulnerable.

Against this background, the Poor Law Act (1838) was designed to relieve the distress of the 'deserving' poor in Ireland. The system initially consisted of 130 Poor Law Unions, which were essentially workhouses aimed at providing accommodation, food and medical care to the poor of the area. Despite the establishment of several new asylums for the treatment of the mentally ill throughout the early decades of the nineteenth century,[68] many of Ireland's mentally ill entered these workhouses during the Famine.[69] Ballinrobe Poor Law Union in County Mayo was located in one of the areas most affected by Famine and examination of its records and minutes demonstrate clearly the challenges in relation to physical and mental disorders during this period.[70]

BALLINROBE POOR LAW UNION

The Ballinrobe Poor Law Union was administered by local Guardians, who met regularly to attend to the administration of the workhouse, review accounts and correspond with the national Poor Law Commissioners. The proceedings of these meetings were carefully recorded by the clerk in the minute book. Meetings generally took place every one or two weeks, though attendance varied significantly. For six consecutive weeks from 20 August 1846 to 24 September 1846, for example, the minutes record that 'the clerk having waited more than one hour, and no Guardians having attended, the meeting was adjourned'.

When meetings went ahead, the Guardians addressed a broad range of issues. At each meeting, the books of accounts and Medical Officer's Book were presented and approved. Personnel issues occupied a significant proportion of the time. On the 26 March 1846, for example, the porter had to be dismissed 'in consequence of having been absent for a considerable time without leave' and a replacement porter was appointed.

Other habitual concerns included the provision of clothing and supplies to 'paupers' in the workhouse. In November 1846, 'the clerk and master again called the attention of the Board to the state of the clothing and bedding, reporting that a large quantity of clothing is wanted for the paupers in the house and that all the bedding is in use'. The Poor Law accounts record that the Guardians were not always in a position to accede to these requests, owing to 'the state of the country' throughout much of the 1840s.

The Board of Guardians was also concerned with matters of discipline in the workhouse. On 30 December 1854, it was recorded that one inmate who was 'registered as a Protestant' had obtained leave 'to attend Divine Service in the Church of Ballinrobe' but 'instead of doing so the Master saw him walking through the town at 1pm'. The inmate 'was called before the Board and cautioned that if he again neglected to attend Divine Service, the Board would order his discharge from the workhouse'.

Similar disciplinary measures were applied to staff. For example, when the workhouse school mistress got married in January 1855 she received a stern lecture from the Board of Guardians:

> The school mistress was … informed that the Board would require of her to pay the strictest attention to her school duties for the future, and also to absent herself from the workhouse as seldom as possible. The school mistress was further informed that the Board will not allow her husband to be a constant visitor to the school, and that his visits when made should only be by the permission of the Workhouse Master.

MEDICAL CARE IN THE WORKHOUSE

Medical care in the workhouse was provided by the medical officers who were appointed and paid by the Board of Guardians. At a meeting of the Ballinrobe Poor Law Union on 5 November 1846 'it was resolved that a cheque for twenty pounds' be drawn up in favour of the medical officer as his 'half years salary'. On 4 March 1847, however, the Guardians heard that the same medical officer 'was dangerously ill of fever, that the master had died of fever, and that the clerk had died of fever'. Some days later, the unfortunate medical officer had also died. A replacement medical officer was persuaded to take the position at an enhanced salary of £80 per year.

In response to the increasing number of persons dying of 'fever', the Board 'resolved that a fever hospital [was to] be attached to Ballinrobe Union Workhouse for the use of the Pauper Fever Patients'. The cost of this 'was not to exceed four hundred and fifty pounds'. By 15 July 1847, however, another medical officer was already critically unwell and 'having attended the Board and his health appearing very delicate it has been thought advisable to allow him leave of absence'. On this occasion, the doctor recovered and the following week, 'having appeared before the Board, reports himself able to take charge of the Hospital'.

The 'hospital' was the workhouse infirmary, in which the 'paupers' were treated for illnesses ranging from 'fever' to mental disorder to 'cancer of the ear'. On 16 April 1846, for example, the 'medical officer reported that there were fifteen paupers under medical treatment in the infirmary'. Happily, that number had fallen to ten by October of that year.

As well as treating patients in the infirmary, the medical officer had responsibility for the overall health of inmates. On a number of occasions, the medical officer recommended that the Board stop admitting people to the workhouse owing to the insanitary conditions. On 14 January 1847, the medical officer told the Board 'that it would be dangerous to admit more paupers' owing to 'the present state of the house' and 'the want of a proper supply of bedding and clothing'. By 8 April 1847 the situation was again critical and it was 'resolved that on the representation of the Medical Officer and the report of the assistant commissioner as to the state of the house that no more admissions take place for the present'.

The medical officer was also responsible for approving the dietary intake of inmates in the workhouse. The daily diet changed from time to time, and each change was clearly outlined in the minutes and approved by the Board of Guardians. In 1847, the basic diet included 'two pints of new milk' and up to one loaf of white bread per day, supplemented by one pint of buttermilk in the period immediately following admission. When the workhouse was short of milk, beer was considered an appropriate substitute. Other components of the diet included meat, Indian meal, cornflour, porter and whiskey.

In general, medical officers lived on the grounds of the workhouse or else nearby. In addition to the medical officer and his assistant, the workhouse employed a variable number of nurses who, among other duties, oversaw a nursery for children at the workhouse. The workhouse, however, suffered from a chronic shortage of rooms for the inmates, medical officers, nurses and other employees. At the Board meeting of 12 April 1855, the medical officer complained 'that the nursery is too small to accommodate the 18 infants and 4 nurses in one unit'. In response to this concern, the Board ordered 'that the nurses be transferred to the Women's Day Room and that the room off the Laundry be used as a day room for the women'. Such reorganisations were frequent occurrences throughout the lives of most Irish workhouses.

MENTAL DISORDER IN THE WORKHOUSE: THE CHALLENGES OF CARE

Many of the 'lunatics' who were admitted to the workhouse were undi-agnosed, homeless persons from the streets. Others were referred directly following discharge from asylums. The minutes from 22 October 1896, for example, record that a woman 'was transferred on a Removal Warrant from the Lunatic Asylum, Perth, Scotland. She was seven years in Scotland and is insane'.

Providing accommodation and treatment to the mentally ill at the workhouse presented particular challenges. On 20 August 1846, a man 'who was confined to the workhouse as a cured patient from the Castlebar Lunatic Asylum took his discharge and went to his home'. There is no record of any attempt, or necessity, to retrieve him. Earlier that year, another inmate had not only become 'insubordinate' and 'used threats and threw stones', but had also 'accused the Master of beating him which he did not do'. The inmate in question was discharged immediately and the Board of Guardians did not pursue formal charges.

Persons who were thought to be 'lunatics' were generally examined by the medical officer as soon as possible after admission. At the Board meeting on 10 September 1896, for example, 'the sum of one pound was ordered to be paid to [the] medical officer of Ballinrobe No. 1 Dispensary District, for his services examining a lunatic'.

In terms of managing psychiatric illness, the Poor Law Union often focused on providing practical support for both the mentally ill and those with disabilities. At a basic level, the workhouse aimed to provide accommodation, food and medical care. Persons with mental disorder often required additional attention and supervision, however, generally in the form of specially employed 'minders'. In October 1896, for example, the Ballinrobe workhouse employed 'a woman at a shilling a day to mind … a woman who is insane'. This individual attention appears to have been the exception rather than the rule.

In addition, occasional attempts were made to find accommodation and occupational placements for 'deserving' persons who came to the attention of the Board. On 8 October 1896, for example, the minutes recorded a letter from a local man who sought assistance for his son, who was deaf and dumb:

> I beg to call your attention to the case of my son … who has been an inmate of the Cabra Institution for the Deaf and Dumb for the past six years and who left there a few weeks ago. I considered he had learnt enough of the saddlery business while there to enable him to earn his own living, but I find he would not be taken in any shop unless on payment of a fee of £20.

The man offered to pay one-third of the fee if the Board of Guardians would pay the remaining two-thirds. The Board agreed to the plan and ordered the payment of £13 to enable the boy to commence his apprenticeship.

Little is recorded about the outcome of mental or medical disorders in the workhouse. Occasionally, inmates left the workhouse to rejoin their families, often travelling to England to follow those who had already emigrated. On 12 April 1855, for example, the Board of Guardians ordered that a female inmate of the workhouse 'who has applied for her discharge, [should] get a blanket and sheet, she being about to proceed to England'. The journey to England was an arduous one, especially for inmates who were not in good health and lacked resources to pay for train travel.

For most inmates at the workhouses, the outcome of medical or mental disorders was not formally recorded. The records indicate, however, that the Board of Guardians required a steady supply of coffins from Ballinrobe town, indicating that death was a common occurrence. The precise causes of death are not known, however, as they were not recorded in the workhouse records. Possible causes of death were legion, and would have included a range of infections and non-infectious diseases, exacerbated by poor general health and the unsanitary conditions of workhouses. The effects of chronic mental disorder, prolonged starvation and habitual homelessness would have further reduced life expectancy both during the Famine and in the years that followed.

MENTAL DISORDER IN THE WORKHOUSE: THE BROADER CONTEXT

The mentally ill and intellectually disabled ended up in workhouses for myriad reasons, including the challenging socio-economic conditions in nineteenth-century Ireland and, especially, the Famine. In addition, the provision of dedicated accommodation and care to the mentally ill was inconsistent and unreliable throughout Ireland and most of Europe during the opening decades of the nineteenth century.[71] For the majority of persons with mental disorder who did not access the few asylum beds that were available, care in the community was nonexistent. At the end of the eighteenth century in Ireland, for example, there was official provision for only 250 persons with mental disorder and virtually no other form of care outside of that.[72] While additional treatment and accommodation were available in St Patrick's Hospital in Dublin[73] and in a scattering of private asylums throughout the country, most of Ireland's mentally ill and intellectually disabled were living with poverty-stricken rural families, consigned to remote huts, wandering the roads or incarcerated in prisons. A similar situation pertained in other parts of Europe.

Throughout the nineteenth century, however, attempts were made to improve the situation, with reformers such as Hallaran adapting the principles of moral management and assuming an ostensibly caring approach to the mentally ill.[74] Despite the progress in centres such as Cork, however, the overall standard of care throughout Ireland was inconsistent and, in many places, formal psychiatric care was still nonexistent. In 1804, in response to this very visible problem, a parliamentary committee recommended the establishment of asylums throughout Ireland and by 1830 asylums had been completed in Dublin, Derry, Belfast, Armagh and Limerick.[75]

In the middle of the nineteenth, century, however, the development of a system of mental health care in Ireland was disrupted by the Famine. It is likely that more people died of disease than of starvation during this time,[76] and many of these diseases, such as vitamin B deficiencies, had neuropsychological complications. Hospitals were overwhelmed and newly founded charitable organisations (such as soup kitchens) were unable to meet the enormous needs of the starving sick. Even the Poor Law Union, with its network of workhouses, lacked adequate resources to contain the crisis. In 1848, workhouse accommodation was expanded to cater for 150,000 people and by 1851 it had been expanded again to cater for a total of 300,000, but even this was not sufficient. Records from Ballinrobe workhouse clearly indicate considerable difficulties maintaining even basic standards of hygiene, let alone mental health care.

In general, little is recorded about the plight of the mentally ill during the Famine. The formal asylum system provided mental health care to some but not all 'lunatics', many of whom inhabited workhouses for prolonged periods.[77] Despite its very obvious limitations, the workhouse system attempted to address inmates' practical needs in terms of accommodation, food, supervision and refuge from a life of vagrancy. Little, however, is known about the outcomes for workhouse inmates with mental disorders.

Overall, it is apparent that despite the development of a network of asylums in the early part of the nineteenth century, many of the mentally ill did not have access to adequate treatment or accommodation, especially during the Famine. It is also clear that mental disorder was strongly linked with homelessness in nineteenth-century Ireland, and stable, sanitary accommodation was one of the main unmet needs of the destitute mentally ill. The workhouse system attempted to address this need, with limited success. Today, over a century and a half after the Famine, the problem of homelessness amongst the chronically mentally ill remains an important one: studies in both Ireland and the United Kingdom still report serious mental disorder in over one third of the homeless population.[78]

On a global level, the WHO confirms that there is still a need to improve mental health services in countries affected by conflicts and natural disasters, like the Irish Famine.[79] Interestingly, many of the barriers to effective care today are essentially the same as those experienced in Ballinrobe workhouse in the nineteenth century, including the provision of effective care based on limited resources, recruitment and retention of staff, alleviation of homelessness amongst the chronically mentally ill, and recognition of the effects of natural disasters on population mental health.

All of these challenges were very apparent to Hallaran and his colleagues. The main societal response to these challenges at that time, however, was the creation of a large network of asylums to house the increasing numbers of mentally ill and intellectually disabled.

Against this rather bleak background, the next chapter in this book, Chapter 2, examines the legal underpinnings of Ireland's emergent asylum system.

2

Creating the Asylums and the Insanity Defence

INTRODUCTION

The problems faced by the mentally ill and intellectually disabled in nineteenth-century Ireland were both common and commonly known. Notwithstanding the relatively enlightened ideas of Hallaran and colleagues in England and France, the main societal and professional response to these challenges was the building of large networks of asylums to house the mentally ill and intellectually disabled. While there were subsequent problems with high committal rates in many countries, including England, France, and the United States, Ireland's admission rates were especially high at their peak, and especially slow to decline.[1]

This chapter examines the legal underpinnings of Ireland's asylum system, the widespread belief that 'insanity' was increasing uniquely quickly in Ireland, and the kind of asylums that emerged from these concerns in the 1800s and early 1900s. This chapter also examines the emergence of the idea of criminal insanity in Ireland, Europe and the United States, with particular emphasis on the insanity defence as it relates to the types of mental and physical disorders explored throughout this book.

BUILDING IRELAND'S ASYLUMS

The nineteenth century was a time of intensive legislative reform in relation to the management of mental disorder in many countries, including the United Kingdom of Great Britain (then including Ireland). Prior to 1821, there was scant specific legislative provision for individuals with mental disorder in Ireland. The 1700s had seen the establishment of a network of workhouses and houses of industry for the destitute poor and, in the absence of dedicated asylum accommodation, many individuals with mental disorder spent significant periods in workhouses and houses of industry, although this was generally inadequate and inappropriate to needs. In 1944, an anonymous psychiatrist, writing in *The Bell*, an Irish literary periodical, highlighted the disturbing and distinctly custodial history of early mental health care in Ireland:

> In 1728 cells were erected in the Dublin House of Industry, and later similar provisions were made in houses of industry throughout the country. These, however, could not be classified as institutions. The term 'cells' is sufficiently informative.[2]

The dearth of accommodation for the mentally ill was also related to the absence of a strong tradition of private asylums in Ireland. This contrasted with the situation in England, where a significant number of individuals with mental disorders were housed in private asylums and others admitted as private patients in large public asylums, such as Bethlem.[3] In the absence of dedicated public or private provision, the mentally ill in Ireland tended towards lives of vagrancy, homeless and destitution. This situation changed slightly in the middle of the eighteenth century with the opening of St Patrick's Hospital, Dublin in 1757, following a bequest by the author Jonathan Swift.[4] By 1817, St Patrick's Hospital had 150 inpatients, including ninety-six 'paupers'.[5] This development was welcome but isolated, and there remained serious deficiencies in provision for the mentally ill, both in Dublin and throughout Ireland for most of the 1700s.

The first systematic change occurred in 1787, when the Prisons Act empowered Grand Juries to establish lunatic wards in houses of industry, and dictated that such wards would be subject to inspection by the inspector general of prisons. The response to the 1787 legislation was relatively modest, however, and by 1804 lunatic wards had only been established in Dublin, Cork, Waterford and Limerick. In addition, however, in Cork, Hallaran founded the Cork Lunatic Asylum in 1791, an important step in establishing dedicated services for the mentally ill in this region.[6] This period also saw a steady expansion in private provision with the opening of a private asylum in Cork in 1799 and establishment of further private facilities in Bloomfield, Donnybrook (1810), Farnham House, Finglas (1814) and Hampstead House (1826).[7]

In general terms, however, there was still a paucity of accommodation and treatment facilities for the mentally ill, especially the destitute mentally ill. These deficiencies resulted in substantial pressure on existing facilities, especially the houses of industry, at the start of the 1800s. Public and governmental concern grew steadily as the century progressed, fuelled in large part by a widespread belief that rates of mental disorder were increasing rapidly, placing further stress on facilities that were already over stretched and inappropriate to the needs of the mentally ill.[8] Much of the formal response to this situation was underpinned by an extraordinary period of legislative activity, which commenced in earnest with the Lunatic Asylums (Ireland) Act of 1821.

THE EARLY ASYLUMS IN NINETEENTH-CENTURY IRELAND

The period between 1820 and 1898 was a time of especially intensive legislative activity in relation to mental disorder and psychiatric institutions in Ireland. The need for extensive and systematic reform had been highlighted in 1804 by a Select Committee of the House of Commons which recommended the establishment of four provincial asylums dedicated to the treatment of the mentally ill, so as to minimise the numbers residing in prisons and houses of industry.[9] This was also a time of substantial reform in England[10] and, while progress was slow in Ireland, the Richmond Asylum in Grangegorman, Dublin eventually opened its doors in 1814.

The Richmond Asylum operated under the direction of a Board of Governors which had powers

> for the regulation, direction and management of themselves and of the said asylum and of all the patients therein and of all and every physician, surgeons, apothecaries, housekeepers, nursetenders, and other attendants, officers and servants of what nature and description soever of or belonging to the same.[11]

The Board was answerable to the lord lieutenant (the chief administrator of the British Government in Ireland), the Duke of Richmond, in whose honour the asylum was named.[12] Patients were admitted to the asylum on the basis of a certificate of insanity which had to be signed by a medical practitioner, clergyman or magistrate.[13]

The prevailing therapeutic paradigm at the new asylum was that of moral management as espoused by Esquirol in France[14] and Hallaran in Cork.[15] In Ireland, moral management constituted the prevailing therapeutic paradigm in the early decades of the nineteenth century and was introduced enthusiastically at the Richmond.[16] The Richmond was, however, quickly overcrowded and it was soon apparent that systematic reform at national level was needed in order to meet the needs of the mentally ill both in Dublin and throughout the rest of the country. Following considerable discussion in parliament,[17] a bill to establish such a system of asylums was presented by William Vesey Fitzgerald and passed on 11 July 1817. This legislation, which was amended in 1820, 1821, 1825 and 1826, represented the first substantive step in the establishment of Ireland's extensive system of district asylums, many of which were to remain in use for over 150 years.

More specifically, the Lunatic Asylums (Ireland) Act 1821 empowered the lord lieutenant to direct the erection of asylums throughout Ireland and specified that these were to be funded by both central government (nationally) and grand juries (locally). The establishment and planning of asylums were to be directed centrally by 'Commissioners for General Control and Correspondence' but local responsibility for directing asylum activity resided with boards of governors for each asylum.[18]

In 1825, the first asylum was established in Armagh and, over the following ten years, a further seven asylums were opened in Limerick, Belfast, Derry, Carlow, Portlaoise, Clonmel and Waterford, at a total cost of £245,000.[19] The design of these asylums was largely influenced by the evolution of various therapeutic paradigms throughout the 1800s. For example, as the emphasis on isolation and classification in the early part of the century yielded to moral management,[20] asylums assumed a 'panoptic' or radial design that was deemed consistent with the principles underlying moral management.[21]

As this period of asylum building continued, the numbers in Irish asylums increased significantly: by 1851 there were 3,234 individuals in the asylums and by 1891 this had increased further to 11,265.[22] The Lunacy (Ireland) Act 1821 directed that applications for admission needed to be accompanied by a medical certificate of insanity and a statement from next of kin confirming poverty; applications were then considered by the physician and manager of the asylum, and presented to the Board for acceptance.[23]

The 1821 legislation also directed that individuals who were insane at the time of a crime could be acquitted in court but detained in indefinite custody at a psychiatric institution 'at the pleasure' of the lord lieutenant. Individuals who were insane at time of indictment could also be so detained. To facilitate this, the Central Criminal Lunatic Asylum was opened in Dundrum, Dublin in 1850 under provisions of the Central Criminal Lunatic Asylum (Ireland) Act (1845, 1846) to provide 'a central asylum for insane persons charged with offences in Ireland' and detained indefinitely under this legislation.[24] The case of one such individual, Edward, is presented here, based on an examination of his original medical records at the Central Criminal Lunatic Asylum.

The Case of Edward, Detained 'at the Lord Lieutenant's Pleasure'

Edward was a 37-year-old man admitted to the Central Criminal Lunatic Asylum in the late 1860s having been charged with the murder of a fellow patient in a large district asylum. He was found to be 'insane on arraignment' and detained in the Central Criminal Lunatic Asylum 'at the Lord Lieutenant's pleasure'. On admission, Edward's level of education was recorded as 'nil' (i.e. he could neither read nor write) and he had 'no occupation'. Admission notes describe Edward as 'intemperate' and his 'mental state on admission' was one of 'recurrent mania with dementia'.

Medical notes record that Edward 'denies his crime [and] states that he is unjustly detained here'. He showed symptoms of 'chronic mania and dementia' and was 'constantly talking to himself and imaginary people'. It is important to note that, in the nineteenth century, the meaning of the term 'dementia' differed from its contemporary meaning; in the nineteenth century, 'dementia' meant any severe mental disorder with delusions and hallucinations (e.g. schizophrenia), whereas currently the term refers to certain chronic brain syndromes chiefly seen in later life (e.g. Alzheimer's disease). These changes in the uses of psychiatric terminology over time add greatly to the difficulty in interpreting clinical diagnoses from the nineteenth century and render it extremely difficult to establish systematically the contemporary equivalents of psychiatric disorders recorded in medical notes from that period.

In accordance with the principles of moral management, Edward was put to work as a 'division cleaner' and while he was 'quiet and well conducted as a rule' he was also 'excitable at times'. Some twenty-seven years after his admission, Edward was still a 'very quiet and well behaved patient' and a 'useful and obliging worker'. He was, however, 'in a weakly state of health [and] slightly depressed'. Edward's heart was 'weak' and late one evening six years later, the asylum doctor found Edward 'in great pain, in a state of almost complete prostration, his heart weak and fluttering'. Edward recovered from this episode but remained 'very weakly'. Some months later he again 'suddenly became collapsed, had an attack of vomiting' and 'sank fast'. Edward died later that night and an inquest confirmed he 'died from heart disease'. Aged 70 years at his death, Edward had spent thirty-three years in the Central Criminal Lunatic Asylum.

The case of Edward illustrates many of the features of both the criminal justice system and forensic psychiatric services in nineteenth-century Ireland. Edward was charged with the murder of a fellow-patient in a district asylum and detained for an indefinite period at the Central Criminal Lunatic Asylum. His subsequent detention was lengthy but by no means unique; many patients experienced detentions in excess of several decades during this period.[25] Like many others, Edward displayed strong signs of mental disorder (e.g. talking to imaginary people). Edward's death at the asylum was not unusual either: all Irish asylums experienced significant mortality rates during the nine-teenth century, owing chiefly to illnesses such as syphilis, dysentery, heart disease, epilepsy and tuberculosis.[26] (The challenges presented by many of these disorders are explored more fully in later chapters in this book.) Finally, the emphasis placed on Edward's performance as a 'division cleaner' was also typical of the times and reflects the importance that moral management accorded to gainful occupation as a key component of treatment.[27]

OTHER LEGISLATIVE INITIATIVES IN IRELAND THROUGHOUT THE 1800s

There was considerable legislative activity in relation to the mentally ill in Ireland as the nineteenth century progressed. The Criminal Lunatics (Ireland) Act 1838, for example, provided a separate form of admission to district asylums for individuals who were considered to be dangerous: such individuals could be detained indefinitely by two justices of the peace, who had the option of using medical evidence to inform their decision. The involvement of the judicial authorities in this way was by no means unique to Ireland: similar laws were introduced at around this time in Canada,[28] Australia,[29] Switzerland[30] and France, with the 1838 French law establishing 'official committal' as the normal means of committal for individuals who were deemed to represent a danger to public safety or order.[31] In Ireland, it was soon apparent that the 'dangerous lunacy' procedures were commonly misused[32] and in 1867 the Lunacy (Ireland) Act made it mandatory to seek a medical opinion prior to committal to a district asylum.

Further legislative activity towards the end of the nineteenth century aimed to address overcrowding in district asylums by decanting patients from asylums into workhouses. The relevant implications of the Lunatic Asylums (Ireland) Act 1875 were outlined by William Dillon, law adviser to the Richmond Asylum Joint Committee in Dublin in 1907:

> By Section 9 of the Lunatic Asylums (Ireland) Act, 1875, it is provided that the Guardians of any Poor Law Union in Ireland may, with the consent of the Local Government Board and the Inspectors of Lunatics, and, subject to such regulations as they shall respectively prescribe, receive into the workhouse any chronic lunatic, not being dangerous, who may have been received into a district asylum, and who may be certified by the Resident Medical Superintendent as fit to be so removed, and upon such terms as may be arranged between the union and governors (not the Committee), and such lunatic shall remain on the books of the Asylum as a patient and the expenses of such patient shall be paid by the governors of such district asylum. This section does not compel the Guardians to receive such lunatic; it makes it optional with the Guardians to accept or refuse the custody of a patient.[33]

In fact, it was the number of patients from workhouses presenting to the asylum that generated greatest cause for concern at this time and, by 1907, workhouse residents accounted for some 30 per cent of all admissions to the Richmond Asylum.[34] Moreover, Dillon advised the Richmond Asylum Joint Committee that 'under Section 9 of the Local Government (Ireland) Act [1898], it would appear that the Joint Committee is liable for the maintenance of all the lunatic poor in the City and Counties comprising the district, and they are bound to receive all insane persons into the asylum'. The 1898 Act, however, also presented a solution to the capacity problems presented by workhouse populations, according to Dillon:

> By the Local Government (Ireland) Act, 1898, aforesaid, Section 76, power is given to Asylum Committees to take over a workhouse or other suitable building from the Guardians of a Union, or to erect buildings themselves under Section 9 of said Act for the reception of chronic

lunatics who, not being dangerous to themselves or others, are certified
by the Resident Medical Superintendent of the Committee's Asylum not
to require special care and treatment in a fully equipped lunatic asylum.

The resident medical superintendent, Dr Conolly Norman, however,
opposed the establishment of auxiliary asylums, noting that 'attempts
have been made in several countries, notably in Germany and in the
State of New York, to establish "chronic" or "incurable" asylums as
distinct from acute asylums, but the system has failed ... It was found that
the notion of incurability attached to an asylum demoralized patients
and staff'.[35]
    There were several other pieces of legislation introduced throughout the
1800s that were not primarily directed at the emerging asylum system but
occasionally had significance for it. The Prison (Ireland) Act of 1826, for
example, required that private asylums be inspected by the inspector general
of prisons. In 1842, more specific legislation relating to private asylums was
introduced, in the form of the Private Lunatic Asylums (Ireland) Act. From
that year onwards, private asylums had to be granted licences on an annual
basis; patients could only be detained following receipt of a certificate
signed by two doctors; and private asylums were subject to visits from the
inspectors of lunacy.
    Throughout the century, the number of private asylums continued
to increase and, by 1844, there were fourteen registered private asylums
in Ireland, of which seven were in the Dublin area.[36] Further legislation
was passed later in the century (e.g. the Private Lunatic Asylums (Ireland)
Act 1874) and by 1893 there were 644 inpatients in twenty private asylums
throughout the country.[37] In addition, the Lunacy Asylums (Ireland) Act
of 1875 permitted the admission of paying patients to district asylums; this
was a thought-provoking legislative change that had a significant effect on
public perceptions of asylum care.[38]

THE END OF THE NINETEENTH CENTURY

By the time the nineteenth century drew to a close, mental health care in
Ireland had been transformed: at the start of the century there had been
minimal provision for the destitute mentally ill and, 100 years later, there
were large district asylums dotted throughout the country, most of which
were filled to capacity. There had also been a significant increase in private

accommodation, with some twenty private asylums registered in 1893, located chiefly in Dublin and its surrounding towns.

These sweeping changes were, for the most part, attributable to extensive legislative and administrative reforms over this period, including the period of extraordinary legislative activity that resulted in the introduction of the Lunatic Asylums (Ireland) Act 1821 and the Criminal Lunatics (Ireland) Act 1838. There were also significant changes in therapeutic paradigms over this time including, most notably, the emergence of moral management as the dominant therapeutic paradigm.[39] Edward's case is particularly instructive, as it not only illustrates many features of the nineteenth-century institutional experience (lengthy detention, ongoing symptoms of mental and physical illness, etc) but also highlights the first of many fundamental tensions that were to shape mental health services in subsequent decades: the tension between medical and non-medical actors in health service planning and provision.

More specifically, the emphasis placed on Edward's performance as a division cleaner reflected the importance placed on gainful occupation as a key component of treatment. This broad, humanistic approach of moral management contrasted sharply with the traditional medical approach, which tended to focus on physical treatments such as bloodletting and the use of physical devices such as circulating swings.[40] Moreover, within the asylum, moral managers tended not to be medical doctors, further highlighting the contrasts between the moral management approach and the traditional medical paradigm.

The tensions resulting from this divergence of approaches in the nineteenth century prefigured many of the fundamental tensions that were to characterise mental health care in subsequent decades, including the tension between psychological and biological approaches in the twentieth century[41] and the tension between medical autonomy and external, non-medical management in the twentieth and twenty-first centuries.[42]

At the start of the twentieth century in Ireland, however, there were also further problems with morale, stemming from a range of sources, including intractable overcrowding in the asylums and a perception that rates of mental disorder were increasing in the population.[43] Many of these issues dominated the Conference of the Irish Asylums Committee that convened at the Richmond Asylum, Dublin in 1903.[44] The exchanges at this meeting, along with continued public and governmental concern about the mentally ill, led to further substantive reform as the twentieth century progressed, culminating in the introduction of the Mental

Treatment Act 1945 (Chapter 5). This was an effort to stem the ever-rising tide of admissions and provide more appropriate, acceptable care to individuals with mental disorder.

DEALING WITH 'THE INCREASE OF INSANITY IN IRELAND'

These increases in institutional provision for the mentally ill in nineteenth-century Ireland coincided with increased concern about an apparent rise in the number of individuals with mental disorder. As early as 1810, Hallaran had lamented the 'hurried weight of human calamity' for which he sought to provide accommodation in Cork Lunatic Asylum.[45]

This concern intensified as the century progressed, and as the nineteenth century drew to a close the Inspectors of Lunatics (1893) reported that 'the number of the insane [receiving treatment] has increased from 249 per 100,000 of the population in 1880, to 839 per 100,000 in 1892'.[46] Dr Daniel Hack Tuke (1827–1895), a prominent physician and mental health reformer, reviewed official statistics in the 1890s and published an influential paper titled 'Increase of Insanity in Ireland' in the *Journal of Mental Science*:

> Now, taking first the number of certified lunatics and idiots in the asylums of Ireland during each of the 19 years 1875 to 1893 inclusive, I find that the rate of increase during the last over the first quinquennium is as high as 60 per cent, after allowing for the decrease of population. In England and Wales during a corresponding period the rise did not exceed 22 per cent. If next we ascertain the total number of lunatics and idiots in Ireland on January 1st, 1875, and subsequent years (except those 'at large'), and the rate of increase we find that the rate of this increase during the last over the first quinquennium has been 53 per cent.[47]

After careful consideration of further statistics and possible confounding issues, Tuke was 'disposed to admit [that] there is ... some actual as well as apparent increase of mental disorder'. Tuke's concern was widely echoed in both public and professional circles.[48]

While it is beyond doubt that the perception of increased rates of mental disorder was a real and significant concern in the nineteenth century, it is substantially less clear to what extent such an increase truly occurred and, if it did occur, what factors produced it. It is likely that a variety of factors were relevant, including (a) increased recognition and diagnosis of mental disorder; (b) mutually re-enforcing patterns of asylum building and psychiatric committal, underpinned by legislative change; (c) changes in diagnostic practices; and (d) possible epidemiological change owing to socio-demographic changes and/or unidentified biological factors. Difficulties in establishing the precise relevance of each of these factors make it virtually impossible to establish whether or not there was a true increase in rates of mental disorder at this time. Nonetheless, closer examination of these four areas is useful in understanding nineteenth-century concerns about rates of mental disorder and the response of the authorities in terms of institutional provision for the mentally ill.

INCREASED RECOGNITION AND DIAGNOSIS OF MENTAL DISORDER

The end of the eighteenth century saw substantial changes in societal attitudes to mental disorder throughout Europe. In a detailed examination of rates of schizophrenia in Ireland over the past two centuries, Walsh notes the relevance of the 'humanitarian climate of the nineteenth century' which may have led to increased efforts to provide care to individuals with mental disorder, resulting in an apparent increase in population rates of disorder.[49] This change in attitude was evident at several locations throughout Europe in the late eighteenth and early nineteenth centuries.

In 1796, William Tuke, a Quaker tea merchant, founded the York Retreat in England, with the explicit intent of providing care for the mentally ill in a humane and nurturing setting.[50] In 1801, Pinel, at the Salpêtrière Hospital in Paris, independently published an influential textbook promoting similar principles and many of his proposals were later championed by Esquirol in Charenton, Paris and at the Salpêtrière. These changes in attitudes resulted in greater recognition that mental disorder was a significant problem for which society had a responsibility to provide solutions for, in terms of both treatment and accommodation for the mentally ill.

These changes in attitudes led to considerable efforts at systematic, governmental reform in many countries, including the United Kingdom.[51] In Ireland, a Select Committee of the House of Commons in 1804 recommended the establishment of four provincial asylums dedicated to the treatment of the mentally ill.[52] In 1815 one such establishment, the Richmond Asylum, finally opened its doors in Dublin.[53] While it

is difficult to quantify the precise effects of these changes in professional
and public attitudes to mental disorder, it is likely that they contributed
to increased recognition and diagnosis of mental disorder and, in turn,
increased presentations to the newly established asylums.

Increased recognition and diagnosis of mental disorder may also be
attributable to societal or political factors. Hallaran, in his 1810 textbook,
emphasised the roles of warfare and social unrest in increasing presentations
to asylums:

> To account therefore correctly for this unlooked for pressure of a public and
> private calamity, it appears to be indispensably requisite to take into account
> the high degree of corporeal as well as of mental excitement, which may
> be supposed a consequence of continued warfare in the general sense ...
> Such I know to have been but too frequently the tragical events of the late
> unhappy disturbances, which it is to be confessed, have added but little to
> the character of this country; and to which may be ascribed in a principal
> degree, the enormous augmentation to the lists of insane persons who have
> within the last ten years been received into our public Asylum.[54]

The latter part of the nineteenth century was also a time of industrialisation,
resulting in significant changes at community and societal levels in many
European countries. Changes to the structure of communities owing to
industrialisation may have increased the visibility of individuals with mental
disorder in communities, resulting in increased presentations to asylums and
an apparent increase in rates of mental disorder.[55]

Tuke, in his 1894 paper, also notes the emphasis that Norman at the
Richmond placed on social attitudes in producing increased rates of presentation to asylums:

> Although the number of persons under treatment in the Dublin Asylum
> has risen from 1,055 in 1883 to 1,467 at the end of 1892 (or 412 more) the
> medical Reporter, Dr Conolly Norman, observes: 'At the same time, as the
> result of much consideration, it is not thought that the facts warrant the
> conclusion that there has been during the period any very marked increase
> in the tendency to insanity among the inhabitants of the district'. So far
> as there is an apparent increase, Dr Norman attributes it to: (1) Decreased
> prejudice against asylums; (2) The friends of patients being less tolerant of
> having insane persons in their midst; (3) Poor-Law Authorities being more
> sensible of the unsuitability of most workhouses to provide for the insane;

(4) The fact that the increase is almost confined to Dublin itself, where the population is increasing [*sic*]. The death-rate and the recovery-rate have also decreased, and will largely account for the accumulation of cases, though, as I have already said, not for the rise in admissions.[56]

These changes in social attitudes, societal structures and patterns of presentation, as well as changes in diagnostic practices (see below), represented significant changes in the interpretation and experience of mental disorder at both individual and societal levels. At the same time as these attitudinal changes were taking place, an elaborate process of legislative reform and asylum building began and inexorably gathered pace as the nineteenth century progressed.

LEGISLATIVE CHANGE, ASYLUM BUILDING AND PSYCHIATRIC COMMITTAL

The nineteenth century was a time of unprecedented legislative activity in relation to mental health in Ireland. The Lunatic Asylums (Ireland) Act 1821, in particular, authorised the establishment of a network of district asylums throughout the country and within fifteen years there were large public asylums established in Armagh, Limerick, Belfast, Derry, Carlow, Portlaoise, Clonmel and Waterford.[57] The reports of the inspectors of lunacy demonstrate that these asylums were filled to capacity soon after opening.[58] This trend continued for the remainder of the nineteenth century: in 1851 there were 3,234 individuals resident in asylums and by 1891 this had increased to 11,265.[59]

There can be little doubt that the sudden availability of hundreds of asylum beds led to increased rates of presentation by mentally ill individuals who had previously lived with families, lodged in workhouses, or been homeless – and had not, therefore, been counted in official estimates of the number of the mentally ill. The Great Irish Famine of the 1840s is also likely to have played a role in increasing social need and pressure for accommodation and food. It is unclear, however, what proportion of admissions to the new asylums was truly suffering from mental disorder and what proportion was admitted for other reasons (e.g. intellectual disability, social problems). Prior draws particular attention to the misuse of 'dangerous lunacy' procedures which offered several practical advantages to families seeking to have family members committed to psychiatric institutions; e.g. the asylum could not refuse to admit a 'dangerous lunatic'.[60]

The true diagnostic mix in admissions to Irish asylums during this period is not clear and undoubtedly merits further systematic study. It is clear, however, that the rapid overcrowding in asylums was related not only to increased rates of presentation, but also to prolonged length of stay or 'accumulation by non-discharge'.[61] Between the years 1850 and 1890, the excess of admissions over discharges was approximately 200 annually; i.e. there were, potentially, 200 new long-stay patients created in Ireland's asylums each year. The type of patients that generated some of these statistics are demonstrated by the cases of Brian and Christopher, which are outlined here based on their case records from the Central Criminal Lunatic Asylum.

The Case of Brian: 'Epileptic Insanity'

Brian was a 28-year-old Irish man charged with murder in the mid-1880s. He was 'acquitted on the grounds of insanity' and detained at the Central Criminal Lunatic Asylum 'at the Lord Lieutenant's Pleasure'. Brian was a married shopkeeper who was able to 'read and write'.

Admission notes record that Brian was 'subject to epilepsy' and the cause of his mental disorder was 'drink'. He had a family history of epilepsy and problems with alcohol: his 'father died in an epileptic fit; one sister died in [an] asylum; and two brothers are epileptics … the two epileptic brothers are intemperate'. Brian's admission diagnosis was 'epileptic insanity'. Medical notes shortly after admission record that 'epileptic attacks and fits of violent maniacal excitement now began to occur frequently and his face has assumed a congested and demented appearance. [His] language [is] incoherent and violent'.

Over time, Brian's symptoms subsided and ten years after admission he was 'quiet and well conducted; works on the land. Health good. Mental condition has much improved'. Some twenty years after admission he was 'quite harmless and easily managed'. Later that year, Brian was transferred back to a district asylum close to his home – the same asylum in which his sister had died many years earlier. There is no further record of Brian's clinical course or outcome, but it is likely that his stay in the district asylum was a lengthy one: residence within an Irish asylum for more than five years almost invariably meant that the individual would spend the rest of their lives behind asylum walls.[62]

Christopher: 'A Case of Recurrent Mania'

Christopher was a 33-year-old Irish man charged with the murder of his wife in the early 1870s. He was found to be 'insane on arraignment' and detained at the Central Criminal Lunatic Asylum 'at the Lord Lieutenant's Pleasure'. Christopher was a tinsmith with eight children and could read but not write.

Admission notes record that the cause of Christopher's mental disorder was 'syphilis' and that he had two previous admissions to his local asylum, including one 'for attempted suicide by cutting his throat'. There was a family history of 'phthisis' and 'scrofulous', both of which refer to tuberculosis, which was a common problem in both general[63] and asylum populations at this time.[64]

On admission, Christopher was diagnosed as

> a case of recurrent mania. Patient has had syphilis and states that on two occasions he has suffered from Delirium Tremens. [He] suffers from hallucinations and delusions, voices, 'poisoned by medicine in his food', 'conspiracy against him'. [He] is noisy and talkative at night; has a peculiar way of making up his bed; states 'it is to keep the bad air out and the electricity from playing on him'.

Despite these symptoms, Christopher was 'quiet and well behaved [and] makes himself generally useful ... is possessed of marked ability and is very clever with his hands'.

Notwithstanding these positive observations, Christopher's detention at the Central Criminal Lunatic Asylum was a lengthy one, owing to a combination of psychiatric symptoms, physical illnesses and a paucity of discharge options. Some four decades after his original committal, Christopher's physical health had become the chief focus of concern. He was 'confined to bed almost continuously during the winter and is very feeble. He suffers from chronic bronchitis and rheumatic arthritis'. The following year, Christopher 'developed hemiplaegia [paralysis] on right side of his body' and died some days later, owing to an 'effusion of blood on the brain'. Christopher was 74 years of age at his death and had spent forty-one years in the Central Criminal Lunatic Asylum.

The cases of Brian and Christopher demonstrate the complex tangle of legal, psychiatric and medical problems that presented substantial challenges to discharge from psychiatric care. This paucity of discharge options undoubtedly contributed to 'accumulation by non-discharge',[65] which, in turn, compounded the apparently intractable overcrowding in Irish asylums throughout the nineteenth century.

CHANGES IN DIAGNOSTIC PRACTICES

Diagnostic practices in psychiatry are continually changing and there are significant difficulties in establishing the contemporary equivalents of diagnoses made in the nineteenth century, especially when retrospective diag- nostic endeavours are based on inconsistent, incomplete medical records.[66] There were, for example, four nineteenth-century terms that correlated with diagnoses that are now known as 'functional psychoses' (i.e. schizophrenia and bipolar affective disorder): mania, melancholia, mono-mania and dementia.[67] The confusion and conflation of these terms in the literature of the times adds greatly to the difficulties of interpreting statistics provided for admissions and discharges throughout the 1800s. Some of these diagnostic challenges, along with the difficulties in separating mental disorder from socio-economically driven concerns, are demonstrated by the case of Dorothy.

The Case of Dorothy with 'Chronic Melancholia'

Dorothy was a 40-year-old housekeeper with seven children who was charged with the manslaughter of her 4-year-old child in the mid-1890s. She was 'acquitted on the grounds of insanity' and detained at the Central Criminal Lunatic Asylum 'at Her Majesty's Pleasure'. Dorothy's admission diagnosis was 'chronic melancholia' which was attributed to heredity; admission notes record that she had a sister in a district asylum.

Medical records note that Dorothy's 'expression of face, attitude and gestures are characteristic of melancholia; she is emotional at times. [She] does not exhibit any delusion'. Her notes, however, also record that 'she takes an interest in her surroundings and associates with the other patients; readily enters conversation. Appetite good, sleeps well, clean and tidy in dress and person. [She] is bad tempered and inclined to sulk if corrected. [She] does needlework and house cleaning'. Subsequent notes confirm that Dorothy was consistently 'well-behaved, quiet and respectable' and 'an excellent worker'. Much of this is not consistent with a diagnosis of 'chronic melancholia'. Indeed, notes from almost two years after her admission specify that Dorothy 'will cry when meditating on her misfortunes'; this reaction would appear understandable, at least in part, given Dorothy's situation (the loss of her child, indefinite detention, etc.)

Notes from six years after Dorothy's admission record that 'this patient is perfectly sane and is most anxious for her discharge but there is some difficulty as her husband is in a workhouse and she has no friends sufficiently well off to provide for her'. Some arrangement must have been reached, however, as two years later Dorothy, then described as 'perfectly harmless', was 'discharged … in care of her daughter'. In this case, the diagnosis of 'chronic melancholia' appears, by today's diagnostic criteria, to be largely unsupported by the clinical details recorded in the notes from her stay in the Central Criminal Lunatic Asylum.

Notwithstanding these difficulties with the interpretation of clinical records, some general conclusions can still be drawn about changes in diagnostic practices throughout the nineteenth century. There is, for example, strong evidence to suggest there was a significant diagnostic shift from intellectual disability ('idiots') towards mental disorder ('lunatics') during the latter part of the century. In 1893, for example, the Inspectors of Lunatics presented findings from the General Report of the Census Commissioners demonstrating a fall in the number of 'idiots' (from 7,033 in 1861 to 6,243 in 1891) and a rise in the number of 'lunatics' (from 7,065 in 1861 to 14,945 in 1891).[68] There are many possible reasons for these changes, not least of which is the sudden availability of hundreds of asylum beds for individuals with mental disorder, which may have prompted a reclassification of certain intellectually disabled individuals as 'lunatics' in order to secure easier access to long-term asylum accommodation.

EPIDEMIOLOGICAL CHANGE?

The possibility of true change in the incidence of mental disorder in nineteenth century Ireland is virtually impossible to resolve definitively, owing to the absence of reliable data about both the incidence of mental disorder and the precise population of Ireland in the 1800s. Even at the time, it was recognised that epidemiological analysis of the population of the United Kingdom (which then included Ireland) was hampered by the absence of reliable data. Dr Richard Powell, in a paper read to the Royal College of Physicians in London in 1810, noted that:

> In order to form a correct judgement respecting the increase or decrease
> of any particular disease, it is not sufficient merely to ascertain the number

of cases in which it occurs within any given period or periods, but it is further necessary to examine the relative population of the country at exactly the same time, and to compare under the same dates the numbers of each. Now upon this subject our data are very deficient.[69]

There were similar problems with data collection in Ireland, with the result that precise epidemiological analysis of the incidence of mental disorder is essentially impossible. It is apparent, however, that certain demographic factors and changes in population structure may have played a role in producing, at the very least, an apparent increase in the rate of mental disorder. There were, for example, substantial increases in life expectancy around 1800 and these may have increased the survival of individuals prone to develop schizophrenia.[70] This would have increased the prevalence of mental disorder (and therefore burden of care) but not necessarily the incidence. In addition, increased preoccupation with quality of life, rather than mere survival, may have further increased rates of presentation to asylums, further increasing the burden of care without truly increasing incidence.

Notwithstanding these arguments, many medical directors in the nineteenth century believed there was a true increase in rates of mental disorder, and cast doubt on arguments suggesting this phenomenon were entirely attributable to accumulation of patients in asylums, decreased stigma, incarceration of individuals with alcohol problems, transfers from workhouses, heredity, the return of emigrants with mental disorder, or a number of other factors.[71] Torrey and Miller argue, in fact, that there has been an epidemic of mental disorder over the past three centuries and that while this has gone largely unnoticed owing to its gradual onset, it represents an important but neglected force in world history.[72] While the evidence they present is persuasive in many respects, it remains exceedingly difficult to determine, with any degree of accuracy, how much of the pressure on asylums in nineteenth-century Ireland was due to true epidemiological change and how much was due to other factors, such as changes in diagnostic practices and societal circumstances (e.g. the Famine and conflict). The matter is further complicated by the fact that societal circumstances may well produce a true increase in rates of certain disorders, and not just an apparent increase due to increased rates of presentation.

In any case, while the causes of any true increase in the incidence of mental disorder (if such truly did occur) are unclear, there is little doubt that the perception of such an increase had a decisive influence on both mental health policy and mental health legislation in Ireland. This perception was, in particular, associated with a remarkable and extensive asylum-building programme and a steady increase in asylum populations over the course of the 1800s. This accumulating inpatient population presented particularly urgent challenges to the managers of Irish asylums at the start of the twentieth century.

INTO THE TWENTIETH CENTURY: 1903–1944

Issues relating to overcrowding in Irish asylums were to the fore of the agenda at the Conference of the Irish Asylums Committee, convened at the Richmond Asylum in 1903.[73] By that time, it was felt that the increase in admissions was related in large part to heredity rather than poverty, adversity, religion or mental anxiety – a conclusion which contrasted with the emphasis Hallaran had placed on political turmoil a century earlier in his influential textbook.[74] Within a few short years of the 1903 conference, however, Norman at the Richmond expressed cautious optimism that the number of individuals presenting with mental disorder was finally in decline. In 1907, he reported to the Richmond Asylum Joint Committee that:

> The number of patients in the asylum has actually undergone a slight decrease since this time last year. It is, therefore, perhaps, possible, without being unduly optimistic, to indulge the expectation that the rate of increase may have reached its summit, and that the difficulty of dealing with the question may not progressively be augmented.[75]

Sadly, Norman was indeed 'unduly optimistic': Ireland's overall asylum population continued to rise throughout the first half of the twentieth century, with just two short lived declines during the two world wars; by 1945 there were 17,708 individuals resident in Irish asylums.[76] The extent of official concern about these trends was reflected by the establishment of three separate inquiries that dealt, to greater or lesser extents, with issues related to mental disorder: the Viceregal Commission on Poor Law Reform in Ireland (1906), the Royal Commission on the Care and Control of the Feeble-Minded (1908) and the Royal Commission on the Poor Laws and Relief of Distress (1910). Notwithstanding the reports of these bodies,[77] there was little real change in the management or conditions of district asylums in the opening decades of the twentieth century. In 1924, E. Boyd Barrett SJ (Society of Jesus; i.e. a Jesuit priest), writing in *Studies: An Irish Quarterly Review*, noted that:

One would suppose that it should be the first aim of asylum staffs to apply the best methods of treatment that science has evolved, and to keep au courant with psycho-therapeutic investigations. But there is little sign of this. The Medical Superintendent finds himself so engrossed in administrative duties (which should be done by a manager or steward) that he has little time to attend to patients. The zeal which, as a doctor, he should have for a generous outlay of money on medical requirements is chilled by his anxiety as an administrator to cut down expenses ... There should be strong public demand for immediate reform of the asylum system, and the complete segregation and scientific treatment of curable cases should be insisted upon. Suitable asylums should be built – healthy, bright, beautiful homes, where patients would be enticed by every art to renew their interests in things. Nerve clinics should be opened in every populous district, where advice and treatment should be available for ordinary cases of nerve trouble and incipient insanity.[78]

In 1925, another governmental commission was established to examine the nature and level of provision for the sick and destitute poor in Ireland, with a particular focus on individuals with mental disorder. This commission's report highlighted serious problems with overcrowding and lack of treatment in Irish asylums, and proposed the development of outpatient services and short-term admission facilities in general hospitals.[79] Reform of the asylum system was, however, excruciatingly slow and another two decades were to elapse before voluntary admission procedures were introduced, in the Mental Treatment Act of 1945. Voluntary admission processes had been already introduced many years earlier in several other jurisdictions, including Switzerland[80] and France (in 1876).[81]

In the opening decades of the 1900s, however, the Irish asylums remained large, overcrowded institutions, filled with detained patients and generally poorly therapeutic and unhygienic. The situation was epitomised by conditions in Ireland's largest asylum, the Richmond, at Grangegorman in Dublin.

THE RICHMOND ASYLUM, DUBLIN IN 1907

The Richmond Asylum in Grangegorman, Dublin (later known as Grangegorman Mental Hospital and St Brendan's Hospital) was established in the early 1800s to help address the unmet needs of the mentally ill, especially the destitute mentally ill, in nineteenth-century Ireland.[82]

The opening of Richmond in 1814 heralded the beginning of the extraordinary period of asylum building which persisted throughout the latter half of the nineteenth century in Ireland.[83] The Richmond is particularly interesting because it was one of the earliest asylums to open in Ireland, was one of the largest residential institutions of any kind in the country, and, arguably, served as a model for the development and management of other psychiatric institutions for the remainder of the century.

From its foundation, the Richmond focused on the moral management paradigm[84] and this remained in evidence for several decades following its establishment. By 1846, the asylum had 289 inpatients and the Inspector of Lunatic Asylums gave a positive report:

> It is unnecessary for me to add that the general business [of the asylum] is most satisfactorily performed ... The asylum continues to maintain its high character as being one of the best-managed institutions in the country; and also for the great order, regularity, and state of cleanliness in which is it kept.[85]

As the asylums expanded during the 1800s, however, attention shifted from the person-focused approach of moral management to a more institution-focused approach, prioritising the administrative requirements of the increasingly large, complex institutions themselves over the needs of individual patients.[86] By the early 1890s, the Richmond Asylum had almost 1,500 patients in accommodation designed for 1,100[87] and in 1893 the inspectors provided a distinctly less positive report, focussing chiefly on the by now chronic overcrowding.[88]

In the mid-1890s the Richmond acquired additional land at Portrane, North Dublin and commissioned a new asylum there, Portrane Branch Asylum, in an effort to alleviate the overcrowding. The proceedings of the Richmond Asylum Joint Committee, governing both the Richmond and Portrane, provide fascinating insights into asylum management and the practical challenges presented by the inexorable expansion in patient numbers. The Committee minutes from 1907 are especially interesting because in that year the Committee appointed a Special Committee to 'enquire into the Question of Provision for Workhouse Lunatics', and Norman, as medical superintendent, was directed to perform a diagnostic segregation of all asylum patients, in order to clarify which patients really needed to be in the asylum and which could be discharged or accommodated elsewhere.[89]

The challenges the Committee faced during this period were myriad, and can be usefully grouped into four key areas:

(a)   Managing the patient populations within the asylums
(b)   Staffing and management issues
(c)   Challenges presented by workhouse populations
(d)   Clinical segregation of patients by Norman.

(a)   Managing the patient populations within the asylums

Given the chronic problems with overcrowding, the Richmond District Asylum Joint Committee was regularly provided with a census of inpatients in Richmond and Portrane. At the meeting of 17 January 1907, for example, the Committee was informed that there were 2,924 patients (1,505 male, 1,419 female) in the asylums, of whom 1,321 (728 male, 593 female) were at Portrane. Over the course of 1907 this figure did not change significantly, with a total of 2,914 patients in the asylums in December 1907.

While the overall number of inpatients varied little from month to month, there were still significant numbers of admissions and discharges. For example, at the Committee meeting of 18 December 1907, Norman reported that over the previous month 'twenty-two men and twenty-two women have been admitted, making a total of forty-four … Fourteen were admitted from the various workhouses within the district, and eleven were cases of readmission'. In December 1907, Norman reported on three particularly challenging admissions of women from the nearby Mountjoy Prison, who 'were more or less habitual drunkards … It is a pity that there is not some mode of dealing with people of this class besides sending them to ordinary district asylums. Ordinary asylum care and treatment have little or no permanent effect, and seem to be as inoperative almost as imprisonment with a view to effecting any real cure'.

Overall, the numbers in Richmond itself had been increasing steadily throughout the late 1800s and early 1900s: in 1890 there were 1,368 inpatients and by 1900 this had risen to 2,254.[90] In Ireland as a whole, the asylum population had also increased substantially over preceding decades: in 1851 there were 3,234 individuals in asylums; by 1891 this had increased to 11,265; and by 1914 this had increased to 16,941.[91]

There was long-standing concern that this increase in the asylum population reflected a true increase in the rates of mental disorder in Ireland.[92] This concern dated from well before Hallaran's 1810 lament about 'the extraordinary increase of insanity in Ireland'[93] and persisted even after Tuke's insightful 1894 paper in the *Journal of Mental Science* which incorporated Norman's views on the matter and speculated about the role of emigration in producing this trend.[94]

This rise in admissions resulted in acute problems for many asylums and the Richmond was no exception.[95] At the Committee meeting on 31 January 1907, the chairman outlined the extent of the problem, noting that:

> for the year 1898, preceding the date on which we took office, the daily average number of patients on our books was 1,958, as compared with 2,878, the daily average number resident during 1906. In a period of eight years, therefore, there has been an increase of no less than 920 patients ... I say it with all deliberation and intense regret, and with experience of the last ten years, that we have already reached a grave and alarming crisis. Richmond is overcrowded. Portrane, provided at a capital charge of £370,000 is full.

Overcrowding at Richmond was also a concern for the Irish Inspectors of Lunatics, who commented, in 1893, that:

> During the year no relief has been obtained as regards the overcrowding ... It is therefore not to be wondered at that the general health of the institution is far from satisfactory, and that the death-rate, as compared with other Irish asylums, is high, amounting to 12.5 per cent, the average death rate in similar institution in this country being 8.3 per cent. Constant outbreaks of zymotic disease have occurred. Dysentry has for many years past been almost endemic in this institution – 73 cases with 14 deaths occurred last year, and it may be mentioned that in no less than three of these cases secondary abscesses were found in the liver.[96]

These problems with overcrowding were compounded by increasing recognition of the large number of individuals with mental disorder living in workhouses which were poorly equipped to meet their medical and social needs.[97] The pressure presented by the workhouse populations, allied with the constant challenges within the large asylum itself, resulted in myriad staffing and management challenges for committees at the Richmond and elsewhere.

(b) Staffing and Management Issues

The Richmond had an extensive staff, including doctors, nurses, porters, attendants, keepers and, from 1855, teaching staff. Various tradesmen were also employed, including carpenters, engineers, tailors, shoemakers and others. The Richmond District Asylum Joint Committee, Richmond

Visiting Committee and Portrane Visiting Committee regularly discussed matters related to employment, salaries and discipline, as well as issues pertaining to supplies of foodstuffs, water, hay, straw (for bedding) and structural supplies for developments at the asylums.

The consumption of excessive quantities of alcohol by a minority of staff members was a recurring problem.[98] At the Committee meeting on 13 June 1907, Norman reported that two weeks earlier one of the attendants 'was noticed at the patients' breakfast to be under the influence of drink. I saw him shortly before 9am when he was under the influence of drink. I ordered him to leave the wards and go to his bedroom and stay there. I saw him again about 2pm. He was still under the influence of drink. He boasted that he had not carried out my orders and he disputed my authority. I then suspended him.' On considering this report, the Committee was 'of opinion that he should be dismissed from the services of the Asylum'.

Alcohol abuse was also a problem among patients: at the meeting of the Richmond Visiting Committee on 12 December 1907, Norman noted that 'since the last meeting of this Committee, eighteen male and twenty-four female patients have been admitted, making a total of forty-two. In at least nine of the male and seven of the female admissions, drink was a main factor in producing insanity'. On 10 January 1907, Norman reported that on the previous Christmas morning (1906), he found one male patient 'extremely drunk' and, on investigating the matter further, was concerned about the role of one particular male attendant whose 'conduct in the matter is very suspicious'. Later that day another patient was 'under the influence of drink. The patient got a fit when he was being removed from the dining room, and was subsequently highly excited. Next day he said he had taken some of the attendants' beer (apparently heel taps left in the tumblers)'.

Norman noted that 'it is a very serious matter giving a patient drink, or allowing him to get drink'. The Inspectors of Lunatics took a similar view and requested the 'RMS to report such matters to them in future within three days of their occurrence'. At the meeting of the Richmond Visiting Committee, on 14 February 1907, Norman suggested that there was 'only one way to prevent such lamentable occurrences, and that is to have a staff on whose good feeling and sense of duty one can depend'. This was a constant challenge at the Richmond.

One of the other challenges that confronted asylum authorities was the provision of adequate medical care to an increasing numbers of inpatients. At the meeting of the Richmond Visiting Committee on 11 April 1907, Norman reported that 'the London County Council Asylums spend a good deal more than we do on the junior medical staff'. He noted that 'a famous foreign reformer writing in French fifty years ago laid down the axiom that there should be one Medical Officer for every hundred patients ... In Ireland the proportion is generally low, often dangerously so'. The numbers of patients and assistant medical officers in Irish asylums (1906) and asylums in London County Council area (1904) are shown in Table 1 and support Norman's concerns that levels of staffing in many asylums, including the Richmond, were well below the standard he outlined.

Table 1

Numbers of patients and assistant medical officers in Irish asylums (1906) and asylums in London County Council area (1904):

Location	Asylum	Number of patients	Number of assistant medical officers
Ireland	Antrim	567	1
	Armagh	522	1
	Ballinasloe	1,340	2
	Belfast	1,108	2
	Carlow	441	1
	Castlebar	676	1
	Clonmel	785	1
	Cork	1,570	4
	Downpatrick	723	2
	Ennis	409	1
	Enniscorthy	500	1
	Kilkenny	465	1
	Killarney	577	1
	Letterkenny	704	1
	Limerick	642	1
	Londonderry	519	1
	Maryborough	536	1
	Monaghan	848	2
	Mullingar	925	1
	Omagh	739	1

	Richmond	1,498	5
	Portrane	1,332	2
	Sligo	687	1
	Waterford	548	1
London County Council Area	Banstead	2,451	5
	Bexley	2,087	6
	Cave Hill	2,109	5
	Claybury	2,394	6
	Colney Hatch	2,153	5
	Hanwell	2,559	6
	Horton	1,964	5

Source: Richmond Asylum Joint Committee Minutes (1907).[99]

Regarding the Richmond, Norman noted that:

> The difficulty of attending to admissions and also paying the necessary visits to the wards in the afternoons is often considerable ... Thus I hope the Committee will agree with me in holding, as I do most respectfully but most strongly, that the Richmond Asylum cannot be worked with a staff of less than four junior officers, allowing for relief and providing that there will be always one actually on duty in each house.

Following consideration of Norman's request, the Committee agreed to appoint a 'clinical assistant' for six months, but declined to fill a vacancy created by the recent departure of one of the Richmond's other doctors, Dr Samuels.

The challenges faced by these doctors were substantial and varied. In addition to mental disorder and alcohol addiction, asylum patients presented with a range of medical and surgical problems including infective diseases and self-injury. On 10 January 1907, Norman reported that one male patient 'admitted on December 31, suffered from an extensive incised wound of the throat, self-inflicted'; that 'a case of dysentery [inflammation of the intestine] has occurred in the female house'; and that 'an old patient, a deaf mute ... died on December 30 somewhat suddenly and unexpectedly. There was time to summon medical assistance before he expired. On post mortem examination extensive fatty disease of the heart [coronary disease] was found to have existed. The Coroner was notified, but did not consider an inquest necessary'.

The obstetric needs of female patients presented particular challenges. On 10 January 1907, Norman reported that a female patient 'admitted on January 3, was delivered of a female infant on January 6. Her husband removed the child home from the asylum at once'. On 14 February, Norman reported that a 'female patient … an unmarried woman, who was pregnant when admitted on February 1, and suffered from uraemia [kidney disease], died on February 10, having given birth to a still-born child'.

Illness and injury to staff working in the asylum were brought to the attention of the Richmond Asylum Committees on a regular basis. On 9 May 1907, Norman reported that a nurse 'who has recently been appointed, has contracted very serious and acute lung trouble'; despite medical intervention, this nurse 'died of acute tubercular consumption on May 26th.' At this time, consumption (pulmonary tuberculosis) was a common cause of death accounting for almost 16 per cent of all deaths in Ireland in 1904[100] and over 25 per cent of deaths in Irish asylums in 1901;[101] similar problems were reported in asylums elsewhere.[102]

Other illnesses reported in Richmond and Portrane included general paralysis (tertiary or advanced syphilis), maniacal chorea (mental disorder with neurological features), acute rheumatism, 'extensive valvular disease of the heart', epilepsy and erysipelas (a skin infection). On 6 March 1907, Norman himself was reported to be suffering from 'a rather severe cold and lumbago' and on 13 June 1907 Dr Cullinan was 'ill with a sharp attack of rheumatic fever'.

There were also reports of injuries to staff. On 14 March 1907, Norman reported 'a lamentable casualty to one of the female employees' who 'accidentally set fire to her clothes' and was 'sent to the Mater Misericordiae Hospital, where she died the next day. It is to be observed that this poor woman's petticoats and undergarments were made of that very dangerous material, flannelette.' Minutes from the meeting of 21 March 1907 note receipt of a 'letter on behalf of the attendants and nurses … making an appeal on behalf of the four orphan children' of the nurse 'who was accidentally burned on the 3rd inst. A sum of money had been collected which would be applied to the relief of the orphans if the Committee would be so kind as to defray the funeral expenses, which amounted to £6 6s 6d'. The Committee paid the funeral expenses.

Patients also suffered injuries: on 4 December 1907 the Portrane Visiting Committee heard that one male patient 'who was assisting in repairing the roof of the boot-shop' had 'overbalanced himself, and fell through one of the glass lights to the floor, a distance of perhaps some seventeen feet. He was stunned, but happily seems to have received no serious injury. Dr Donelan rightly points out the danger of putting patients to work on roofs, a practice which certainly must be discontinued.' Norman reported that another male patient 'was thrown down by another patient ... and sustained a fracture of the right thigh bone. As he is a feeble old man, and this is a serious injury, he will probably die.'

The Richmond Asylum Joint Committee minutes from 1907 record various initiatives to improve safety and working conditions in the asylums, including improvements to fire alarm systems and the introduction of electric lights, as well as ongoing discussion about insurance and compensation schemes. Norman was also concerned about the general conditions of the asylums from the patients' perspective, and at the meeting of 4 December 1907 wondered if the Committee would 'take into consideration the question of painting the wards generally? The walls are now in a condition in which this could be done properly ... May I suggest to the Committee to make a small grant for cheap pictures to decorate the wards? Such objects have a very beneficial effect upon the patients, and tend to bring about the spirit of contentment and tranquility.'

While the Committee considered Norman's suggestions, they deferred clear decisions to future dates. There is some evidence, however, that a certain amount of consideration was given to the experiences of patients in the day-to-day running of the asylum: a meeting of Richmond District Asylum Joint Committee on 19 September 1907, for example, records receiving a letter from a patient in Portrane 'suggesting that the substitution of a dinner of corned beef instead of curry dinner on Mondays would prove a most acceptable change to the patients'.

Significant emphasis was placed on games and sporting activities for both patients and staff in most asylums at this time.[103] This was also the case at the Richmond: at the meeting of the Richmond Visiting Committee on 14 March 1907, Norman lamented the departure of

Dr Samuels, who has been about a year and nine months clinical assistant, has been appointed third Assistant Medical Officer to the Warwick Asylum ... Dr Samuels will be really a loss to the Institution, as he was not only an excellent medical worker, but was most enthusiastic in promoting games and sports and entertainments among the patients and staff, with whom he was universally and deservedly popular.

Notwithstanding these initiatives, however, problems continued to mount at the Richmond, not least of which was the challenges presented by individuals presenting from the workhouses, seeking admission.

(c)   Challenges Presented by Workhouse Populations

At the Richmond District Asylum Joint Committee meeting on 31 January 1907, the Chairman noted:

> a large number of our admissions come here direct from workhouses. I have looked up the exact numbers and find they average about thirty per cent of total admissions. During the last four financial years 709 patients came from workhouses. I do not think I would be very much in error in estimating that fifty per cent of these 709 admissions would come under the head of Chronic and Harmless Lunatics, and probably at the present time there are not far short of 700 or 800 cases in the whole institution who could be so classified. The 76th section of the Local Government Act of 1898 provides for the establishment of auxiliary asylums for such cases.

The matter was again brought to the attention of the Committee on 15 August 1907 when they received correspondence from the guardians of the North Dublin Union Workhouse 'enclosing a report from Dr Courtenay, Inspector of Lunatics, in which he states that the lunacy wards of the workhouse are overcrowded and the condition of the insane there deplorable'. On 26 September 1907, the Committee held a special meeting 'on the question of dealing with the lunatics at present housed in the different workhouses of the Asylum District'. The Committee's law adviser provided a response to the Committee's 'query as to the liability of the County to maintain all the lunatic poor of the Asylum District. In my opinion under Section 9 of the Local Government Act, 1898, the Committee are bound to maintain them, and if the Union authorities of each asylum district were to send every weak-minded person in the workhouse to the asylum, the Committee would be bound to accept the custody of such patients'.

Increasingly alarmed, the Joint Committee appointed a special committee to 'enquire into the question of provision for workhouse lunatics'. The 'special committee', accompanied by Norman, duly visited asylums at Youghal, Cork and Downpatrick, and inspected Union Workhouses in North and South Dublin. They examined patient numbers, clinical conditions and financial arrangements and reported back to the Joint Committee at the Richmond on 19 December 1907.

The special committee noted that Youghal Asylum had 410 patients and was 'kept entirely apart from the Cork Asylum, the connection of the latter being limited to the filling up of vacancies and providing the funds to meet expenditure'. In addition, 'patients who become violent are transferred back to the parent asylum'. In Cork, the 'special committee' was 'much pleased with the brightness and management of the various wards'. Downpatrick Asylum was of particular interest, however, because 'Down County Council in 1901, after the fullest examination into the fiscal aspect of the question, decided to enlarge the Downpatrick Asylum for the reception of the insane then located in the workhouses'. The 'special committee' presented details of the accommodation at Downpatrick and concurred with the Inspector of Lunatics who, on 16 November 1906, concluded that 'this county is amongst the few in Ireland which has made full provision for all the insane chargeable to it … Nowhere are the insane better housed in bright, cheerful, well-furnished and well-heated wards, where they are properly cared for, well fed, and well clothed.'

The special committee also visited North Dublin Workhouse, where they found 'that the provision for the inmates of the lunatic departments is truly deplorable. The overcrowding is very marked, and calls for prompt relief.' The female ward for 'healthy lunatics' is 'little more than a dungeon, ventilation is inadequate, and the beds are laid upon wooden trestles. The patients are obliged to take their meals in this repellent place'. The male wards 'are much overcrowded … Forty-two of the patients are confined to bed, twenty of them being of the dirty class. Ten patients have to be spoon-fed'. The special committee' concluded that 'all buildings occupied by the lunatic patients are deficient in light and air' and 'all lunatic inmates of the North Dublin Union Workhouse ought to be removed as speedily as possible'. Dr Fottrell at the workhouse 'supplied us with a list of sixty patients, twenty males and forty females, with an urgent request that these be provided for without delay'. The special committee also visited South Dublin Union Workhouse, where their 'experiences were much more agreeable'.

The special committee made four recommendations to the Richmond District Asylum Joint Committee. First, they urged the Committee 'to assume the full responsibility imposed upon them by the Local Government Act of 1898 with respect to pauper lunatics within the district'. Second, they recommended 'that provision for the 600 patients should be made by the erection of suitable buildings at Portrane, where ample space for that purpose is

available'. Third, they concluded that 'a thorough classification and segregation of our existing inmates at Richmond and Portrane would secure an
immediate reduction in our cost of maintenance'. Finally, 'inasmuch as the
condition of things in the North Dublin Union Workhouse requires prompt
remedy', they recommended 'that the Portrane Committee be instructed
to make immediate provision in the temporary buildings at their disposal
for the patients whose removal is applied for by Dr Fottrell'. The Joint
Committee adopted all four recommendations on 19 December 1907.

The Joint Committee was not alone in its concern about the mentally ill in
Irish workhouses at this time.[104] In 1894, Tuke reported that between 1871 and
1891 the number of mentally ill individuals in Irish workhouses had increased
by no fewer than 1,500.[105] Official figures confirmed that in 1851 there were
494 'lunatics' in workhouses and by 1891 this had risen to 2,787.[106] Workhouses
were designed for the relief of poverty and were clearly unsuited to meeting the
medical and social needs of the mentally ill.[107] One of the key steps identified to
address this problem at the Richmond was the clinical segregation of patients in
the Richmond and Portrane requested by the Committee in 1907.

(d)   Clinical 'Segregation' of Patients by Norman

One of the recurring difficulties in planning mental health services for
patients from workhouses related to diagnostic problems. As the Richmond
District Asylum Joint Committee's law adviser informed the Committee on
26 September 1907, 'the legal definition of the term "lunatic" is very wide
and would seem to include any feeble-minded person'. Official figures
confirm that workhouses contained large numbers of both 'lunatics' and
'idiots' in the latter half of the nineteenth century.[108] As a result, diagnostic
issues in both asylums and workhouses were of considerable concern to the
Richmond Committee. On 31 January 1907, the chairman duly requested
'an exhaustive report from our Medical Superintendent on the segregation
of patients at present in the asylum'.

In his subsequent report, Norman noted that:

There are now (24 September 1907) in the Richmond Asylums
(Dublin and Portrane) 2,894 patients and, according to the latest official
statistics at my disposal, there are in the various workhouses in the district
618 persons of unsound mind of various classes. Thus a total of 3,512
persons have to be considered ... I hope I shall not be deemed anxious
to minimize the very serious state of things thus revealed, if I point out

that there are some indications that the increase in the number of cases
of mental disease coming under official cognisance, which has been so
alarming of recent years, may be drawing to a close ... the great increase
in the asylum population in this district of late years was rather among the
old and those past middle age than among the young ... This appears to
show that the increase of total numbers was not due to racial degeneration,
but to altered social and other conditions, together with accumulation.

Given that the census returns for 1901 showed the population for the district
to be 574,850, 'it will be seen that the proportion of the insane to the general
population is very high – 1 to 163.6. This is no doubt partly accounted for by
the large floating [homeless] population in Dublin'.

Norman was particularly concerned about the number of individuals
with learning disability (then termed 'idiots and imbeciles') in the asylum.
He believed that 'an institution specially equipped for teaching the
teachable and improving the improvable is essential. It is neither wise nor
humane to neglect this class as they are neglected in this country'. Norman
felt 'every effort should be made to force this matter upon the attention of
Government' and hoped 'that the forthcoming Report of the Commission
on Imbeciles will contain some proposal for dealing comprehensively with
the idiots of the country'.

Regarding treatment, Norman had clear proposals for reforming the
management of patients who were:

fairly orderly and capable of work [through] the establishment of a proper
system of family care [which] is cheaper than institutional treatment, not
only through the saving in capital cost, but also because maintenance
charges are less. This has been found everywhere, but I may exemplify
Scotland ... If 20 per cent of the chargeable insane in this district were
thus provided for the necessity for accommodating in asylums no less
than 700 patients would be removed ... The attempt was made in the
Department of the Seine in France, where 82 patients were placed in
family care in 1892. Within fourteen years the number in family care had
risen to 1,500. This shows how rapidly the system can, with energy and
determination, be adapted to a country where it is perfectly new.

Not all patients, however, were 'fairly orderly and capable of work' and
appropriate care needed to be provided for 'the old, the feeble, the demented',
as Norman pointed out:

Experience, however, has taught that the most hopeless class are also those that really require most careful nursing, and this means expense. The classes that are most neglected in workhouses are the senile, the bedridden, the unclean, the utterly demented, and the paralytic, and they cause us the most anxiety in an asylum ... From what I hear, and from the Inspectors' reports, it is evident that many of the workhouse cases belong to this category. I fear it will be impossible ever to accommodate them cheaply and yet with that humanity which I know every member of the Committee would be anxious to extend to this most pitiable class.

Interestingly, Norman opposed the idea of segregating these patients to an 'auxiliary asylum', noting that 'attempts have been made in several countries, notably in Germany and in the State of New York, to establish "chronic" or "incurable" asylums as distinct from acute asylums, but the system has failed, and has in both instances been given up. It was found that the notion of incurability attached to an asylum demoralized patients and staff, and led to all kinds of abuses'. Instead of establishing an 'auxiliary asylum', Norman recommended that the Committee look towards developments in the Down District, where 'this question was considered very carefully, and the Committee eventually decided that it would in the end be cheaper to put up additional buildings of a very economical structure on the asylum property. This was done, and the result seems very satisfactory.'

Notwithstanding all of these reports and discussions, proposals and plans, the Richmond Asylum, like other asylums throughout the country, continued to expand during the early decades of the twentieth century. Many of the issues highlighted by Norman in 1907 were highly relevant to this process, and many remain relevant over a century later, especially in relation to the merits of 'family care' or 'home care' for certain patients;[109] the challenges presented by 'the large floating [homeless] population' in Dublin;[110] the often 'unsatisfactory' therapeutic results in individuals with alcohol problems;[111] and the need to provide improved services for individuals with intellectual disability.[112]

There was, however, one additional issue which Norman did not highlight in 1907, and which contributed significantly to Ireland's asylum population: the emergence of the insanity defence during the 1800s and its subsequent impact on the nature and number of admissions at another iconic Dublin asylum, the Central Criminal Lunatic Asylum in Dundrum.

CRIMINAL INSANITY AND THE INSANITY DEFENCE

The insanity defence has a rich and complex history in most societies for which there is recorded history, stretching from ancient Greece and Rome to contemporary Europe and the United States.[113] In 1838, Dr Isaac Ray (1807–81), an American physician and graduate of Harvard Medical School (1827), became one of the founding fathers of forensic psychiatry in the United States, following the publication of his Treatise on the Medical Jurisprudence of Insanity.[114] In his preface to the first edition, Ray lamented the state of contemporary medical jurisprudence of insanity:

> Few, probably, whose attention has not been particularly directed to the subject, are aware how far the condition of the law relative to insanity is behind the present state of our knowledge concerning that disease … Insanity itself is an affection so obscure and perplexing, and the occasions have now become so frequent and important when its legal relations should be properly understood, that an ampler field of illustration and discussion is required …[115]

By the time his book was published, Ray had devoted considerable attention to this topic, having visited medical facilities throughout Europe and studied literature on insanity and the law from Great Britain, Germany and France:

> In all civilized communities, ancient or modern, insanity has been regarded as exempting from punishment of crime, and under some circumstances at least, as vitiating the civil acts of those who are affected with it. The only difficulty, or diversity of opinion, consists in determining who are really insane, in the meaning of the law.[116]

The remainder of the nineteenth century was to see a considerable increase in pubic and professional interest in reform of insanity legislation in the United States, Europe and elsewhere, much of which was attributable, at least in part, to the prescient observations of Ray. Many aspects of this history can be demonstrated by both summarising key historical moments in the evolution of the insanity defence and examining selected case histories drawn from the archives of the Central Criminal Lunatic Asylum in Dublin.

The Evolution of Criminal Insanity Legislation in Ireland, the United States and Elsewhere

The first clear legislative provision for the mentally ill in Ireland was in the Prisons Act of 1787 which led to the establishment of 'lunatic wards' in poorhouses (workhouses), with the aim of providing accommodation for individuals with mental disorder ('lunatics') and individuals with intellectual disability ('idiots').[117] Admission required certification by two magistrates, and the lunatic wards were subject to inspection by the inspector-general of prisons. Local implementation of these measures was generally inadequate, however, and, in 1810, Hallaran drew particular attention to the lack of facilities for the mentally ill, noting that it was 'at times a source of extreme difficulty to contrive the means of accommodation for this hurried weight of human calamity!'[118]

Widespread concern about 'this hurried weight of human calamity' led to the development of legislation, presented to parliament in 1817 (and amended in 1820, 1821, 1825 and 1826) which directed the establishment of a network of 'district asylums' throughout Ireland.[119] In 1838, the same year in which Ray published his Treatise on the Medical Jurisprudence of Insanity in the United States,[120] an additional piece of legislation, the Criminal Lunatics (Ireland) Act 1838, was passed in Ireland, largely in response to the killing of a director of the Bank of Ireland by an individual with apparent mental disorder. This legislation permitted the transfer of an individual from a prison to an asylum if they were considered to be dangerous and either mentally ill or intellectually disabled; the relevant order had to be made by two justices of the peace who could use medical opinion to inform their decision.[121] This 'dangerous lunacy' procedure soon became the admission pathway of choice for many families in Ireland, because it dispensed with the need for a certificate of poverty and gave the police full responsibility for transporting the individual to the asylum, which was then under an obligation to admit them. As a result, the 'dangerous lunacy' procedure was widely abused throughout the nineteenth century.[122]

In international context, Ireland's Criminal Lunatics (Ireland) Act 1838 was by no means an isolated development, but formed part of a broader trend toward reform of legislation providing for the mentally ill and, especially, mentally ill offenders. In most jurisdictions, these laws accorded substantial roles to justices of the peace, magistrates and/or the police in initiating or approving committal orders. In February 1838, the first lunacy law in the canton of Geneva, Switzerland, directed the involvement of the police or authorities of justice in all committals.[123] In June of the same year, France introduced new legislation making *placement d'office* ('official committal') the usual means of committal for individuals with mental disorder who presented a danger to public order or safety.[124] In many countries, subsequent amendments increased the role of medical authorities in the committal process: in Ireland, for example, the Lunacy (Ireland) Act of 1867 made it a requirement that medical opinion be sought prior to committal to a district asylum.

Notwithstanding these amendments, or possibly because of them, there was a perceived need for legislation that prioritised the individual's status as patient rather than offender. In the United States, Ray published an influential paper in 1869 which outlined the necessity for mental health laws that facilitated treatment, optimised confidentiality and protected from wrongful imprisonment.[125] Also at around this time, in 1868, the Association of Medical Superintendents in the United States developed a 'model mental health law' which required medical certification as part of the committal process, with a magistrate attesting to the reputability of the certifying physician.[126]

The emergence of these new ideas about mental disorder and laws to deal with the mentally ill soon necessitated the development of new institutions in many countries, including the United States, Canada and Ireland. In South Carolina, for example, the South Carolina Lunatic Asylum opened its doors in 1828, inspired by therapeutic optimism and new approaches to treatment that were largely European in origin.[127] In Toronto, a temporary asylum located at Toronto Gaol was vacated in 1841 and the permanent Toronto Provincial Asylum was opened in 1850.[128] Similar developments took place at multiple locations in the United States, Canada, Europe and beyond, resulting in substantial expansions of asylum capacity as the nineteenth century progressed.[129]

Notwithstanding these expansions in accommodation and treatments for the mentally ill, individuals with mental disorder and offending behaviour continued to present particular problems in many jurisdictions. In response to these concerns in Ireland, the Central Criminal Lunatic Asylum was opened in 1850 in Dundrum, Dublin.[130] From the outset, the nature and role of the Central Criminal Lunatic Asylum was to be defined by the interplay between psychiatry and the law during the nineteenth century and, in particular, the emergence of the insanity defence in the courtrooms of Great Britain, Ireland and the rest of the world.

The Emergence of the Insanity Defence

While the insanity defence has a long and varied history in many cultures,[131] its recent history is dominated by the case of Daniel McNaughtan, a man with apparent mental disorder who attempted to assassinate the British Prime Minister, Sir Robert Peel, in 1843.[132] Following careful deliberation on the case, the British House of Lords defined a set of formal criteria for criminal insanity that soon become known as the McNaughtan Rules:

> The jurors ought to be told in all cases that every man is presumed to be sane, and to possess a sufficient degree of reason to be responsible for his crimes, until the contrary be proved to their satisfaction; and that to establish a defence on the ground of insanity, it must be clearly proved that, at the time of the committing of the act, the party accused was labouring under such a defect of reason, from disease of the mind, as not to know the nature and quality of the act he was doing; or, if he did know it, that he did not know he was doing what was wrong.[133]

Ray's Treatise on the Medical Jurisprudence of Insanity[134] provided a critical basis for McNaughtan's courtroom defence and, therefore, played an important role in shaping the McNaughtan Rules.[135] These rules were to prove hugely influential as the insanity defence became more widely understood and used in the courtrooms of Great Britain, Ireland, the United States and elsewhere.[136]

In the United States, various versions of the insanity defence had been used prior to the McNaughtan case, with such influential figures as William H. Seward and Edwin M. Stanton (cabinet members), and Abraham Lincoln (future president) presenting insanity defences prior to 1843.[137] While the emergence of the McNaughtan Rules in 1843 brought some clarity and consistency to the insanity defence; however, difficult, controversial cases still came before the American courts[138] and significant differences of clinical and public opinion in relation to insanity and criminal responsibility persisted throughout the remainder of the nineteenth century,[139] as they do today.[140]

In nineteenth-century Ireland, individuals who were found to be mentally ill at the time of an alleged offence could be detained at the Central Criminal Lunatic Asylum 'at the Lord Lieutenant's pleasure' or 'at her Majesty's pleasure'.[141] As was the case in many other jurisdictions, however, a finding of mental disorder tended to result in lengthy detention, as is illustrated by the case of Brendan, a 59-year-old soldier charged with 'shooting … with intent' and detained at 'her Majesty's pleasure' in the Central Criminal Lunatic Asylum, in the early 1890s.

On admission, Brendan was diagnosed as having 'mania with delusions' but had also been 'drinking heavily at time of crime'. He had been 'out shooting blackbirds with a small pistol' when 'he saw a cat sitting at the door of a shop, had a shot at the cat but hit a Mrs [X], who was coming out of the shop at the time'. Admission notes record that Brendan was a widower whose wife had 'died of phthisis' (pulmonary tuberculosis). His pension had been 'stopped by the War Office [and] he is much dissatisfied at this'. Brendan was 'a silent morose man' who was 'subject to delusions of suspicion'. Three years after admission, Brendan developed persistent 'iritis in his left eye', but generally declined treatment 'considering that there is a conspiracy to destroy his sight.'

Nine years after admission, Brendan was working 'on the farm' but 'has a delusion that people in this asylum mean to take his life … but he is so smart that they are unable to obtain a chance'. Some thirteen years after admission, this 'quiet old man', now aged 72 years, was transferred back to his local district asylum. There is no further record of Brendan's outcome, but there is every likelihood that he spent many years in the local district asylum and, ultimately, died there.[142]

Overall, individuals found to be mentally ill at the time of their alleged offence tended to remain at the Central Criminal Lunatic Asylum for a mean of 14.5 years, and 42 per cent of such individuals eventually died in the asylum.[143] Women committed following infanticide or child murder tended to have shorter durations of detention (9.3 years), although this varied widely (from 3 months to 38 years).[144] Overall, however, the trend toward shorter detentions for women is consistent with those observed in other jurisdictions in both forensic and general psychiatric settings: in Canada, for example, 10 per cent more women than men were discharged from the Toronto and Hamilton asylums between 1851 and 1891.[145]

As with most asylums in Ireland, the longer an individual was detained at the Central Criminal Lunatic Asylum, the greater was the likelihood they would live the rest of their lives behind the asylum walls; individuals who died in the Central Criminal Lunatic Asylum had been there for a mean of 19.6 years at time of death, which was notably longer than the overall mean duration of stay (14.5 years).[146] Similarly, in Irish district asylums, once an individual was committed for more than five years, they almost invariably died there.[147] This trend was also apparent in other jurisdictions, with data from Robben Island Lunatic Asylum in South Africa demonstrating that once an individual had been detained there for four years, it was exceedingly unlikely they would ever be discharged.[148] This trend towards prolonged institutionalisation resulted in multiple problems for asylum staff and patients, many of which were related to intractable overcrowding and resultant physical ill health amongst patients.

OVERCROWDING, ILLNESS AND DEATH IN NINETEENTH-CENTURY ASYLUMS

Throughout the nineteenth century, professional and governmental considerations of the problems of insanity in many countries were dominated by the belief that rates of mental disorder were increasing rapidly.[149] In Ireland, this belief was outlined in vivid terms by Hallaran at the start of the century[150] and became an article of faith as the nineteenth century progressed, finding support in the reports of the Irish Inspector of Lunatics[151] as well as professional psychiatric opinion. This included Dr Daniel Hack Tuke, an influential British psychiatrist who studied the relevant statistics and concluded that there was indeed 'some actual as well as apparent increase of mental disorder' in Ireland.[152]

While the reasons underlying this perception of increasing rates of insanity are myriad and complex, there is little doubt that this period saw the emergence of significant problems with overcrowding in Irish asylums, including the Central Criminal Lunatic Asylum.[153] In the case of the Central Criminal Lunatic Asylum, these problems were compounded by the particularly high numbers of individuals found to be mentally ill in Irish courtrooms during the 1860s, 1870s and 1880s.[154] While the overcrowding generated a broad range of issues for asylums, problems with physical health were amongst the most concerning.[155] Infectious diseases presented particular challenges, especially at large asylums such as the Richmond.[156]

The roots of these problems lay, in large part, in the overcrowded conditions of asylums, lengthy detention periods and the chronic or recurring physical illnesses experienced by many patients.[157] Some of these factors are illustrated by the case of Henry, a 77-year-old farmer who was charged with murder but found 'insane on arraignment', and detained 'at the Lord Lieutenant's pleasure' in the Central Criminal Lunatic Asylum, in the early 1890s. On admission, Henry was diagnosed with 'chronic mania' and described as 'intemperate' (as opposed to sober). He had 'delusions of injustice and persecution' and believed he had 'God in his stomach'. Henry also 'vomits frequently after his meals' and had 'some chronic intestinal trouble but I am unable to discover the exact nature thereof.'

Seven years after admission, the medical officer observed that 'this impulsive old man' was 'delicate and losing strength' but will not allow me to touch him or prescribe for him in any way'. Soon, Henry became 'very weakly' and was 'confined to bed'. He was diagnosed with 'pleurisy of the left side' and 'his breathing is much affected'. Notwithstanding the doctor's prescription of 'whiskey, 4 ounces', Henry 'got rapidly worse ... his breathing is distressed to a very great extent, his lips and fingers are much cyanosed, and his heart is very weak'. As Henry's condition became critical, his niece informed the medical officer that over the course of Henry's life he had spent 'over fifty years in lunatic asylums'. A couple of days later, Henry died of pulmonary infection, at the age of 84 years, having spent the last seven years of his life at the Central Criminal Lunatic Asylum.

Pulmonary infections, tuberculosis in particular, presented especially challenging public health problems in nineteenth-century Ireland and by 1904 tuberculosis accounted for almost 16 per cent of all deaths in the Irish population.[158] Staff and patients in asylums were at particular risk of infection and by 1901 tuberculosis accounted for 25 per cent of deaths in Irish asylums.[159] Similar problems were reported in other countries, with tuberculosis recorded as the leading cause of death in South Carolina Lunatic Asylum at the turn of the century.[160] In Ireland, problems related to tuberculosis were slow to resolve, although the start of the twentieth century saw renewed public health initiatives,[161] dedicated legislative measures, such as the Tuberculosis Prevention (Ireland) Act of 1908,[162] and changes in socio-political circumstances helped alleviate matters somewhat.[163]

Notwithstanding these developments, death rates in Irish asylums still presented considerable cause for concern. In 1893, the Inspector of Lunatics (1893) reported a national death rate of 8.3 per cent in Irish district asylums; this figure was derived by dividing the number of deaths in Irish district asylums over the course of 1892 (995 deaths) by the daily average number of asylum residents during the year; on 1 January 1893, that number stood at 12,133.[164] Of those who died in district asylums, 198 (19.9 per cent) underwent post-mortem examinations which were, in the opinion of the Inspector of Lunatics, 'of so much importance for the protection of the insane and for the furtherance of the scientific study of insanity'.[165]

Certain asylums, such as the Richmond Asylum in Dublin, reported death rates (12.5 per cent) that were higher than the national average, possibly related to particular problems with overcrowding and infective illnesses at the Richmond.[166] Comparable death rates were reported in other jurisdictions, however, with a 14 per cent death rate in South Carolina Lunatic Asylum between 1890 and 1915.[167] Similarly, 33 per cent of men and 21 per cent of women admitted to the Toronto Asylum between 1851 and 1891 died there.[168] At the Central Criminal Lunatic Asylum in Dublin, some 42 per cent of individuals who were detained following a finding of mental disorder in court between 1850 and 1995 died in the asylum[169] and 27 per cent of women committed following infanticide or child murder between 1850 and 2000 died there.[170] This difference in outcome between men and women may be related to several factors, including increased discharge rates amongst women as well as various factors stemming from differing understandings of criminal responsibility in women as opposed to men.

NINETEENTH-CENTURY VIEWS OF CRIMINAL RESPONSIBILITY IN WOMEN WITH MENTAL DISORDER

Throughout the nineteenth century, women with mental disorder were treated differently to men by the Irish criminal justice and psychiatric systems.[171] Following committal to the Central Criminal Lunatic Asylum, women generally experienced shorter periods of detention and were more likely to be discharged than men.[172] Some of these differences may be attributable to the nature of offences committed by women: 54.2 per cent of women committed to the Central Criminal Lunatics Asylum between 1868 and 1908 were convicted of killing, of whom a majority were convicted of child killing.[173]

In some cases, women charged with child killing were sent from prison to the Central Criminal Lunatic Asylum, even prior to trial if they demonstrated features of mental disorder while in prison. Pauline, for example, was a 25-year-old woman charged with infanticide in the mid-1890s and incarcerated at a provincial Irish prison to await trial. The prison medical officer noticed that Pauline appeared 'a little weak-minded' and then became 'unmanageable' before 'finally becoming insane' while in prison.

Pauline was transferred to the Central Criminal Lunatic Asylum prior to trial, and on admission it transpired that, nine years earlier, she had been 'confined in [her local] district asylum as a dangerous lunatic for five months'. Recently, however, she 'became pregnant by a man with whom she kept company for some time'. The child was born 'in the absence of the patient's mother, nobody else being present. She asserts that the child was dead when born; that she lay on a bed for 2 or 3 hours after the birth; and then rose and threw the child out of the house.'

On admission to the Central Criminal Lunatic Asylum, Pauline was diagnosed with 'recurrent insanity' and noted to suffer from 'amenorrhoea'. She was generally 'quiet and well-conducted' but 'in consequence of a constant broad good-humoured grin on her features, she gives one the idea of a certain lack of intelligence'. Two months after admission, medical notes recorded that Pauline 'has shown no symptoms of insanity since admission ... keeps herself clean and tidy, and works in the laundry'. Two years after admission, the medical officer reported that 'this patient is slightly weak minded and has suffered from two attacks of mania' but 'she might keep well if the relative to whom she is discharged would keep her under [her] care'. Notwithstanding this positive assessment, Pauline spent three years at the Central Criminal Lunatic Asylum before being transferred back to prison 'to await trial'.

While there is no accessible record of the outcome of Pauline's trial, there was a general tendency on the part of the Irish courts to take an ostensibly lenient approach to infanticide, which was, in theory, punishable by the death penalty. Juries tended to reach verdicts other than infanticide (e.g. manslaughter) in order to avoid the possibility of capital punishment and no woman in Great Britain or Ireland has been executed for infanticide since 1849.[174]

Overall, in terms of criminal responsibility, there is strong evidence that issues related to menstruation, pregnancy and childbirth were significant factors in determining how women were viewed in many jurisdictions, including Ireland, Great Britain and the United States. In Ireland, for example, Dr Fleetwood Churchill, wrote that, 'if a very slight deviation from bodily health distorts or upturns [the] mental operations' of men, then:

> How much more exposed must women be to such disturbances, who, in addition to the causes common to both, possess a more delicate organi-sation, more refined sensibilities, more exquisite perceptions, and are, moreover, the subjects of repeated constitutional changes and develop-ments of a magnitude and importance unknown to the other sex.[175]

In Churchill's view, 'menstruation, conception and pregnancy, parturition and childbed, and lactation' could all produce 'disturbance' that 'may amount to incoherent action or insanity'. In Great Britain, Dr Henry Maudsley pinpointed irregularities of menstruation' as 'recognised causes of mental disorder' which could generate a 'suicidal or homicidal impulse' in women.[176]

The medical emphasis on the role of menstruation is demonstrated by the case of Úna, an 18-year-old woman charged with 'the manslaughter of her illegitimate child' but found 'insane on arraignment' and detained 'at the Lord Lieutenant's pleasure' in the Central Criminal Lunatic Asylum, in the late 1880s. Diagnosed with 'chronic mania, Úna was described as "incoherent, noisy and refractory … dirty in her habits".'While the medical officer felt Úna was 'the subject of tubercular diathesis, probably', medical notes repeatedly recorded that she became 'very excited and violent at each menstrual period' and 'was quiet but for these attacks'. Ultimately, some fourteen years after admission to the Central Criminal Lunatic Asylum, Úna was transferred back to her local district asylum and there is no further record of her clinical outcome.

In the United States, a similar emphasis was placed on menstruation as a cause of disturbed behaviour and/or mental disorder in women.[177] In 1865, for example, a female defendant was found insane at the time of a shooting, owing to paroxysmal insanity resulting from being 'crossed in love and suffering from painful dysmenorrhea'.[178] Ray, in his Treatise on the Medical Jurisprudence of Insanity, described an apparent link between menstruation and fire setting, citing several cases 'in which the incendiary propensity was excited by disordered menstruation, accompanied in some of them by other pathological conditions'.[179]

One case involved a 22-year-old woman who 'committed three incendiary acts' but 'had had a disease two years before, that was accompanied by violent pains in the head, disordered circulation, insensibility, and epileptic fits; and that since then menstruation had ceased'. This case was not unique:

> That the evolution of the sexual functions is very often attended by more or less constitutional disturbance, especially in the female sex, is now a well-established psychological truth … Any irregularity whatsoever of the menstrual discharge, is a fact of the greatest importance in determining the mental condition of incendiary girls.

Ray's concern with female menstrual and reproductive functions was by no means limited to 'incendiary girls', as he also described a link between 'the propensity to steal' and 'certain physiological changes' in women, including pregnancy. He outlined in particular detail the case of one 'pregnant woman who, otherwise perfectly honest and respectable, suddenly conceived a violent longing for some apples from a particular orchard … and was detected by the owner in the act of stealing apples'. The woman was duly 'convicted of theft' but a 'medical commission was appointed' to consider her case:

> Their enquiries resulted in the opinion that she was not morally free, and consequently not legally responsible while under the influence of those desires peculiar to pregnancy; adding that if Eve had been in the condition of the accused, when she plucked the forbidden fruit from the tree, the curse of original sin would never have fallen on the race.

Medical and judicial views on menstruation, pregnancy and childbirth were to remain highly relevant to issues of criminal responsibility in women throughout the remainder of the nineteenth century, especially in relation to infanticide.[180] Interestingly, some of these issues retain psychological and legal significance today, not only in relation to infanticide and mental disorder,[181] but also in relation to the use of premenstrual syndrome as a defence or mitigating factor in court.

CRIMINAL INSANITY TODAY

Many of the issues related to criminal insanity that presented challenges to doctors, jurors and judges in the nineteenth century continue to present challenges to psychiatric and judicial systems today. The use of the insanity defence, so hotly contested in the nineteenth century, still generates considerable controversy two centuries later.[182] This point is usefully demonstrated by comparing the case of Daniel McNaughtan in 1843 with that of John Hinckley in 1981.[183] While McNaughtan attempted to assassinate Sir Robert Peel in nineteenth-century England, Hinckley attempted to assassinate President Ronald Reagan in the United States in 1981, and both McNaughtan and Hinckley were found to be insane. The McNaughtan and Hinckley cases bear many similarities: both involved the attempted assassination of heads of states by individuals with apparent mental disorder; both attracted controversy in their respective eras; and both formed important legal precedents in their own jurisdictions and beyond.

One of the most enduring controversies generated by the insanity defence in the nineteenth century, however, centred on arguments about clinical and legal definitions of insanity,[184] and this issue continues to present challenges to legislators today. Controversy also persists in relation to the correct balance between treatment and punishment for offenders with mental disorder. One of the most important legacies of nineteenth-century medical jurisprudence in Ireland and Great Britain was the de facto abandonment of capital punishment for the crime of infanticide, albeit replaced by indefinite and commonly lengthy detention in the Central Criminal Lunatic Asylum.[185]

While capital punishment has now been abolished in many countries (including Ireland), the use of capital punishment in individuals with mental disorder in certain jurisdictions still generates controversy,[186] as evidenced by the case of Larry Robison, a 42-year-old man with paranoid schizophrenia who was executed in Texas in January 2000 for killing five people in 1982.[187] Overall, there is strong evidence of high rates of mental disorder, neurological insult and intellectual limitation amongst prisoners on death row in the United States[188] and this further deepens controversy about the appropriateness of capital punishment in this group.[189]

Finally, as the cases presented in the chapter demonstrate, the consideration of criminal responsibility in women during the nineteenth century was shaped in large part by issues related to menstruation, pregnancy and childbirth. While the overall societal context has changed considerably over the intervening centuries, some of these issues retain psychological and legal significance for women today, not only in relation to infanticide and mental disorder,[190] but also in relation to the use of premenstrual syndrome as a mitigating factor in court. Interestingly, while premenstrual syndrome is generally unsuccessful as a legal defence in the United States,[191] it has been used with some success in England to support a defence based on diminished capacity.[192] In Canada, the legal potential of premenstrual syndrome has yet to be explored fully, but it has already been recognised as a mitigating factor in sentencing in certain cases.[193]

Overall, it is likely that the use of premenstrual syndrome as a substantive defence will remain controversial and will be both limited and defined by evolving medical and psychological understandings of the syndrome.[194] A similar proviso applies more generally to the relationship between mental disorder and the law, especially as it pertains to criminal responsibility: for as long as psychiatric knowledge continues to develop, and legal practice continues to change, it is likely that the psychiatric and medico-legal controversies that troubled doctors, jurors and judges throughout the nineteenth century will continue to challenge medical, judicial and social services for many years to come.

Women in the Central Criminal Lunatic Asylum, Dublin, 1868–1948

The plight of the mentally ill in nineteenth-century Ireland was generally grim, as many were either homeless or placed in workhouses or one of the few asylums that existed at that time (Chapter 1). The central element in society's response to this situation was the creation of a remarkable network of asylums, underpinned by the widespread belief that insanity was increasingly uniquely quickly in Ireland, constant legislative change, the emergence of psychiatry as a profession and increased use of the 'insanity defence' as the 1800s drew to a close (Chapter 2).

Chapter 3 explores these themes in greater depth by focusing on one specific group within Ireland's asylum system: women committed to the Central Criminal Lunatic Asylum (later Central Mental Hospital) in Dundrum, Dublin between 1868 and 1948.[1] Most of these women had been charged with crimes, deemed insane by the courts, and sent to the Central Criminal Lunatic Asylum for indefinite periods of custody and care. This chapter uses original archival case records to examine the clinical and social characteristics of these women, and presents histories of mental disorder, social deprivation and infanticide (the killing of infants). These discussions place particular emphasis on the clinical dimensions of these cases, unearthing and decoding, as best as possible, signs and symptoms of mental disorder in this troubled, troubling group.

This chapter commences with a case history of infanticide, followed by systematic considerations of women committed to the Central Criminal Lunatic Asylum between 1868 and 1908, and between 1910 and 1948.

These women are divided into these two chronologically defined groups so as to facilitate examination of patterns of admission and changes in clinical characteristics over time.

INFANTICIDE IN NINETEENTH-CENTURY IRELAND

Infanticide is the killing of an infant (under 1 year of age).[2] Cases of infanticide are described in almost every human society for which there is recorded history[3] and appear in the mythology, folklore and literatures of myriad cultures.[4] Societal responses to infanticide have involved varying mixtures of judicial and psychiatric measures aimed at punishing and/or treating perpetrators, and protecting children. Many of these features are demonstrated by the case of Dora, drawn from the archives of the Central Criminal Lunatic Asylum.[5]

The Case of Dora: 'With a Delusion that She is Lost'

In 1892, Dora, a 34-year-old servant from Dublin, was charged with the murder of her 8-month-old child and sent to Grangegorman Prison in Dublin. Eight days later, she transferred to the Central Criminal Lunatic Asylum, where she was detained at the 'Lord Lieutenant's pleasure'. On admission, Dora was described as 'pale and pasty, hair brown, eyes grey'. The admitting officer recommended she have a 'hot bath and be put to bed'. Dora was 'nervous; given to crying on the least provocation; a heavy sleeper, subject to bad dreams'. She was diagnosed as 'a case of melancholia, with a delusion that she is lost – no heaven for her. She is here for drowning her child eight-months old and attempting to drown herself.'

> [Dora] had five children [and] all died young. Her last child was very delicate. Some weeks before the crime, she had been drinking more than usual. For the last seven years she has neglected her religious duties entirely; this upset and worried her greatly – she thought she was lost with no hope of being saved. Some days before the crime, she suffered from a violent pain in the head. She felt as if the top of her head was splitting open – she was very depressed and unable to attend her household duties. The loss of her family with very little hope of the last child living, together with her religious troubles, weighted on her mind so that she determined to drown herself and the child. On the morning of the crime, she took the

child in her arms and left the house. She wandered off some distance from home, did not know where she was or what she was doing. She imagined that she was followed by a large crowd of soldiers and people. She had no idea of drowning the child when she left the house that morning [and] is now sorry that she did not drown herself – but wishes the child was alive.

Five months after admission, Dora was 'careless and untidy in her dress and person; takes no interest in her surroundings; does not associate with the other patients. She works in the laundry but is much inclined to sit about brooding over her troubles.' The initial diagnosis of melancholia with nihilistic (deeply depressive) delusions was supported by the observation that, when Dora's husband visited, 'she does not appear to take any pleasure or interest in the visits [and] will not enter conversation with him'. In 1895, three years after admission, Dora displayed clear 'delusions of infestation and had treatment. She works in the laundry but if anyone also there employed turns their back to her she imagines they are laughing at her.'

By 1895, Dora had developed 'ptosis [drooping] of the right eyelid which has of late almost become complete. This is due no doubt to some central nervous lesion'. This diagnosis was further supported by a marked coars-ening of Dora's speech: toward the end of 1896, she was confined to bed because 'for some weeks past … her language has been of such an obscene and disgusting character that it is impossible to allow her to associate with the other patients … She is under the belief that other patients wear her clothes and she now refuses to put them on.' Throughout 1897, Dora continued 'as above, only that she manages to control her language somewhat and is not confined to bed for more than two days at any time, but this occurs about three times per month'.

The following year, Dora began 'to suffer from attacks of spasm of the glottis with laryngeal stridor [choking]. She has been attacked by this several times during the past few days and always after eating. These sudden attacks taken in conjunction with the ptosis of the right eyelid seem to indicate a central nervous lesion probably due to a neoplasm' (a brain tumour). In January 1899, Dora 'fell down on the ground "working" her arms and legs violently, but after a short time she recovered completely' (a severe epileptic-type seizure). These attacks continued regularly and the medical officer noted that 'after such an attack the patient is morose and bad tempered, requiring considerable tact to get her to carry out her ordinary work'. As with the episodes of coarsening of language, these attacks occurred in episodic clusters: 'This patient seems to get "fits" about every fortnight or three weeks and then she generally gets three or four in the twenty four hours. She gets very much cyanosed [blue] and there appears to be a "spasm of the glottis". They last only some seconds and end usually by a spasmatic cough lasting about five minutes.'

Dora was treated with a combination of mercury and potassium iodide. This treatment was commenced in 1895, when the drooping of her right eyelid became complete, further suggesting a brain tumour. In 1898, when Dora developed 'attacks of spasm of the glottis with laryngeal stridor', medical notes recorded that 'she has already been treated for ptosis with mercury and potassium iodide without result, but we have again recoursed to the same treatment'. A note from January 1899 records that 'the potassium iodide is being continued'. In March 1899, with 'fits' occurring in clusters every few weeks, Dora was 'tried with mercury'. In April 1899 notes record that 'she is on mercury at present and some improvement seems to have taken place'. This improvement was sustained until at least the following year, when she was working the laundry and 'the fits which were fairly constant last March have now almost departed and her general health is very fair'.

Later in 1900, however, Dora's overall condition deteriorated and in August 1900 she was 'very silent and almost morose and often very difficult to get her to speak at all ...' By 1901, Dora was:

> demented and it is almost impossible to get her to speak. What a change for the worse has taken place: in 1894 she was a well-conducted and well-spoken woman and often in good spirits, laughing and generally well pleased with herself and those round her. Now she is miserable and demented, never speaks, takes no interest in anything and stands about in a semi-dazed condition. The fits from which she suffered some months ago have disappeared but it is thought she has a cerebral [brain] tumour.

Dora's mental state remained generally unchanged throughout the remainder of her time in the Central Criminal Lunatic Asylum. In 1906, she was transferred to Richmond Lunatic Asylum in Dublin and there is no further information available about her progress or outcome.

INFANTICIDE: INCIDENCE AND RESPONSES

The incidence of infanticide varies between countries and over time.[6] In London, for example, it is estimated that 1,130 babies under the age of 2 years were killed between 1856 and 1860,[7] although recent epidemiological evidence suggest that the incidence of infanticide is now very much lower, at least in developed countries.[8] As there is a paucity of systematic data about infanticide in Ireland in the past, it is extremely difficult to estimate the incidence of infanticide in nineteenth-century Ireland, although it may well have been relatively high, especially during times of economic hardship. Generally, infanticide in Ireland has been associated with poverty and illegitimacy, and tended to occur when women felt that society afforded them no alternative course of action.[9] Similar trends are in evidence today in the United States, with neonaticide (the killing of an infant within hours of birth) most frequently committed by mothers who are young, unmarried, poor and received little prenatal care.[10]

It was not until 1949 that Ireland's Infanticide Act recategorised infanticide from a crime equivalent to murder into a crime equivalent to manslaughter, thus tilting the balance toward psychiatric rather than purely judicial responses. As Dora appeared in court several decades earlier, however, she was charged with murder and sent to prison, followed by transfer to the Central Criminal Lunatic Asylum.[11] Overall, sixty-four women were admitted to the Central Mental Hospital following infanticide and child murder between 1850 and 2000: most were either 'guilty but insane' or 'unfit to plead', and most went on to stay for indefinite periods at the asylum.[12]

Medical records clearly demonstrate the challenges faced by staff in making medical and psychiatric diagnoses at the Central Criminal Lunatic Asylum. Dora, for example, received an admission diagnosis of melancholia with nihilistic delusions, but it is clear that her evolving symptomatology prompted staff to consider the possibility of a brain tumour. The possibility of a physical or organic basis for her illness might have been suggested by her original presentation, when she complained of 'a violent pain in the head' as if 'the top of her head was splitting open'. The possibility of an altered state of consciousness is also suggested by the observation that 'on the morning of the crime, she ... wandered off some distance from home, did not know where she was or what she was doing ...' Despite these vague symptoms, some of which are consistent with various organic brain disorders (e.g. migraine, temporal lobe epilepsy), Dora received the diagnosis of melancholia, which was the most common diagnosis amongst women charged with infanticide or child murder and admitted to forensic psychiatry inpatient care in Ireland during this period.[13]

In Dora's case, clinical notes also suggest the possibility of epilepsy (possibly owing to a brain tumour) or a movement disorder, such as Tourette syndrome. During her stay in the Central Criminal Lunatic Asylum, Dora developed further signs of an organic lesion: drooping of the right eyelid, episodes of coarsening of language, episodes of 'spasm of the glottis with laryngeal stridor' and, eventually, episodic clusters of epileptic-type seizures. The possibility of a cerebral tumour was mentioned in the notes in 1901, and Dora's final recorded mental state was one of possible dementia, consistent with end-stage organic brain disease, such as a brain tumour.

Dora's management at the Central Criminal Lunatic Asylum involved a range of treatments, including elements of 'moral management' and administration of mercury and potassium iodide. The 'moral management' approach emphasised daily activity, rigorous exercise and adherence to a healthy diet.[14] In Dora's case, it is clear that medical authorities placed considerable emphasis on her working in the hospital laundry and regarded her return to work there as a sign of improvement.

Medical staff also prescribed mercury and potassium iodide at various stages in the course of Dora's illness. In the late nineteenth century, both mercury and potassium iodide were widely used in the treatment of a number of disorders, including syphilitic disorders of the nervous system.[15] The use of mercury for the treatment of syphilis had a particularly long history: the seventeenth-century English physician Thomas Sydenham, in particular, recommended the use of mercury to induce free salivation, believing that it was the salivation, rather than the mercury itself, that produced a cure.[16] Syphilis was a particular problem in certain places: at the Sainte Anne Asylum in Paris, for example, 'general paralysis' (severe syphilis, affecting the brain) accounted for 30 per cent of voluntary male admissions between 1876 and 1914.[17] In Ireland, however, it appears that syphilis accounted for a smaller proportion of admissions[18] and available clinical records do not suggest that Dora's illness was attributable to syphilis.

Overall, Dora spent fourteen years in the Central Criminal Lunatic Asylum. Between 1850 and 2000, the length of stay following infanticide or child murder varied between three months and thirty-eight years, with an average of 9.3 years.[19] Ultimately, 27 per cent of women were, like Dora, transferred to a local asylum after they left the Central Criminal Lunatic Asylum, while 41 per cent were released to the care of another institution or their families. Women tended to have shorter hospital stays than men: men who were declared 'guilty but insane' in Ireland between 1850 and 1950 had an average 'time to discharge' of twelve years, while women had the shorter average time of nine years.[20]

A similar pattern was evident in other, non-forensic Irish asylums at this time, as short-term female patients spent shorter periods in asylums compared to short-term male patients. There was, however, little difference for long-stay patients: once an individual was in an asylum for five years, it was highly likely they would remain behind asylum walls for life, regardless of gender.[21] There are no systematic data available to indicate the ultimate outcome for individuals who, like Dora, were discharged from the Central Criminal Lunatic Asylum back to local asylums. While some of these women may have been later released to the care of their families, it appears likely that many lived in psychiatric hospitals or other institutions for the remainder of their lives.

WOMEN COMMITTED TO INPATIENT FORENSIC PSYCHIATRIC CARE IN IRELAND, 1868–1908

The case of Dora is just one example of a woman committed to the Central Criminal Lunatic Asylum in late nineteenth-century Ireland. Was her case typical? Were there many others like her? What diagnoses did these women receive? For how long were they detained?

Dora's case was certainly typical to the extent that she, like so many other women committed at this time, experienced significant social exclusion and denial of opportunities to return to life outside the walls of the asylums.[22] This experience of forensic psychiatric institutionalisation was related to myriad societal and historical factors, not least of which was a strong belief in the ability of contemporary treatments to cure individuals of their insanity.[23] In addition, women tended to have different institutional experiences than men in the nineteenth century, indicating that gender is an important issue in this context.[24]

Against this background, it is worth examining in some depth the clinical and social characteristics of women committed to inpatient forensic psychiatric care in the late nineteenth and early twentieth centuries. The remainder of this chapter examines women so committed over two time periods (between 1868 and 1908,[25] and between 1910 and 1948[26]) and compares the two groups in order to identify changes in admission patterns over time.

Between 1868 and 1908, seventy women were admitted to the Central Criminal Lunatic Asylum. Female admission rates increased throughout the 1870s and 1880s and reached a peak in the early 1890s: in the five-year period commencing in 1868, there were two female admissions while in the five-year period commencing in 1893 there were twenty-two female admissions (Figure 1). Female admission rates started to decline in the mid-1890s, with ten female admissions in the five-year period commencing in 1903.

Figure 1

Female admission rates to the Central Criminal Lunatic Asylum, Dublin, 1868–1908

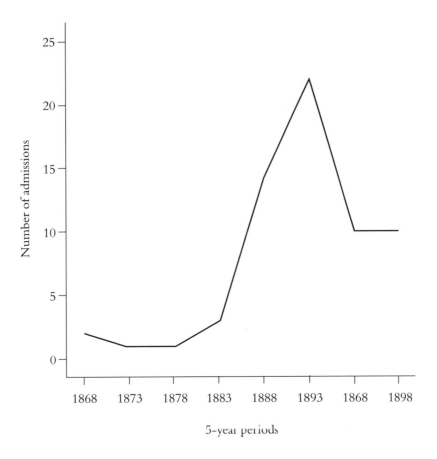

5-year periods

Note for Figure 1

In order to identify overall admission trends (rather than year-on-year fluctuations), this figure presents female admission rates aggregated into 5-year periods: i.e. in the 5-year period commencing in 1868 there were two female admissions; in the 5-year period commencing in 1873 there was one female admission; etc.

These data were extracted from archival medical case records at the Central Criminal Lunatic Asylum (now the Central Mental Hospital), Dundrum, Dublin, Ireland.

Table 2

Characteristics of women admitted to the Central Criminal Lunatic Asylum, Dublin, 1868–1908

Characteristic	n	Percentage
Marital status		
Single	38	58
Married	22	33
Widowed	6	9
Nationality		
Irish	66	97
English	2	3
Religion		
Roman Catholic	57	83
Church of Ireland	6	9
Episcopalian	3	4
Presbyterian	2	3
Atheist	1	1
Occupation		
Servant	17	30
Housekeeper	14	25
Prostitute	11	20
Dealer	3	5
Farm worker	2	4
Attendant	1	2
Ballet dancer	1	2
Cook	1	2
Dress-maker	1	2
Home business	1	2
Laundry worker	1	2
Nurse	1	2
Pauper	1	2
Tailor	1	2

Note for Table 2

These data were extracted from archival medical case records at the Central Criminal Lunatic Asylum (now the Central Mental Hospital), Dundrum, Dublin, Ireland.

Table 3

Crimes committed by women admitted to the Central Criminal Lunatic Asylum, Dublin, 1868-1908

Crime	n	Percentage
Murder	26	37
Manslaughter	11	16
Larceny	8	11
Assault with intent to murder	6	9
Malicious wounding	3	4
Malicious injury	2	3
Attempted suicide[i]	2	3
Obtaining goods by false pretences	2	3
Obtaining money by false pretences	1	1
Infanticide[ii]	1	1
Drunk and disorderly	1	1
Theft	1	1
Placing stones on railway	1	1
Malicious damage	1	1
Forgery	1	1
Wandering and doing actual bodily harm	1	1
Breaking and entering	1	1
Assault	1	1

Notes for Table 3

(i) Suicide was a crime in Ireland until 1993
(ii) In the cases of many women charged with child killing, the crime

was recorded as murder or manslaughter rather than infanticide, consistent with the legal practice in late nineteenth-century and early twentieth-century Ireland

These data were extracted from archival medical case records at the Central Criminal Lunatic Asylum (now the Central Mental Hospital), Dundrum, Dublin, Ireland.

The average age of women at time of admission was 33 years but ranged from 17 to 63. The majority of women were Irish in nationality and Roman Catholic in religion (Table 2). More than half were single (i.e. never married) and a third were married at time of committal. Number of children was not recorded for thirty-five women and five were childless; among the remainder, the average number of children was three, although this ranged from one to twelve. Occupations were recorded for fifty-six women, most commonly servant, housekeeper and prostitute. Unfortunately, records do not specify if these are current occupations or occupations dating from any previous time in the woman's life.

Thirty-eight women (54 per cent) had been charged with killing: twenty-six (37 per cent) were charged with murder, eleven (16 per cent) were charged with manslaughter and one (1 per cent) was charged with infanticide (Table 3). Women charged with killing had an average age of 30 years at time of committal, compared to an average age of 36 years for women committed for reasons other than killing. The two groups did not differ in terms of marital status or level of education, but differed significantly in terms of sentencing: 86 per cent of women charged with killing were detained 'at the Lord Lieutenant's pleasure' (i.e. indefinitely), compared to 50 per cent of women charged with other offences.

The identity of the victim was recorded in the cases of thirty-three women charged with killing. Twenty-three cases (70 per cent) involved child killings; the next most common victim was the woman's mother (9 per cent) or a fellow patient in an asylum (9 per cent). Other victims included a mistress, another family member and a friend. The twenty-three women charged with child killing did not differ from women charged with killing other people in terms of age, level of education or sentencing, but were more likely to be married.

The twenty-three child killings in this sample included twenty cases with one child victim, two cases with two child victims and one case with three child victims. The ages of child victims were not recorded in all cases, but at least thirteen child victims were below the age of 1 year, including seven newborn babies. In the cases of many women charged with child killing, the crime was recorded as murder or manslaughter rather than infanticide, consistent with legal practice in late nineteenth-century and early twentieth-century Ireland.

Overall, between 1868 and 1908, forty-seven women (69 per cent) were sentenced to be detained 'at the Lord Lieutenant's pleasure'. Two women (3 per cent) received life sentences and nineteen women (28 per cent) received sentences of specific durations. The majority of women who were detained 'at the Lord Lieutenant's pleasure' had been charged with either murder (53 per cent) or manslaughter (13 per cent); the average duration of detention in this group was fourteen years, although this ranged from less than one year to forty-six years. Women who received sentences of specific durations were detained for shorter periods (ranging from less than one year to seven years) and the two women who received life sentences spent an average of thirty-eight years in detention.

Medical notes indicate that eight women (11 per cent) were considered to be sane on admission. Some of these women had previously shown evidence of 'recurrent insanity', 'puerperal mania' (mental disorder following childbirth), 'transitory mania after birth' or 'senile decay' (age-related mental disorder) prior to admission. One had been 'hysterical' at time of trial and another had been 'drinking' at time of offence. Twenty-nine women (41 per cent) were assigned a diagnosis of 'mania' (possibly bipolar affective disorder); eighteen (26 per cent) had 'melancholia' (possibly depression); six (9 per cent) had intellectual disability, of whom three also showed evidence of mental disorder; five (7 per cent) had 'dementia' alone; two (3 per cent) had 'epileptic insanity'; one (1 per cent) had 'puerperal insanity'; and one (1 per cent) had 'delusional insanity'.

There are no systematic records of treatments provided to these women during their time in the Central Criminal Lunatic Asylum. Medical notes indicate that many were employed within the hospital in household tasks such as laundry. At the end of their periods of detention, almost half of women (49 per cent) were transferred to local asylums; others were transferred to prison (12 per cent) or released to the care of family (14 per cent), friends (6 per cent), a Prison Aid Association (1 per cent) or a convent (1 per cent). Ten women (14 per cent) died in detention; causes of death were recorded in nine cases and included 'heart disease' (four women), 'cancer' (two), 'senile decay' (dementia) (one), 'phthisis' (pulmonary tuberculosis) (one) and 'uterine tumour' (cancer of the womb) (one).

Many of these facts and figures are demonstrated more vividly through the case histories of three women committed to the Central Criminal Lunatic Asylum during this period: Kathleen, Linda and Niamh.

The Case of Kathleen:
'Very Nervous, Shy and in a Highly Strung Condition'

Kathleen was a 24-year-old, unmarried, Roman Catholic servant admitted in 1905, having been charged with murder and detained 'at the Lord Lieutenant's pleasure'. Kathleen was described as sane on admission and not deemed to be a danger to others. The prison surgeon confirmed that Kathleen had 'been under my observation as to her mental condition; I consider she is of sound mind'.

Medical notes from the Central Criminal Lunatic Asylum recorded that Kathleen was 'in here for the murder of her illegitimate child'. Kathleen had given birth in a workhouse in the west of Ireland and 'ten days after, she … threw her baby into the river. She was quite well aware that she was committing murder but she made her mind up while in the [workhouse] that she would do away with child as she was not in a position to care for it and bring it up. This is her own statement.'

Kathleen was 'very nervous, shy and in a highly strung condition. She cries freely when spoken to and deplores her terrible fate in being sent to a Criminal Asylum. At present she shows no signs of insanity … Her father and mother are dead and she has no relations.' One month after admission, Kathleen had settled in to hospital life and was working 'daily in the laundry, is quiet and well conducted, and gives every satisfaction'. One year after admission, Kathleen was released to the 'care of Prison Aid Association'.

The Case of Linda:
'A Case of Simple Melancholia' Resulting from 'Intemperance'

Linda was a 31-year-old, married mother of five who was charged with murder and detained 'at the Lord Lieutenant's pleasure'. She was charged with 'cutting her child's throat in the yard of the workhouse' and diagnosed as 'a case of simple melancholia' resulting from 'intemperance'. Medical notes confirm that alcohol produced a 'state of wild excitement, with intense melancholia, thinking she was to be done away with, suspicious of every one, crying and lamenting her offence. It appears that this attack was due to her having obtained alcoholic liquor.'

After three years in the Central Criminal Lunatic Asylum, Linda had demonstrated 'no signs or symptoms of insanity at present but is somewhat irritable and bad tempered (easily put out). She is most industrious with her needle'. It was customary for patients to receive 'porter' (beer) at dinner time, but Linda's porter was stopped 'on account of her alcoholic tendency' and she appeared 'to have better control over herself since the porter was stopped'. The medical superintendent noted that 'for nearly two years has been free from mental disease. She has taken the pledge and if she persists in abstinence from alcohol, I do not anticipate a relapse'. More than four years after admission, Linda was 'discharged' back to prison and there is no further record of her progress.

The Case of Niamh:
'Greatly Worried Over Her Five Little Children'

Niamh was a 38-year-old, Roman Catholic housekeeper admitted in 1906 having been charged with 'obtaining goods under false pretences' and detained 'at the Lord Lieutenant's pleasure'. A married mother of five children (aged between 2 and 9 years), Niamh 'was never in prison before this'. She was sane on admission. According to medical notes, Niamh's husband was 'a labouring man and in delicate health' and they were 'very poorly off. From her own statement which by the depositions I see is correct, she went to a shop and asked for two pairs of shoes, saying she was sent by a Mrs [Y] for them; this was not true, as she took the shoes for her own children. I have had several conversations with this woman and I can find nothing wrong with her mind.'

Niamh was 'greatly worried over her five little children and she says there is no one at home to look after them … This woman tells me she is now eight weeks away from her house and thinks that is punishment enough for the stealing of two pairs of shoes. She is in good health and works in the laundry'. Medical notes indicate that Niamh was consistently 'very quiet' and showed 'no signs of insanity' at any point. Niamh spent more than five months at the Central Criminal Lunatic Asylum before being discharged to the 'care of her husband'.

Understanding the Statistics and Stories of Women
Committed Between 1868 and 1908

One of the striking features of these statistics and case histories is that, between 1868 and 1908, almost one woman in ten was considered sane at time of committal to the Central Criminal Lunatic Asylum, despite having previously shown signs of mental disorder at time of offence or trial. It is likely that these women had spent some time in prison after their trials, awaiting transfer to the asylum. For some, it is likely that their psychiatric symptoms subsided during this period, suggesting that these women may have just experienced short-lived episodes of illness, possibly related to alcohol misuse, infection or other physical factors. For others, it is possible that their symptoms were not especially marked at any stage and did not constitute mental disorder at any point in the clinical opinion of prison surgeons or admitting officers at the Central Criminal Lunatic Asylum. For these women, it is possible that findings of insanity at trial may have been driven by legal rather than clinical factors. There is strong evidence of generally excessive use of 'dangerous lunacy' procedures in nineteenth-century Ireland[27] and it is possible that there was similar excessive use of committal to the Central Criminal Lunatic Asylum as a convenient disposal in Irish courts. This merits further study from the perspective of Irish legal history.

It is likely that poverty and destitution also played substantial roles in creating the context for the committal of certain patients. Kathleen, for example, showed no significant signs of mental disorder at any point, although it is recorded that she was a servant, unmarried mother and orphan with no relations. After giving birth to her child in a workhouse in the west of Ireland, she felt 'she was not in a position to care for it and bring it up'. The challenges Kathleen faced were very real: even within the impoverished workhouse populations of the west of Ireland, unmarried mothers faced the greatest number of difficulties, including social exclusion and stigma, as well as reduced prospects for future marriage and employment.[28]

In terms of psychiatric diagnoses, cases of infanticide often present particular diagnostic difficulties, owing chiefly to the combination of psychological, psychiatric, socio-economic and developmental issues that contribute to the killing of a child. Today, it is clear that at least some women who kill their children suffer from mental disorders, such as personality disorder and psychosis,[29] but it is also clear that there are still strong links between child killing and marital and social circumstances.[30] The relevance of such a diversity of factors demonstrates the difficulties involved in piecing together the circumstances and events that contributed to any particular case of infanticide, especially when more than a century has passed since the infanticide occurred.

As a result, it is difficult retrospectively to establish definite psychiatric diagnoses for many of the women charged with child killing in nineteenth-century Ireland and committed to the Central Criminal Lunatic Asylum.[31] In the present study, the most common recorded diagnoses included mania, melancholia, intellectual disability and dementia. Even in these cases, however, the true diagnosis is not clear, as the contemporary diagnostic equivalents of conditions such as dementia are by no means clear. For example, it is likely that the 'dementia' included both cases of psychosis (e.g. schizophrenia) and organic mental disorder (e.g. cerebral neoplasms). In addition, it is likely that certain cases presented ongoing diagnostic difficulties at the time, as further psychiatric and organic symptoms emerged throughout the course of the women's stays at the Central Criminal Lunatic Asylum.[32]

There is particular difficulty with the diagnosis of postpartum psychosis (i.e. severe mental disorder following childbirth) in the Central Criminal Lunatic Asylum in the 1800s and 1900s, owing to the absence of systematic data on the intervals between childbirth, date of onset of mental disorder, date of offence, age of infant/child and date of arrest. Historical studies based in general (non-forensic) asylums offer greater opportunities to determine the population incidence of postpartum psychosis during this period: at Royal Edinburgh Hospital in Scotland, for example, the incidence of puerperal psychosis within ninety days of childbirth between 1880 and 1890 was 0.34 cases per 1,000 childbirths.[33] This is identical to the rate reported at Denbigh Asylum in North Wales between 1875 and 1924.[34] At present, it is not possible to calculate a comparable rate for Ireland.

From an historical perspective, diagnostic practices in relation to postpartum mental disorder have been substantially influenced by myriad factors, including social environments and prevailing moral contexts, suggesting that variance in diagnostic rates may reflect combinations of biological and societal trends rather than true medical or psychiatric differences.[35] Interestingly, it is nonetheless possible that incidence of postpartum psychosis may have been higher in the late nineteenth/early twentieth centuries than the late twentieth/early twenty-first centuries.[36] The explanation for this possible trend is unclear, but may relate to changes in psychiatric admission practices, changes in obstetric and birthing practices, or improved standards of prenatal care.

Sentencing Practices for Infanticide in Nineteenth-Century Ireland

From a legal perspective, punishment for infanticide in Ireland varied significantly throughout the nineteenth century. While the death penalty was associated with murder (including child murder) in the early part of the century, no woman in Ireland or Great Britain was executed for infanticide since 1849.[37] As the nineteenth century progressed, juries tried to convict women of crimes other than infanticide, especially when the deceased child was less than 1 year old at time of death. On this basis, many women charged with child killing were charged with murder or manslaughter, rather than infanticide. Ultimately, many of these women were detained 'at the Lord Lieutenant's pleasure' in the Central Criminal Lunatic Asylum. While their periods of detention were often lengthy, the alternatives to the Central Criminal Lunatic Asylum were similarly bleak and included the death penalty (although this was increasingly unlikely) or detention in other settings, such as district asylums or prisons (which was, ironically, the ultimate fate of many women anyway, following their time in Central Criminal Lunatic Asylum).

These changes in conviction and sentencing practices may account, at least in part, for the increased rates of admission to the Central Criminal Lunatic Asylum towards the end of the 1800s. There was, in particular, a notable increase in the number of 'guilty but insane' verdicts in Irish courts during the 1880s.[38] Admissions for infanticide or child murder also peaked in the 1880s and declined gradually over the following decades.[39] It is unlikely, however, that this rise in admissions to the Central Criminal Lunatic Asylum was solely attributable to changes in conviction and sentencing practices in Irish courts: all Irish asylums experienced relentless increases in admission rates during this period.[40] These trends generated substantial problems with overcrowding in most institutions, including the Central Criminal Lunatic Asylum,[41] further diminishing the quality of life of detained women.

This was the rather bleak picture for women detained at the Central Criminal Lunatic Asylum between 1968 and 1908. Did the dawn of the twentieth century herald significant reform? Did the women committed in the second period to be examined in this chapter (1910–48) differ in any significant way from those committed in the earlier period (1868–1908)?

WOMEN COMMITTED TO INPATIENT FORENSIC PSYCHIATRIC CARE IN IRELAND, 1910-48

Two of the key determinants of patterns of forensic psychiatric committal in the opening decades of the twentieth century were the continued emergence of forensic psychiatry as a medical discipline and the continued evolution of the insanity defence in Great Britain, Ireland and elsewhere.[42] Particular controversy accompanied the emergence of the insanity defence in Victorian courtrooms, centred largely on medical objections to the legalistic rather than medical approach that determined, in large part, the contents of the McNaughtan rules governing criminal insanity (Chapter 2).[43] The resultant tension between medical and legal professions was largely attributable to the relatively recent renewal of medical interest in insanity, which challenged entrenched legal views of issues related to criminal responsibility.[44]

An increased role for medical evidence was encouraged, nonetheless, by the introduction of defence lawyers who sought expert medical opinion to support insanity defences in British courts.[45] In France, there were similar competing points of view, but certain shared perspectives also emerged among judges, psychiatrists and various others empowered to apply new penal strategies.[46] In the United Kingdom, the eventual emergence of similar shared perspectives (especially the establishment of the McNaughtan insanity defence and its increased use in Victorian courtrooms) was a critical factor in the emergence of a distinct speciality of forensic psychiatry and the establishment of dedicated asylums for individuals who demonstrated offending behaviour in the context of apparent mental disorder (Chapter 2).[47] In Ireland the number of 'guilty but insane' verdicts duly increased in the late 1800s, consistent with international trends.[48]

But what about the early 1900s? Did rates of committal of women to the Central Criminal Lunatic Asylum continue to rise in the early decades of the new century, in line with overall asylum committal rates?[49] Did the hectic pace of legal reform in the 1800s persist into the new century? Did the social and diagnostic profiles of committed women change?

Interestingly, the early years of the twentieth century had brought little legislative change in relation to mental disorder, despite several commissions of inquiry into provision for the mentally ill. The 'Commission on the Relief of the Sick and Destitute Poor including the Insane Poor' (1927) had called for a system of auxiliary mental hospitals to be established in old workhouses and recommended the introduction of a voluntary admission status, as well as outpatient clinics.[50] The need for administrative and legislative reform and, in particular, a voluntary admission status to district asylums, was emphasised by an anonymous psychiatrist writing in *The Bell*, an Irish literary periodical, in 1944:

> Many cases reach institutions at least one year too late to have a reasonable hope of recovery. In many of these the delay is due to the existing laws regarding admission of patients to public Mental Hospitals. Before admission, each case must be certified by one or two doctors, and one or two Peace Commissioners or a District Justice. In its simplest form, certification of a patient needs one doctor and one PC (Peace Commissioner), and unless the case is a bad one, relatives are slow to take action. It is not too much to hope that legislation in the near future will remedy this and provide for the admission of voluntary patients.[51]

Many of these reforms were not to occur until the introduction of the Mental Treatment Act of 1945 (Chapter 5).[52] In the meantime, during the 1910s, 1920s, 1930s and early 1940s, committal to district asylums and the Central Criminal Lunatic Asylum continued to be largely governed by laws and practices dating from the nineteenth century.

Female Admissions to the Central Criminal Lunatic Asylum, 1910–48

Between 1910 and 1945, forty-two women were admitted to the Central Criminal Lunatic Asylum.[53] Interestingly, female committal rates at the asylum decreased steadily between 1910 and 1945: in the five-year period commencing in 1910 there were twelve female committals while in the five-year period commencing in 1940 there was one female committal (Figure 2). Female committal rates rose again with the introduction of the new Mental Treatment Act in 1945; in the three years following the introduction of the 1945 Act there were seven female committals.

Figure 2

Female Admission Rates to the Central Criminal Lunatic Asylum, Dublin, 1910–1948

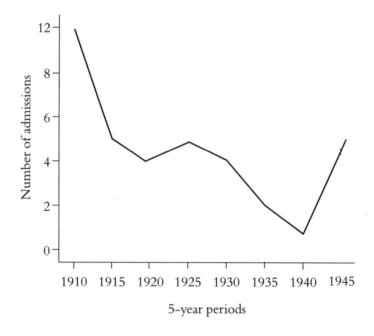

5-year periods

Note for Figure 2
In order to identify overall admission trends (rather than year-on-year fluctuations), this figure presents female admission rates aggregated into 5-year periods; i.e. in the 5-year period commencing in 1910, there were twelve female admissions.

These data were extracted from archival medical case-records at the Central Criminal Lunatic Asylum (now the Central Mental Hospital), Dundrum, Dublin, Ireland.

Table 4

Characteristics of Women Admitted to the Central Criminal Lunatic Asylum, Dublin, 1910–1948

Characteristic	n	Percentage
Marital Status		
Single	8	28
Married	15	52
Widowed	6	21
Nationality		
Irish	34	97
English	1	3
Religion		
Roman Catholic	35	85
Church of Ireland	3	7
Jewish	1	2
Presbyterian	1	2
Atheist	1	2
Occupation		
Housekeeper	10	38
Servant	5	19
Housewife	2	8
Farm Worker	2	8
Prostitute	2	8
Factory Worker	1	4
Shopkeeper	1	4
Waitress	1	4
Weaver	1	4
Tramp	1	4

Note for Table 4

These data were extracted from archival medical case-records at the Central Criminal Lunatic Asylum (now the Central Mental Hospital), Dundrum, Dublin, Ireland.

The average age of women committed was 36 years, and this ranged from 21 to 65. As in the period between 1868 and 1908, the majority of women were Irish in nationality and Roman Catholic in religion (Table 4). Married women accounted for over half of admissions. Number of children was not recorded for twenty-three women and three were recorded as being childless. Among the remainder, the average number of children was again three (this ranged from one to nine). The most common occupations recorded were housekeeper and servant.

Thirty-six women (86 per cent) were admitted to the Central Criminal Lunatic Asylum after being charged with a crime; the remaining six women (14 per cent) were transferred to the Central Criminal Lunatic Asylum from other psychiatric institutions under the Mental Treatment Act 1945 (see Chapter 5 for details of the Mental Treatment Act 1945). Of the women charged with a crime, twenty-four (75 per cent) were charged with killing; six (17 per cent) were charged with assault; three (8 per cent) were charged with malicious damage; two (6 per cent) were charged with attempted murder; and one (3 per cent) was charged with larceny.

Of the 24 women charged with killing, nineteen (79 per cent) were charged with murder; four (17 per cent) were charged with infanticide; and one (4 per cent) was charged with manslaughter. In twenty-two cases the identity of the victim was recorded: seventeen cases (77 per cent) involved child killing; the next most common victim was another member of the woman's family (18 per cent). In the cases of some women charged with child killing, the crime was recorded as murder or manslaughter rather than infanticide, consistent with the legal practice at the time. Overall, the seventeen child killings included twelve cases with one child victim, one case with two child victims and one case with more than two child victims. The ages of child victims were not recorded in all cases, but at least six child victims were below the age of one year, including three newborn babies.

Legal sentences were recorded for thirty-four of the thirty-six women admitted to the Central Criminal Lunatic Asylum following being charged with a crime. Of these, twenty-nine women (85 per cent) were sentenced to be detained 'at the Lord Lieutenant's Pleasure'. Three women (9 per cent) received sentences of specific durations and two women (6 per cent) received life sentences. The majority of women detained at the Lord Lieutenant's Pleasure had been charged with murder (52 per cent), assault (21 per cent) or infanticide (14 per cent); the mean duration of detention in this group was 5.6 years, with detentions ranging from less than one to 27 years. The three women who received sentences of specific durations were detained for shorter periods (ranging from less than one year to twelve years) and the two women who received life sentences spent an average of 13.5 years in detention. Durations of detention are recorded for two of the six women admitted without being charged with a crime (i.e. transferred from other psychiatric institutions under the Mental Treatment Act 1945); both of these women spent approximately one year in detention at the Central Criminal Lunatic Asylum.

Medical records indicate that three women (7 per cent) were considered to be sane at time of admission to the Central Criminal Lunatic Asylum and it is recorded that two of these women had previously shown signs of depression. This is similar to the proportion of sane admissions recorded for the period between 1868 and 1908 (11 per cent). Between 1910 and 1948, sixteen women (38 per cent) were given a diagnosis of mania or delusional insanity; ten (24 per cent) had melancholia; eight (19 per cent) had intellectual disability, of whom three also showed evidence of mental disorder; one (2 per cent) had 'dementia'; one (2 per cent) had epileptic insanity; one (2 per cent) had neurasthenia; and two (5 per cent) did not have any clear diagnosis recorded.

There are no systematic records of treatments provided at the Central Criminal Lunatic Asylum, although medical notes indicate that many women were employed within the hospital in household tasks such as laundry. Final outcomes are recorded for thirty-two women, of whom nine (28 per cent) were transferred to local asylums at the end of their detention; six (19 per cent) were released to the care of family; five (16 per cent) were released without any further details being recorded; two (6 per cent) were released 'cured'; one (3 per cent) was released to care of friends; one (3 per cent) was transferred to prison; and one (3 per cent) was transferred to a convent. Seven women (22 per cent) died in detention; causes of death were recorded for six women and included heart disease (three women), diabetes (two women) and suffocation following an apparent cerebro-vascular accident (stroke) (one woman).

Diagnostic Challenges in Early Twentieth-Century Psychiatry

These statistics relating to women admitted to the Central Criminal Lunatic Asylum between 1910 and 1948 are notably similar to those for women committed between 1869 and 1908. The only significant change is the declining rate of admission in the opening decades of the 1900s, which was most likely related to broader societal change in Ireland as much as it was to changes to psychiatric or legal practices. Many other factors remained remarkably constant over the two periods. For example, women committed between 1910 and 1948 still tended to present from socially deprived backgrounds and many had additional psychosocial stressors (e.g. single parenthood), just like their counterparts between 1868 and 1908.

The majority admitted between 1910 and 1948 also had, like their counterparts between 1868 and 1908, signs or symptoms of mental disorder recorded in their case notes in detail. During both periods, common diagnoses included mania and melancholia. Notwithstanding these diagnoses, however, and the general clarity of the case notes in which they are recorded, it remains exceedingly difficult to determine the precise current diagnostic equivalents of these used. At least four different terms ('mania', 'melancholia', 'mono-mania' and 'dementia') appear to have been the equivalent of contemporary 'functional psychoses' (schizophrenia and bipolar affective disorder), making retrospective diagnostic classification extremely challenging.[54]

The interpretation of diagnostic categories is further complicated by the fact that diagnostic and institutional practices in nineteenth- and early twentieth-century Irish psychiatry were substantially shaped by social power rather than expertise in relation to lunacy, as social and economic factors were strong determinants of asylum bed usage for much of this period and right into the twentieth century.[55] These social factors may have been particularly relevant to the 'criminally insane', whose predicament and fates were determined not only by the social circumstances in which they lived but also the legal process that unfolded following their offending behaviour.

Perhaps the social force that had the greatest influence on the fate of the women in this study was the inexorable expansion of the Irish asylum system throughout the nineteenth and early twentieth centuries. Not only were these women admitted to the Central Criminal Lunatic Asylum for extended periods, but almost one third of them were released to the care of district asylums at the end of their detention in the Central Criminal Lunatic Asylum. In the context of the United Kingdom, Scull relates the expansion of the asylum system during this period to the role of 'medical men as moral entrepreneurs', the emergence of psychiatry as a profession, and the notion that asylums were benign institutions providing humane care to those in need.[56] Many of these factors were similarly relevant in Ireland, and Walsh draws particular attention to 'the humanitarian climate of the nineteenth century' as well as the increased visibility of the mentally ill as a result of industrialisation and urbanisation.[57] The Great Irish Famine of the 1840s is also likely to have played a role, generating increased numbers of destitute, mentally-ill individuals presenting to Irish workhouses and further increasing pressures to expand the emerging network of district asylums.[58]

The Early Twentieth Century: Ireland's Asylums Continue to Expand

The relentless expansion in asylum capacity in Ireland continued into the twentieth century, notwithstanding the absence of specific treatments for most psychiatric disorders.[59] The therapeutic optimism associated with moral management was in decline and asylums were under increasing pressure for space, owing to the steady accumulation of 'incurable' cases for which no treatment appeared effective. In 1924, Edward Boyd Barrett, SJ MA, drew particular attention to the lack of effective treatment in asylums, in an article in *Studies*, an influential Irish quarterly review:

> Thanks to this indifference of the public, our asylums are in a bad way. They are over-crowded. They are both understaffed and inefficiently staffed. Curable and incurable cases are herded together. There is practically no treatment. The percentage of cures remains at a very low figure. Public money is wasted. The asylums are unsuited for their purpose in almost every respect.[60]

For many patients, admission to an asylum was often the only intervention they received. The very fact of being separated from family and admitted to the asylum setting was often perceived as therapeutic in itself. In 1944, the anonymous psychiatrist, writing in *The Bell*, outlined the importance of rapid admission to institutional settings:

> There are many types of mental disease and it is to be understood that each type has to be treated in its own way. Nevertheless there are certain principles which govern the treatment of all cases. These in the main are: removal from home and relatives; rest; adequate diet; sleep. These can be achieved only in an Institution with a trained staff, and the sooner these can be had the more likelihood of a speedy recovery.[61]

As a result of this persistent belief in the therapeutic power of the asylum, the system of institutional care established in Ireland throughout the 1800s remained the defining feature of Irish mental health services at the start of the twentieth century, as evidenced by the fate of women committed to the Central Criminal Lunatic Asylum. This situation was slow to change. The reluctance to develop alternative models of care may be attributable, at least in part, to the turbulent social, political and economic circumstances of the opening decades of the new century. At this time, Ireland was still part of the United Kingdom, although events in the early decades of the new century were to present significant challenges to this position. Despite ongoing initiatives to develop home rule for Ireland, a group of Irish republicans staged a short-lived uprising in central Dublin in Easter 1916, demanding the establishment of an Irish republic.[62] While the Easter Rising was not a military success, the British response to it deepened sympathy for the Republican cause. The subsequent War of Independence and Anglo-Irish Treaty (1921) were followed by a bitter civil war in the 1920s and, ultimately, the establishment of the Republic of Ireland in 1949. Against this turbulent background, reform of the Irish asylum system may have seemed a low priority.

The early decades of the twentieth century were also a period of significant social and political upheaval in the six counties that were to form the British province of Northern Ireland.[63] While the nineteenth century had seen expansion of asylum capacity in the north of Ireland that was similar to that in the south,[64] the early 1900s also saw economic and political conditions impact significantly on the development of asylum services in the north.[65] Social and economic conditions were also similarly slow to improve in the south, owing to ongoing political unrest, the recession of the 1930s, and a protracted trade war with England. While health service reform was not a political priority in the South during much of this period, the 1940s saw the emergence of several significant initiatives in the area of public health. This was attributable to a range of factors including eventual political stability in Ireland, the emergence of the National Health Service in the United Kingdom, and the influence of Catholic social teaching on political and administrative reform.[66]

This period of reform also saw the emergence of the Mental Treatment Act 1945, which was to prove the most extensive reform of mental health legislation in the entire twentieth century.[67] Details of this legislation are presented in Chapter 5, but, in terms of forensic psychiatry, the central implications of the Mental Treatment Act of 1945 related to Section 207 (permitting the transfer of individuals who are 'unfit to plead' to the

Central Criminal Lunatic Asylum) and Section 208 (permitting transfer of detained patients from a district mental hospital to the Central Criminal Lunatic Asylum).

The analysis of female admissions between 1910 and 1948 presented in this chapter demonstrates some of the effects of these legislative changes on female admission patterns at the Central Criminal Lunatic Asylum: female admissions rose sharply around 1945, reflecting the sudden increase in patients transferred from local asylums under the provisions of the new Act. These women had not been charged with specific criminal offences but were transferred to the Central Criminal Lunatic Asylum from local district asylums owing to difficulties with their management in the district asylum system. Durations of detention were recorded for only two of the six women so admitted in 1945, both of whom spent approximately one year in detention at the Central Criminal Lunatic Asylum. This is significantly shorter than the periods spent there by women who had engaged in offending behaviour including, most notably, infanticide.

Infanticide Committals to the Central Criminal Lunatic Asylum in the Early Twentieth Century

Overall, the majority (86 per cent) of women admitted to the Central Criminal Lunatic Asylum between 1910–48 were charged with a crime. The most common crimes involved killing and the most common victims were a child or children. While ages were not recorded for all child victims, at least six were under the age of 1 year, including three newborn babies. These were, therefore, cases of infanticide.

Until 1949, infanticide was considered equivalent to murder in Ireland but there was a long-standing tendency for juries to reach verdicts other than infanticide in order to avoid the possibility of the death penalty.[68] Notwithstanding these attempts at apparent leniency, women who were charged with killing their children and committed to the Central Criminal Lunatic Asylum spent an average of nine years in the asylum. In addition, discharge of individuals who killed children was particularly challenging and, as the present analysis demonstrates, between a half and a third of these women were sent to district asylums following their time the Central Criminal Lunatic Asylum.[69] It is likely that many of these women spent the rest of their lives behind asylum walls.

The reluctance to use the death penalty following infanticide in the United Kingdom (including Ireland) likely reflected not only the apparent leniency of juries, but also a more broad-based public acceptance of the occurrence of infanticide, which was generally widely reported in Irish newspapers.[70] This trend echoes Wright's arguments in the context of learning disability and, in particular, his emphasis on the role of popular and lay attitudes, rather than medical approaches, in changing diagnostic practices.[71]

In the context of infanticide, Marland also draws attention to the description, in 1820, of the diagnosis of 'puerperal insanity' (i.e. severe mental disorder following childbirth), which further strengthened the association between infanticide and insanity, and emphasised the medical rather than criminal dimensions of the act.[72] This trend was reinforced by the occurrence of infanticide in all social classes and the influence of higher social classes in promoting the more acceptable description of infanticide in medical rather than criminal terms. Finally, ongoing efforts to establish psychiatry as a respected branch of medical practice also contributed to the psychiatric 'appropriation' of infanticide, often via 'puerperal insanity'.[73]

From the analysis presented in this chapter, it is apparent that women committed to the Central Criminal Lunatic Asylum in the late nineteenth and early twentieth centuries generally came from lower social classes and many had evidence of additional psychosocial stressors. This is consistent with patterns observed amongst women committed to British asylums following infanticide[74] and with general patterns of female psychiatric committal in other countries, such as Canada.[75] Coleborne draws particular attention to the policing of sex in nineteenth-century Australia and the use of lunacy charges to facilitate the arrest of women working as prostitutes.[76] Between 1910 and 1948, only two of the forty-two women committed to the Central Criminal Lunatic Asylum were described as 'prostitutes', but the recording of occupations was unlikely to have been systematic, and only twenty-six out of these forty-two women had any occupation recorded at all. The true rate of committal of prostitutes to Irish asylums is not clear.

The role played by gender more generally in the committal process, and in British and Irish psychiatry as a whole during the nineteenth and twentieth centuries, has been explored by a number of authors.[77] Walsh, for example, notes that while a familial basis to insanity was well recognised, insanity was believed to be passed exclusively through the female line, and there was a persistent tendency to ascribe insanity in women to moral rather than physical causes.[78] Notwithstanding this tendency – or possibly because of it – female patients in district asylums tended to have better living conditions, lower death rates and greater chances of permanent discharge, compared to male patients.[79] McCarthy notes, however, that gender ideology interacted with a range of other social, personal and medical factors in determining how each woman experienced her illness and the institutional and societal responses to it.[80]

Various other trends in thought and practice were also relevant in shaping the institutional experiences of women committed to the Central Criminal Lunatic Asylum during these periods. Harris, in her considerations of medicine, law and insanity in *fin de siècle* France, highlights the emergence of the concept of 'degeneration' and the idea that insanity was becoming more common than it had been in the past.[81] This preoccupation echoed similar concerns in the Irish medical community throughout the nineteenth and early twentieth centuries.[82] Harris, however, also notes the relative leniency with which women were treated in French courtrooms, as compared with the severity of approach assumed towards young males whose offences had a political dimension. One of the factors contributing to this tendency was undoubtedly the assumption that women were generally more frail than men and, therefore, more susceptible to mental disorder (Chapter 2).[83]

In addition to gender, religion was another non-medical factor that had a significant impact on understandings of mental disorder and institutional responses to the mentally ill throughout the eighteenth, nineteenth and twentieth centuries.[84] Michael and Hirst, for example, note the pivotal role of the Anglican Church in establishing the list of subscribers for the North Wales Lunatic Asylum in Denbigh; members of the Bible Society were also recruited for door-to-door collections for the cause.[85] In Ireland, evolving tensions between Protestant and Catholic sectors of the population also had a significant impact on asylum life. Up until 1904, for example, all of the staff and physicians at Ballinasloe Asylum were Protestant, while over 90 per cent of patients were Catholic.[86] Regrettably, it is not possible to engage in a detailed examination of religion in the Central Criminal Lunatic Asylum as part of the present analysis, owing to the strong dominance of Roman Catholicism among the women studied and the absence of information about staff. It is highly likely, however, that religious differences were a significant factor in asylum life.

CONCLUSIONS: WOMEN COMMITTED TO THE CENTRAL CRIMINAL LUNATIC ASYLUM, 1868–1948

Women admitted to the Central Criminal Lunatic Asylum between 1868 and 1948 faced substantial social, legal, medical and psychiatric challenges during one of the most politically and economically unstable phases of recent Irish history. While rates of committal of women declined in the early decades of the twentieth century, rates rose again in the 1940s, following the introduction of the Mental Treatment Act 1945 and in line with general committal rates to Irish district asylums.

In the case of women charged with child killing, it is notable that the alternatives to lengthy detention in the Central Criminal Lunatic Asylum included the death penalty or committal to local district asylums. In this respect, the Irish data presented in this chapter support the idea that women who offended in the context of mental disorder following childbirth tended to be treated relatively sympathetically by the authorities, including the medical profession and the courts.[87] Ireland's particularly strong tradition of psychiatric institutionalisation, however, meant that many of these women spent lengthy periods in the Central Criminal Lunatic Asylum and almost one in three was subsequently institutionalised in district asylums throughout Ireland, possibly for lengthy periods of time. It is debatable just how sympathetic this treatment really was for many of these women.

The ultimate fate of most of these women was generally determined by a combination of societal, legal and medical circumstances, as evidenced by both the socio-economic profile of women admitted to the Central Criminal Lunatic Asylum and changes in admission patterns following the introduction of the Mental Treatment Act 1945. The factors contributing to the development of the 1945 legislation and more general reform of Ireland's asylum system in the twentieth century are considered in Chapter 5. First, however, Chapter 4 explores in greater depth the clinical case histories of men and women committed to the Central Criminal Lunatic Asylum in the 1800s and early 1900s, focusing especially on medical and social aspects of their cases. Chapter 4 also places strong emphasis on symptoms of physical and mental disorder, in order to determine, insofar as possible at this remove, the true extent of physical and mental disorder in this group.

4

Clinical Aspects of Criminal Insanity in Nineteenth- and Twentieth-Century Ireland

INTRODUCTION

As Chapter 3 demonstrated, during the 1800s and 1900s, people were committed to asylums for complicated combinations of psychiatric, medical, social and legal reasons. This chapter presents a series of case histories of men and women committed to the Central Criminal Lunatic Asylum in the 1800s and early 1900s, examining all of these diverse aspects of their cases. There is a strong emphasis on symptoms of physical and mental disorder, demonstrating compelling clinical evidence of disorders such as syphilis, intellectual disability and, most fascinatingly, folie à plusieurs, a rare psychiatric disorder which affects several individuals at the same time.

FOLIE À PLUSIEURS

Folie à plusieurs refers to a psychiatric disorder in which one or more delusions (fixed, false beliefs, not amenable to reason) are shared by a number of individuals, often within a family or other close-knit group.[1] Folie à deux is the term used when the disorder affects just two individuals who share similar symptoms, most commonly paranoid delusions.

While there was a number of clinical descriptions of these syndromes throughout the seventeenth and eighteenth centuries, the received view is that the term folie à deux was coined by two French doctors, Ernest-Charles Lasègue (1816–83) and Jean-Pierre Falret (1794–1870), in the 1870s and translated as 'communicated insanity' by William Wotherspoon Ireland (1832–1909), a Scottish adventurer and polymath, in the 1880s.[2] More recently, this syndrome of 'communicated insanity' has been included under the heading 'induced delusional disorder' in The ICD-Classification of Mental and Behavioural Disorders of the World Health Organization.[3] Prior to the standardised descriptive terms and broad categorisations of the ICD, however, folie à deux enjoyed a complex, colourful career in the history of psychiatry.

Identifying the precise point of 'discovery' or first description of any psychiatric symptom or disease is an historiographically complex task.[4] While many authors have written clinical and historical reviews of folie à deux, the precise point of its emergence as a diagnostic entity has still not been fully determined, and the classic description remains that of Lasègue and Falret in the 1870s.[5] As a result of their seminal work, throughout the late 1800s and early 1900s, the term 'folie à plusieurs' came to refer to cases of 'communicated insanity' in which symptoms are shared by three or more individuals. This syndrome was also known as 'induced psychotic disorder' because there tends to be one 'primary' patient whose illness is 'transmitted' to one or more 'secondary' patients.[6]

The majority of cases of induced psychotic disorder occur within families and most commonly involve mother and child, wife and husband, or woman and sibling.[7] Treatment involves identifying the primary patient and treating their mental disorder and physical disorder (if present). The secondary patient may not require specific treatment following separation from the primary patient but in certain cases there may be mental disorder, physical disorder or some form of disability that also requires management.[8] Psychological and social support may also form an important element in the overall management plan.

There have been several reports of forensic complications of communicated insanity,[9] including theft, violence,[10] attempted murder[11] and murder.[12] These complications, rare but important, are well demonstrated in the two sets of cases presented here, drawn from the archives of the Central Criminal Lunatic Asylum: the cases of brothers who all 'became insane at the same time' and a family of parents and children who 'all became insane at once'.

Brothers Who All 'Became Insane at the Same Time'

In 1896, two brothers were admitted to the Central Criminal Lunatic Asylum on the same day. Both were unmarried farmers who lived on a family farm in rural Ireland. Both were charged with the murder of their brother and detained in the Central Criminal Lunatic Asylum 'at the Lord Lieutenant's pleasure'. Liam, the elder, was 36 years of age, and had no history of mental or physical disorder, epilepsy or alcohol abuse.

Admission notes describe Liam as 'industrious, honest ... timid and nervous'. At the time of admission, Liam had 'two brothers and a sister in an asylum' because 'all the family became insane at the same time'. Liam himself was 'timorous and sleepless, watching an insane brother for about 12 days'. He was diagnosed with 'acute delusional mania, convalescent' and the cause of his 'nervous disease' was recorded as 'hereditary'.

While physical examination on admission to the Central Criminal Lunatic Asylum was normal, the prison surgeon's report from four months earlier (when the brothers were detained in prison awaiting trial), noted that they were 'wild and haggard-looking ... conjunctiva [eyes] congested, tongue dry and brown, spoke fairly sensible'. Liam's temperature was 100° Fahrenheit (38° Celsius; slightly raised) with a raised pulse rate of 116 beats per minute. At night the brothers' conditions worsened: Liam, for example, became 'wildly delirious, believed there were devils in his cell, sprinkling bed and cell with water, praying constantly, pupils dilated, voice hoarse, spitting frequently ... hallucinations of sight and hearing, refused food, slept none that night, were placed in muffs ...'

The following day, still in prison, Liam remained acutely unwell, with continued high temperature and fast heart rate. His 'tongue was very dry and brown, conjunctiva much congested' and he 'seemed completely exhausted, still had delusions, slept none at night and had delirium'. Over the following days, he began to recover: 'tongue becoming moist, taking nourishment, some delusions and sleeplessness at night. Prisoner gradually improved from this, he remained in a state of the most extreme collapse for some weeks, tongue white and furred, complained of headache and giddiness. Prisoner was kept quiet in hospital and given plenty of milk, beef tea and two bottles of stout daily'.

It was reported to the prison surgeon that:

> Delirium occurred at night in the different police barracks where [the two brothers] were confined previous to committal to prison. I consider Liam was suffering from acute delirious mania. After due time I certified

prisoner fit for trial. His mental condition seems to have received a severe shock and his trial upset him considerably.

When Liam was 'charged with the murder of his brother' he said that his (now deceased) 'brother was insane for ten days previous'.' At his trial, Liam was charged with murder and then detained at the Central Criminal Lunatic Asylum indefinitely.

Following his arrival at the Central Criminal Lunatic Asylum, medical notes recorded that Liam was:

> quite recovered from the attack of acute mania from which he suffered while in [prison] and for some days previously; he accounts for the insanity in his family (which occurred almost suddenly) being brought on by "some thing" they all partook of while at meals, but is unable to say what the nature of this "something" was. He recognises perfectly the crime that both he and his brothers committed and is fully aware that he was at the time "out of his mind." He has a somewhat down-cast appearance, a slow slouching gait and is depressed in manner and appearance.

Over the following weeks, Liam was generally 'very quiet and has been sent to work on the land'. He played cricket in the evenings. Liam's treatment was described as 'moral supervision and dietetic' and, four months after his initial admission, notes record that 'this patient has never presented any symptoms of insanity'.

Liam's younger brother, James, who was admitted on the same day in 1896, presented with a very similar history. Aged 34 years at the time of admission, James was also charged with murder and detained in the Central Criminal Lunatic Asylum 'at the Lord Lieutenant's pleasure'. On admission, he was described as 'industrious' and 'not sick but timorous and sleepless watching an insane brother for about 12 days'. He was diagnosed with 'acute delusional mania, convalescent' and the cause of his illness was 'hereditary'.

The admission notes record that 'the prison surgeon's report of this patient is identical with the report of his brother'. Like his brother, James experienced high temperature, fast heart rate, hallucinations and delirium while in prison but, by the time he was admitted to the Central Criminal Lunatic Asylum, appeared to have:

> quite recovered from the attack of acute mania from which he suffered at the time of committing the murder of his brother and afterwards while in

[prison]. Patient is very quiet and well-conducted, is in fair health, takes his food well and sleeps soundly. Has been sent with his brother [Liam] to work on the land and they are both satisfied and pleased to do so.

James and Liam could 'only account for the sudden burst of insanity which occurred in their family by their haven eaten some poison or some other substance which was equally obnoxious and having taken it unconsciously in their food. James appears depressed, in very quiet and respectful, is naturally of a slow, quiet and silent disposition'. While James did not show signs of mental disorder at the Central Criminal Lunatic Asylum, he began to lose weight in the year following his admission. Nonetheless, the medical officer could 'discover no organic disease present. Mentally is in excellent health. Sleeps well, works on the land and is well conducted.'

Later in 1896, a third brother, Robert, also charged with the murder of his brother, and was transferred from prison to the Central Criminal Lunatic Asylum to be detained 'at the Lord Lieutenant's pleasure'. Again, Robert was a labourer on the family farm and the cause of his illness at the time of the murder was described as 'hereditary'. Admission notes record him as 'very quiet, well spoken and most respectful; both in manner and appearance he much resembles his brothers ... He presents no symptoms of insanity. I consider him perfectly sane; but like his brothers he suffered from an attack of acute mania while in [prison] ... He is quite unable to in any way account for the insanity which occurred in his family, he feels deeply the great misfortune which has befallen them and is depressed when speaking of his brother ... who was the unfortunate victim of their insanity.'

On admission, Robert had a history of 'phthisis' (tuberculosis) which worsened in the months following admission. In 1897, the medical officers at the hospital wrote to the Inspector of Lunatics stating that Robert was 'suffering from effects of detention and presents symptoms of incipient phthisis. We strongly recommend his discharge on the grounds that his disease will be aggravated by his detention'. Despite treatment with cod-liver oil, medical notes recorded that 'phthisis makes itself more evident each day. Crepitation may be heard at the apex of right lung; owing to constant and continued cough, loss of appetite and sweating, patient has lost greatly in weight.' The medical officers again wrote to the Inspector of Lunatics stating that Robert's 'condition has become critical and that if he is to be discharged, he should be released at once, as in our opinion, he will soon become too ill to be removed. His temperature at night has reached 102 [i.e. 102° Fahrenheit; 38.9° Celsius; raised] and in our opinion he will not survive this winter'. After two more weeks, Robert was discharged to the care of his sister, but died three months later in late 1897.

Neither Liam nor James showed any convincing signs of mental disorder during their time at the Central Criminal Lunatic Asylum. In 1898, the medical officer sent a report to the Inspector of Lunatics stating that both brothers were:

> suitable for discharge. They both have been industrious and extremely well behaved since admission here. The only distinction I wish to make is that detention is having a bad effect on James's health and he may become ill in the same manner as his brother Robert, who died soon after his being released from here.

Four months later, the medical officer sent an additional report in relation to James, stating that he was now 'in very delicate health and threatened with phthisis and we consider that he will die from this disease if not discharged soon. We also certify that he may be discharged with safety to himself and others.' Later that year, James was 'discharged in care of sister' after two years in the Central Criminal Lunatic Asylum. Three years later, Liam was also discharged 'in care of his sister' after more than five years in the Central Criminal Lunatic Asylum. There is no further record of their clinical course or outcome.

Parents and Children Who 'All Became Insane at Once'

In 1888, Bridget, a 40-year-old woman, was charged with the murder of her son and sentenced to be detained in the Central Criminal Lunatic Asylum 'at the Lord Lieutenant's pleasure'. A married mother of five, Bridget was unable to read or write. Admission notes record that 'she, her husband and a number of their children all became insane at once and jointly murdered one of the sons, an imbecile idiot'.

This case was described in further detail by Dr Oscar T. Woods, medical superintendent of the Killarney Asylum, in a case report published in the *Journal of Mental Science* (forerunner of the *British Journal of Psychiatry*) in 1889.[13] In 'Notes of a case of folie à deux in five members of one family', Woods described how five members of one family were admitted to Killarney Asylum in 1888, including a mother (Bridget), three daughters (aged 24, 18 and 15 years) and one son (aged 22). In his paper, Woods presented an account of the aftermath of the killing provided by the local constabulary sergeant:

I saw the dead body of a boy lying in the yard in front of the door; it had no clothing on except a shirt. The nose had disappeared; the front of both cheeks had been removed by violence. When I came in front of the house I saw a number of the family grouped together … They were all evidently insane, jumping about and shouting in an excited way. These patients were brought to the asylum together, where they were seen by two magistrates, who committed all except the father. He, although suffering from hallucinations, was quiet and comprehended all that was said to him.

On admission to Killarney Asylum:

> … the three daughters were in a very violent state of acute hysterical mania, flinging themselves about; could not comprehend anything said to them; pupils largely dilated; pulse quick. Mother and son very excited, but more collected, and able to comprehend what was said to them. All patients were much bruised about the body … Mother and son both fell on their knees and prayed to God and the Virgin Mary and the former made the following statement: 'On Saturday night at cock-crow I took that fairy … he was not my son, he was a devil, a bad fairy … carried him out of the house and threw him into the yard, and then got a hatchet and struck him three blows on the head. I then came back, and we all prayed and went to Heaven'. All had the one dominant delusion that they had been to Heaven, each one describing minutely what they imagined they had seen.

Woods noted that the 24-year-old daughter had 'not been quite herself for about a week' prior to the killing. In addition, the family had recently eaten 'heartily' of 'goat's meat, part of which I found in a tub in the house, which was stinking, green and putrid'. The family had also 'lost their rest the previous week while sitting up minding a sow and young ones'.[14]

Following their admission to Killarney Asylum, the patients remained disturbed and religiously deluded for two or three more days, but were soon 'all quieter, generally improving'. On the fourth day after admission, Bridget was 'willing to talk but pretends to forget everything. Says [her son] is alive, knows where she is, and is very collected … evidently [she] is not speaking the truth and knows everything, but as she now realises her position, wishes to conceal the fact of her guilt'. Regarding treatment, Woods wrote that 'no special medical treatment was found necessary. Aperient [laxative] and tonic medicine with chloral as a night draught during the first week; plenty of nourishing food and out-door exercise was alone required.'

Four weeks after admission to Killarney Asylum, there was general improvement in most family members, with the notable exception of the 24-year-old daughter who had been the first to become unwell. Some ten months after her initial admission to Killarney Asylum, this daughter was 'still an inmate of the asylum, daily becoming more demented'. The others were discharged approximately five months after admission, the delay being due to 'the criminal charges hanging over these patients'.

The trial took place seven months after the killing. Bridget, the mother, was charged with murder and detained in the Central Criminal Lunatic Asylum 'at the Lord Lieutenant's pleasure'. At this point, Bridget's clinical condition had again worsened: she was diagnosed with 'chronic mania' and described as a 'most determined tearer of her clothing and bedding, almost impossible to keep her covered'. She remained generally unwell and episodically disturbed throughout her time at the hospital. In 1892, four years after admission, she was 'very incoherent, noisy and excitable, constantly jabbering and shouting. Very abusive and obscene in her language ... is very violent, kicking, biting and striking the attendants with her head. She is also most destructive, tearing up her bed clothes and wearing apparel; she has in consequence to wear a canvas restraint nearly always'.

In 1893, medical notes record that Bridget 'is demented; no improvement can be hoped for in this case'. By 1894 she was 'quieter and is no longer kept in canvas restraint; is noisy at times and violent, most incoherent and erotic'. The following year, Bridget was 'transferred to Killarney Asylum: a case of chronic mania with occasional attacks of noisy excitement.' There is no further record of her clinical course or outcome.

FORENSIC COMPLICATIONS OF FOLIE À PLUSIEURS

These two sets of cases demonstrate some of the possible forensic complications of folie à plusieurs: both sets of cases involved the killing of one family member and subsequent detention of other family members in Ireland's only forensic psychiatry institution, the Central Criminal Lunatic Asylum.

The case of the three brothers is particularly interesting in light of indications that these patients suffered from an acute organic disorder with many features of delirium (high temperature, fast heart rate, insomnia, visual hallucinations) which is a primarily physical rather than mental disorder. Moreover, it appears that these acute, physical disturbances were short-lived and all three brothers remained in good mental health throughout their time in the Central Criminal Lunatic Asylum.[15] Their treatment while in hospital was described as 'moral supervision and dietetic', a management approach which involved regular exercise, gainful employment and an emphasis on healthy dietary habits.[16] The principles of moral management had a substantial influence not only on psychiatric care in nineteenth-century Ireland, but also on the design of asylums built in Ireland during this period.[17] Moral management focused on the use of reason and emotion, gainful occupation, good diet and physical activity in order to treat mental disorder. Activities in the Central Criminal Lunatic Asylum around this time included ball games, dancing, music, evening parties and reading books and newspapers (for those patients able to read).[18]

Two of the brothers, James and Robert, appear to have had problems with tuberculosis while in the Central Criminal Lunatic Asylum. Tuberculosis was a substantial problem in both general and asylum populations throughout the nineteenth century.[19] The eventual decline in tuberculosis in early twentieth-century Ireland was most likely attributable to a range of factors, including public health measures,[20] legislation[21] and socio-political change.[22] Throughout the 1890s, however, Ireland's asylums were extremely overcrowded[23] and tuberculosis was still a serious problem; at least one of the three brothers in this case series (Robert) eventually died of the disease.[24]

The case of Bridget, who was charged with killing her son after 'she, her husband and a number of their children all became insane at once', also presents several points of interest. In this case, it appears that the 24-year-old daughter was the primary case, as she had 'not been quite herself for about a week' prior to the killing and, some ten months later, was 'still an inmate of the asylum, daily becoming more demented'.[25] Bridget, too, developed further illness and, following her admission to the Central Criminal Lunatic Asylum, was described as 'demented; no improvement can be hoped for in this case'.

In her account of the killing, Bridget stated that her son 'was not my son, he was a devil, a bad fairy'. This is a reference to the folk belief in 'changelings', which were the offspring of fairies or other mythical creatures that were said to be secretly left in place of a human child. Although the precise features of changeling myths vary somewhat across different cultures, changelings were generally said to be vicious, unpleasant creatures that caused considerable alarm.[26] Belief in changelings was strong in the south of Ireland, where Bridget lived, as later evidenced by the emergence of Ireland's best-known changeling story in the mid-1890s – the story of

Bridget Cleary.[27] Changeling myths were also recounted by Lady Francesca
Speranza Wilde in her *Ancient Legends, Mystic Charms, and Superstitions of
Ireland*[28] and William Butler Yeats in his *Irish Fairy Tales*.[29] While there have
been recent explorations of possible links between changeling myths and
intellectual disability,[30] autism,[31] developmental difficulties[32] and Capgras
syndrome (a rare delusional disorder),[33] there is a relative paucity of literature exploring why the changeling myth took such a firm hold on the Irish
imagination.[34]

In his published account of Bridget's case, Woods wrote that:

> Happily, such cases as this have not often to be reported in this country.
> In foreign countries, however, they are not so uncommon; no doubt
> the hereditary taint and the strong superstitious ideas instilled into their
> ignorant minds by the old country women, acting on people whose
> bodily health was somewhat undermined by bad food and loss of rest, had
> much to say to the cause of the attack.[35]

Interestingly, one of the three brothers in the first case series also contended
that their illness was 'brought on by 'some thing' they all partook of while at
meals, but is unable to say what the nature of this something was'.

Woods's 1889 description of folie à plusieurs was especially compelling
and built on the work of W.W. Ireland, who had recently published a
collection of clinical vignettes illustrating both clinical and forensic aspects
of folie à plusieurs or 'communicated insanity'.[36] Presciently, Ireland had
written that:

> It seems likely that, as the same causes produce the same effects, in a family
> equally exposed to unfavourable influences, two or three brothers or
> sisters might become insane at once; and this might especially be thought
> to hold good with twins.

Ireland went on to describe a case of folie imposée (delusions imposed by
one person on another) 'taken from Dr Marandon de Montyel' in which a
woman 'persuaded her husband that their misfortunes were the result of a
plot laid against her; and in 1878 she told him that she heard the voice of
an angel who announced that God called her to high destinies ...' While
experiencing these hallucinations and delusions, the woman 'felt herself
constrained by a superior force to commit eccentric actions. She broke
panes of glass, openly tried to carry away a vase in a church, and struck

the sacristan who opposed her'. Following her admission to an asylum, her husband came to see Dr de Montyel, the superintendent of the asylum, and had 'a violent outburst of anger and threats':

> 'My wife,' he said, 'has never been mad. She looked after her affairs as well as ever; nothing was changed in our home. The strange actions she did were in obedience to the voice of God. Now she wants to get out; the time of trial is over. No one can keep her any longer.'
>   In this case it seems clear that while his wife was insane, the husband was simply weak and credulous. By the superior force of her intellect, and the energy of her character, she was able to lead him into delusions which he alone would never have originated or conceived. It is what the French call folie impose.

Three years after Ireland's chapter appeared, Dr Daniel Hack Tuke (1827–95), formerly of the York Retreat,[37] published a detailed account of the clinical features of folie à deux or 'double insanity' in the leading journal *Brain*.[38] Ireland also noted the clinical importance of this syndrome and outlined the case of 'Sir William Courtenay, Knight of Malta' in order to illustrate 'the influence a religious lunatic may have over stupid and ignorant people'.[39] This case also illustrates the potential forensic complications of imposed insanity. Sir William Courtenay's real name was John Nichols Thom, the 'son of a publican in Cornwall. His mother is said to have been insane.' In 1832 'Sir William' arrived in Canterbury, claimed to be from the Holy Land, and stood for election:

> Failing to pay his election expenses, Sir William was imprisoned for debt. On being released, he appeared as a witness to get off some men accused of smuggling. He was placed on trial at Maidstone for perjury, and sentenced to three months imprisonment and transportation for seven years. He was soon removed from jail to the County Asylum at Barming Heath, as a criminal lunatic, where he was detained for four years.

Following his release, 'Sir William' went to Kent where he started 'denouncing the rich and inciting the rural labourers to claim their share of the land and its produce':

He caused his followers to believe that they were invulnerable to bullet or
to sword. Two constables were sent to arrest him when Courtenay fired
a pistol at one of them, wounded him, and stabbed him with a dagger.
He then declared himself to be the Christ, and administered a sacrament
of bread and water to his followers. Two companies of soldiers were called
who came in sight of him in Bassendean Wood, Courtenay killed a lieutenant with a shot from a pistol, but was himself shot dead, with six of his
followers by the soldiers.

Woods, in his account of Bridget's case in Killarney, paid particular
attention to the role of the psychiatrist when such cases have forensic
complications:

> A question arose during the preliminary investigation on which I would
> be glad to have your opinion – as to whether the medical officer of an
> asylum is right to divulge in a court of law statements made by a patient,
> either when that patient is labouring under delusions or convalescent.
> I think any conversation with an inmate of an asylum should be privi-
> leged, as it is held not with the object of obtaining information, but with
> a view to test the sanity and promote the recovery of the patient. If all
> conversations held with a lunatic could be extracted from a superin-
> tendent in a witness-box his influence over many of the patients would,
> I believe, be lost. I, at all events, refused at the preliminary inquiry to state
> communications made to me by the prisoners, and was not asked to do
> so at the assizes.[40]

Over 100 years since the patients in this case series were admitted to the
Central Criminal Lunatic Asylum, individuals with folie à plusieurs still
present many clinical and ethical challenges to mental health services in
general[41] and forensic mental health services in certain cases.[42] Mela, for
example, provides a detailed clinical account of folie à trois in three incarcerated individuals in the same hospital unit and emphasises the importance
of autonomy and confidentiality in such cases.[43]

The forensic cases of folie à plusieurs from nineteenth-century Ireland
presented in this chapter demonstrate that many of the diagnostic, clinical
and ethical challenges that 'communicated insanity' presents to mental
health and judicial services today were similarly relevant in nineteenth-
century Ireland. The optimal balance between punishment and treatment
continues to be difficult to achieve,[44] while both treatment and community

reintegration present ongoing challenges, especially in cases with substantial forensic dimensions.[45]

INTELLECTUAL DISABILITY

In 2008, the Irish College of Psychiatrists reported that 'the needs of people with learning disability and offending behaviour pose a huge challenge to service providers … The vulnerability of people with a learning disability who come into contact with the criminal justice system is well described and noted'.[46] The College noted that 'the population with learning disability who offend does not easily fit into existing services' and reported that 'the majority of service providers strongly supported the urgent development of a forensic learning disability service'.

The challenges presented by individuals with intellectual disability and offending behaviour are not specific to Ireland[47] or to this period in history.[48] Careful study of the archives of the Central Criminal Lunatic Asylum[49] indicate significant engagement by the courts and forensic psychiatric services with individuals with apparent intellectual disability who engaged in offending behaviour throughout the late 1800s and early 1900s.[50]

The history of institutional care for individuals with intellectual disability is both under researched and troubling.[51] The history of care for individuals with both intellectual disability and mental disorder is particularly difficult to research, owing to myriad factors including the persistent social and historical marginalisation of this group, as well as changes in diagnostic and clinical practices over time. In particular, there was a tendency to classify individuals as either intellectually disabled and/or mentally ill, and to minimise or ignore the co-existence of both conditions in the same individuals.[52] Recent epidemiological work suggests that between 10 per cent and 39 per cent of individuals with intellectual disability also fulfil diagnostic criteria for mental disorder.[53]

The next cases to be explored in this book were selected to demonstrate the challenges faced and presented by individuals who were considered intellectually disabled and mentally ill, and admitted to inpatient forensic psychiatric care in the late 1800s and early 1900s. This subgroup was chosen owing to both the enduring challenges presented by offending behaviour in the context of intellectual disability and mental disorder,[54] and the paucity of literature on individuals admitted to forensic care in Ireland during this period.[55] A majority of cases presented are women, owing, in part, to evidence that the experience of women in Ireland's asylums differed significantly from that of men, highlighting the importance of a gendered dimension in the historical study of institutional mental health care.[56]

Patrick: 'No Improvement in Mental Power is Possible'

In the early 1890s, Patrick, a 35-year-old 'messenger' from the south of Ireland was committed to the Central Criminal Lunatic Asylum having been charged with assault and declared 'insane on arraignment'. Patrick was detained 'at the Lord Lieutenant's pleasure'.

Admission notes record a diagnosis of 'congenital imbecile' and note that Patrick's 'expression of face is characteristic, especially while laughing. His gait is slouching; [he] manages his legs badly ... He has slight nystagmus. Teeth are decayed, irregular and somewhat crowded together. The hard palate is much arched. His speech is indistinct, halting and stammering, and becomes much worse if patient is excited'. Patrick was 'quick-tempered, pettish and requires to be humoured. His memory is bad'. Patrick's 'appetite is large' and he was 'subject to attacks of vomiting after meals due to over-eating'.

Four days after admission, it was apparent that Patrick was adjusting quickly to institutional life and was 'much improved. His expression of face is brighter and more intelligent-looking. [He] is a very good house-cleaner'. Eight months after admission, Patrick was 'much brighter and tidier, and is useful and trustworthy. He presents the usual physical characteristics of imbecility and no improvement in mental power is possible'.

Three years after admission, Patrick was 'very quiet and well conducted' and 'very childish in his ways'. He 'takes part in the cricket and has a very exaggerated opinion of himself on that subject'. Four years after admission, Patrick was 'well behaved ... ready to "laugh at nothing" [and] is perfectly happy'. Eight years after admission, he was taking part 'in all amusements, cricket, football, etc. and enjoys life well'.

During his fourteenth year at the Central Criminal Lunatic Asylum, Patrick reported sick one morning and was diagnosed with 'pneumonia of the right lung'. Patrick's temperature was 102° Fahrenheit (39° Celsius; raised) and pulse was raised at 100 beats per minute. Patrick was initially treated with a combination of milk, beef tea, eggs, digitalis and blisters. Three days later, however, he was 'weaker and has been ordered port wine'. At this stage, Patrick was treated with 'strychnine, digitalis and morphia hypodermically'. His condition continued to decline and six days later Patrick died, at the age of 49 years, having spent his final fourteen years in the Central Criminal Lunatic Asylum. Three days later, an inquest concluded that Patrick had 'died from pneumonia'.

Patrick's case history illustrates many of the characteristic features of life in Ireland's psychiatric institutions in the late nineteenth and early twentieth centuries. There was, for example, a strong emphasis on gainful occupation (Patrick was 'a very good house-cleaner'), consistent with the principles of moral management which had such a decisive effect on institutional thought and practice throughout the nineteenth century.[57] Patrick was also involved in sport ('cricket, football, etc.') consistent with the key role sport played in asylum life in England and Ireland during this period.[58]

Clinical notes suggest that Patrick developed a fatal respiratory infection during his fourteenth year of detention. Physical illness, especially infective illness such as tuberculosis and dysentery, presented substantial problems in all Irish asylums at this time. Most asylums were substantially overcrowded[59] and the Central Criminal Lunatic Asylum was no exception.[60] Tuberculosis was a particularly persistent problem in these overcrowded, unsanitary, poorly ventilated institutions and by 1901 tuberculosis accounted for over 25 per cent of deaths in Irish asylums.[61]

These problems were compounded by the absence of effective treatments for most physical illnesses, including infective illnesses such as Patrick's 'pneumonia'. Over the course of his brief illness, Patrick was treated with 'digitalis and blisters' and, as his condition deteriorated, he also received 'strychnine, digitalis and morphia hypodermically'. Throughout the nineteenth century, blisters, strychnine, digitalis and morphine were all used for the treatment of a wide range of medical conditions: indications for strychnine included 'shock', poor muscle tone, reduced appetite and weak bladder;[62] indications for digitalis included 'shock', 'weak heart' and irregular heartbeat;[63] and indications for morphine included diarrhoea, cough, asthma, pain, gallstones, kidney colic and any condition requiring general anaesthesia.[64] The combination of all of these treatments may well, however, have contributed to Patrick's decline.

Eileen: 'Mentally Deficient Since Birth'

In 1917, Eileen, a 41-year-old single charwoman (cleaner) from Dublin, was charged with attempted murder and, owing to her mental state, detained at 'the Lord Lieutenant's Pleasure' in the Central Criminal Lunatic Asylum.

Admission notes describe Eileen as a:

thin delicate looking woman with a decidedly weak stamp of countenance. She strikes one as being mentally deficient since birth and seems
unable to realize the serious nature of her offence. While her sister was
suffering from an epileptic fit she attempted to kill her by cutting her
throat. Patient tells me she wanted to kill her sister while she was unconscious as she was very troublesome and unable to work.

Eileen settled in well and was soon 'working regularly in the laundry; is neat,
tidy and industrious; has given no trouble. Sleeps and takes her food well'.
Some weeks later, medical notes confirm the initial clinical impression of
Eileen as 'weak-minded and neurotic with delusions and hallucinations'.

Six months after admission, medical notes report that Eileen 'refused to
work for the past ten days. She says her back is strained and tortured at night
by both men and women in the asylum. [She is] a weak-minded patient
with delusions of persecution'. In the following months, Eileen worked
intermittently in the laundry but eighteen months after admission, she
was 'listless and apathetic; takes little interest in anything; does some sewing
occasionally; bodily health only poor'.

Two years after admission, Eileen remained 'weak-minded and extremely
neurotic' and medical notes indicate that 'her mental condition has deteriorated since admission; has done no work for the past twelve months; bodily
health only poor'. After almost three years, Eileen was 'transferred to the
Richmond Asylum' and there is no further record available of her course
of outcome.

Patricia: 'Weak-minded from Birth'

In 1926, Patricia, a 45-year-old woman from the south of Ireland, was
charged with murder and, owing to her mental state, detained at the
'Governor General's Pleasure'. After five weeks in prison, she was transferred
to the Central Criminal Lunatic Asylum.

Medical notes record that:

[Patricia] formerly lived with her brother who is a farmer … She threw
his child aged nine months into a pond and drowned it. She lacks intelligence and has evidently been weak-minded from birth. She is practically
devoid of reason, speaks with difficulty and is incapable of conversing
intelligently. She has given little trouble. She sits in the same pose all day
and stares vacantly. She is indifferent to her surroundings and is unable to

work. Her appetite is good and she is of clean habits. Her bodily health is fair but she is very lame and walks with great difficulty.

Seven months later, Patricia had 'given no trouble since admission and although she seems oblivious to everything, she possesses more intelligence than one would suspect'. Nonetheless, after five years in the hospital, she was generally agreed to be 'incapable of coherent conversation or concentrated effort'.

At around this time, Patricia became 'one of the noisiest patients in the institution. She hammers on the door and shutters of her cell, whistles and in general creates as much noise as she can. Her reason for this tirade is that she is dead and wishes to get out of her coffin ... She requires large doses of paraldehyde ... ordinary hypnotics are useless ...' Despite these disturbances, Patricia continued 'to work daily in the laundry and is in good bodily health'.

These disturbances continued intermittently throughout the remainder of Patricia's time at the Central Criminal Lunatic Asylum. Some fifteen years after admission, she was still 'extremely noisy and abusive during the night' and occasionally 'became very troublesome at dinner in the dayroom. Had to be secluded but this condition passed off in a few days.'

Twenty-five years after admission, Patricia developed epilepsy and records from the following year record that she was not 'at all well during the winter and has spent a while in bed; a bad attack of influenza and bronchitis left her very much deteriorated'. Her mental state was, however, generally unchanged. Hospital records suggest that Patricia remained at the hospital for several more years, but there is no record of her further clinical course or outcome.

Anne: A 'Woman of Low Intelligence'

In 1926, Anne, a 40-year-old 'farm-worker' was convicted of murder in Dublin and sentenced to life imprisonment. After some weeks in prison, Anne was transferred to the Central Criminal Lunatic Asylum, owing to concerns about her mental state.

Anne was a widow with four children, and admission notes describe her as 'a delicate looking woman of low intelligence and she strikes one as being mentally deficient from birth. She had been a widow for several years and lived with her family on her late husband's farm ... She suffocated her illegitimate child on the roadside and then brought it home and buried it.'

Anne's physical health was poor, and six weeks after admission she was 'extremely delicate. She is slowly recovering from a severe cardiac attack complicated by bronchitis. She is taking nourishment fairly well.' Anne remained unwell and deeply distressed throughout the following months: she was 'restless, irritable and very depressed; is constantly in tears and imploring to be sent home; bodily health only poor'.

Eleven months after admission, there had 'been no improvement in this patient. Many efforts have been made to induce her to work in the laundry. She has made several attempts to injure herself and declares that she will "do for herself" on the first opportunity'. Two months later, 'this patient made a determined effort to commit suicide by swallowing a quantity of Jey's Fluid [cleaning detergent]; for several days her condition was precarious but she is now out of danger'. Following this incident, Anne remained 'under continuous supervision' and was described as 'cunning and plausible and is constantly complaining about ill-treatment. She is irritable and emotional and can readily turn to laughter or dissolve into tears.'

Four years after admission, medical notes record that Anne 'attributes her misfortune to her family and neighbours; in fact, to everything and everybody except herself. She is plausible and scheming and requires the closest supervision.' Overall, there was 'little change in this patient'. She was 'always under strict supervision. She is most unhappy and discontented here and frets incessantly because she has not been sent back to her family.' Almost five years after admission, Anne was 'conditionally discharged to-day in care of her son'.

Maura: 'Undoubtedly of Low Mental Capacity'

In 1930, Maura, an unmarried 21-year-old 'servant' from the west of Ireland, was charged with the murder of an infant and 'concealment of birth'. She was detained at the 'Governor General's Pleasure' at the Central Criminal Lunatic Asylum.

Hospital notes record that Maura was:

sent here for the murder of her illegitimate infant and endeavouring to conceal its birth. She is a young delicate looking girl about twenty years old and strikes one as always being weak-minded. Since admission she has hardly uttered a word and either refuses to or is incapable of giving any information about herself. She has been put to work in the laundry and is neat and clean in her habits. Her bodily health is fair.

During her first year, Maura was 'employed daily in the laundry. Her mental condition shows a marked improvement since admission. She answers intelligently when spoken to but is unwilling to converse and is undoubtedly of low mental capacity. She tells me that she killed the baby by choking it. Her bodily health is good.'

Three years after admission Maura was still described as:

> clean, neat and industrious in [the] laundry, but seems somewhat dull-minded or sullen – gives no trouble but said to be obstinate and surly if crossed in anyway. Her rather slow appearance may be due more to the fact of her upbringing being in a very wild and backward district with no schooling or social conditions than to any actual mental deficiency; she seems to have developed fairly well since admission and is probably more intelligent than she appears at first sight. She is said to have known only a little English when coming here, speaking mostly Gaelic.

Notes from 1939 indicate that Maura had remained 'in excellent health' over the nine years since admission, but was 'reported to be suffering from amenorrhoea [i.e. her menstrual periods had stopped] for the past four months. She is looking very well and works every day in the laundry.' The next note, written some months later, provides the only remaining hint about the cause of Maura's amenorrhoea: 'She is very quiet, well behaved and industrious. Works daily in ward making sacks and stockings. Has given no trouble since last year when the cause of her amenorrhea, noted above, became known! She is in very good bodily health.'

Some eleven years after admission Maura was 'most industrious during the year, manufacturing the socks of the institution'. She was 'the best patient in the house ... Takes a keen interest in all activities and well informed on current affairs.' In 1944 she developed a 'slightly puffy appearance but no evidence of hepatitis or albuminuria could be found'. An underactive thyroid gland was suspected but never diagnosed. In the last recorded medical note, Maura was in good health and had gained some liberty from the institutional routine (e.g. taking trips to town for tea).

Helen: 'Mentally Slightly Defective'

In 1930, Helen, a 30-year-old single 'servant', was charged with murder and detained at the 'Governor General's Pleasure' in the Central Criminal

Lunatic Asylum. Admission notes describe Helen as:

> a respectable looking young woman of the farming class. Helen was employed as a domestic servant with the same family for the past two years. She was seduced by a farmer … [She] then went to her married sister who … turned her out and she returned to her mother … with her twin children. Her family was unaware of what had happened. She strangled both babies beside her home and buried them in a neighbouring field. She appears to feel her position acutely and has wept almost continuously since admission.

One month after admission, Helen was 'working daily in the laundry and is neat, tidy and most industrious. Although she exhibits no symptoms of insanity and converses intelligently, I consider her mentally slightly defective.' Two months after admission Helen was 'suffering from intense iritis in both eyes for the past month. She has been seen by Dr Maxwell and is now steadily improving. There is a history of a similar attack about ten years. Her family history is bad, two sisters having died of consumption [tuberculosis] before thirty.'

Helen's health improved and she was soon back 'working in the laundry. She is cheerful, good humoured and converses intelligently but she has probably been always mentally slightly defective.' She remained 'most industrious, neat and tidy; although slightly weak-minded, she is quite intelligent to converse with and has exhibited no symptoms of insanity since admission. Her bodily health is good.' Less than three years after admission, Helen was 'discharged … to care of nuns' in a named convent.

DIAGNOSIS AND CLINICAL MANAGEMENT OF INTELLECTUAL DISABILITY

These six cases (Patrick, Eileen, Patricia, Anne, Maura and Helen) were selected for presentation here because their clinical records contained possible evidence of intellectual disability; i.e. terms such as 'weak-minded', 'devoid of reason', etc. Their clinical records are, however, extremely varied in content and structure, and demonstrate many of the diagnostic and interpretive challenges presented by the study of clinical records from this period.

In all cases, there are difficulties establishing the extent of intellectual disability, if any, that these individuals actually experienced. Clinical notes provide varying levels of detail for each case and terminology is both vague and inconsistent; e.g. Eileen is described as 'mentally deficient since birth' while Patricia was 'weak-minded from birth ... practically devoid of reason'. There was particular uncertainty regarding Patricia, who was initially 'incapable of conversing intelligently'; later thought to possess 'more intelligence than one would suspect'; and subsequently 'incapable of coherent conversation or concentrated effort'. It is conceivable that an episodic psychotic mental disorder or some other relapsing and remitting disorder could account for some or all of these varying clinical descriptions.

In the case of Anne, the clinical impression of intellectual disability is explicitly subjective ('she strikes one as being mentally deficient from birth') and confined to the admission notes, with no further reference to it during the subsequent five years. Clinical information regarding Maura is similarly difficult to interpret: she 'hardly uttered a word' in the days after her admission and 'either refuses or is incapable of giving any information about herself'. Maura's unwillingness to converse was taken to indicate 'low mental capacity' but is also consistent with several other possible diagnoses (e.g. stupor or organic catatonia, which may have been a relatively common feature of post-partum illness at that time). There are similar diagnostic difficulties in relation to Helen, as clinical impressions are explicitly subjective ('I consider her mentally slightly defective') and she was discharged less than three years after admission, to the care of a convent.

In the context of these diagnostic uncertainties, it is useful to note the conceptual framework outlined in the Mental Deficiency Act of 1913. Although this legislation never applied in Ireland, in England it articulated four classes of 'mental deficiency': (1) 'idiot' (unable to protect oneself from common dangers); (2) 'imbecile' (unable to take care of oneself); (3) 'feeble-minded' (requires care to protect oneself); and (4) 'moral defectives' (a broad category, which could include criminals).[65] The cases presented here were selected on the basis of their clinical records which contained some suggestions of possible intellectual disability, although it is notable that none of these individuals were actually described as 'idiots'. In addition, terms such as 'weak-minded' were relatively common in medical records at that time and is likely that some or all of these women would not be classified as 'intellectually disabled' today.

It is noteworthy that three out of these five women discussed here had concealed the births of, and then killed, their illegitimate children. In terms of diagnosis, their post-partum condition makes the clinical picture especially complicated.[66] Diagnostic analysis is rendered even more challenging again owing to the probable role of social circumstances in the presentations of these women to judicial and psychiatric services: the birth of an illegitimate child was deeply contrary to prevailing social mores in the nineteenth and early twentieth centuries in Ireland and often led to distressing, conflictual predicaments for women.[67] Conley, for example, cites the case of one mother who refused to nurse her illegitimate infant, preferring to place the child in a workhouse instead.[68] It is likely that these prevailing social values played a significant role in shaping the context for the judicial, diagnostic and institutional experiences of these five women. It is possible, for example, that subjective labels such as 'weak-minded' or 'defective' may have been more readily applied to women who had given birth outside of marriage compared to women who had not done so; this issue merits closer study in future historical studies of diagnostic and judicial practices during this period.

Medical records clearly illustrate that the man and women whose cases are presented here experienced significant difficulties during the periods they spent at the Central Criminal Lunatic Asylum. These included problems with adjustment to the asylum environment, ongoing symptoms of mental disorder and signs of poor physical health. These were also the central challenges faced by managers of general asylums throughout Ireland during the late nineteenth and early twentieth centuries. Not least amongst these challenges was the spread of tuberculosis throughout the entire asylum system. Helen for example, experienced an apparently innocent attack of 'iritis' but medical notes recorded that her 'family history is bad, two sisters having died of consumption [tuberculosis] before thirty'.

'Consumption' refers to pulmonary tuberculosis which had become a common cause of death in both the general population[69] and asylums by the end of the nineteenth century.[70] The spread of tuberculosis throughout crowded, unsanitary institutions was, however, just one of the myriad problems created by the mass institutionalisation of the mentally ill and intellectually disabled throughout the nineteenth and early twentieth centuries in Ireland. The broader challenges presented by mass institutionalisation of the intellectually disabled in nineteenth- and early twentieth-century Ireland are considered next.

INSTITUTIONALISATION OF THE INTELLECTUALLY DISABLED IN NINETEENTH- AND EARLY TWENTIETH-CENTURY IRELAND

There is strong evidence that individuals with intellectual disability formed a significant proportion of the ever-increasing numbers of individuals committed to Irish asylums during the nineteenth and early twentieth centuries.[71] There was substantial professional and governmental concern about rates of institutionalisation during this period, underpinned by a widespread belief that rates of mental disorder were increasing rapidly in the Irish population.[72] Despite this concern about diagnostic issues, there was a strong tendency to ignore the co-existence of intellectual disability and mental disorder in the same individuals.[73] While there was some limited professional recognition of the occurrence of mental disorder in individuals with intellectual disability,[74] official statistics tended to regard the two conditions as diagnostically exclusive, consistent with the framework later outlined in the Mental Deficiency Act of 1913.[75]

Notwithstanding these complexities, governmental concern eventually focused on the fact that individuals with intellectual disability were increasingly being housed in the extensive network of asylums that had been built to meet the needs of the mentally ill – especially the destitute mentally ill – throughout the 1800s.[76] There was already evidence of this trend in the United Kingdom[77] and official data finally confirmed the same trend in Ireland by demonstrating that the number of individuals with intellectual disability in Irish asylums increased from 202 in 1851, to 1,896 in 1881.[78] Some of this extra pressure on the asylum system may have been related to adverse social conditions experienced by the mentally ill and intellectually disabled during and after the Great Irish Famine (1845–52).[79] In the case of the Central Criminal Lunatic Asylum, it is likely that overcrowding also resulted, at least in part, from the increased numbers of 'guilty but insane' verdicts in Irish courts towards the end of the nineteenth century.[80]

As a result of this mass institutionalisation, medical notes pay considerable attention to traditional institutional values (industriousness, neatness, etc.) amongst long-stay patients, especially the intellectually disabled. At the Central Criminal Lunatic Asylum, Helen was recorded as 'working daily in the laundry' and was 'neat, tidy and most industrious'. Maura was noted to have been 'most industrious during the year, manufacturing the socks of the institution'. There is also evidence of a limited reward system at the hospital, with Maura described as the 'best patient in the house' and taken by staff on a trip to Dublin city centre for tea. In general, however, women admitted to the Central Criminal Lunatic Asylum, especially following infanticide and child murder, tended to remain there for lengthy, indefinite periods, with only approximately 6 per cent serving finite sentence.[81] Their ultimate clinical and social outcomes are not recorded in many cases (e.g. Patricia and Maura).

Overall, these cases highlight the myriad clinical and institutional challenges presented by individuals with intellectual disability and mental disorder at the Central Criminal Lunatic Asylum in the late 1800s and early 1900s. In all of these cases, there was significant difficulty establishing the diagnosis and/or extent of intellectual disability, owing chiefly to the use of suggestive but subjective phraseology (e.g. 'weak-minded') throughout the clinical records. These linguistic issues are compounded by the more general diagnostic difficulties presented by the historical study of clinical materials, dating from a time when clinical record-keeping was both quantitatively and qualitatively different to that of the present era.

Notwithstanding these diagnostic difficulties, the medical records of these individuals demonstrate that they experienced significant difficulties with adjustment to the institutional environment of the Central Criminal Lunatic Asylum and then had ongoing problems with physical and mental health during their time there. These problems were not, of course, unique to this group of patients[82] and many of these issues still present substantial challenges to care providers today,[83] especially in relation to risk assessment[84] and provision of ongoing care.[85] The individuals described here, however, also experienced particular social stresses including, for example, the stigma of giving birth outside of marriage.

Against this background, it is clear that individuals with intellectual disability in the asylums presented a particular set of challenges to physicians and asylum managers. In 1907, for example, Norman reported to the Richmond District Asylum Joint Committee that there was 'in the Asylum about 200 idiots, and this is probably an underestimate. There are stated to be in the workhouses, 143. In the whole island there are said to be between five and six thousand idiots'.[86] Norman noted that 'an ordinary asylum is not a suitable place for them in any way' and recommended that 'an institution specially equipped for teaching the teachable and improving the improvable is essential ... It is neither wise nor humane to neglect this class as they are neglected in this country'.

Notwithstanding Norman's interest and concern, there is a remarkable dearth of information about the experiences of individuals with intellectual disability who were committed to Irish psychiatric institutions throughout the nineteenth century. It is likely that their institutional experiences were similar, in at least some respects, to those of individuals without intellectual learning disability. Both groups were similarly institutionalised and tended to experience lengthy periods of detention in poorly therapeutic facilities, poor mental and physical health, and a high risk of dying in the asylum.[87]

It is also likely that the institutional experiences of individuals with intellectual disability in Ireland were similar to those of individuals with intellectual disability in other jurisdictions during this period.[88] In the United Kingdom, for example, the late 1800s saw the management of individuals with intellectual disability move out of the private, family sphere and into the public, social sphere, thus becoming a 'social problem' and necessitating the development of institutional provisions.[89] The late 1800s also saw the emergence of the principle of segregation of the intellectually disabled from the rest of society and, in particular, permanent segregation, deemed to be in the best interests of both the individual and society.[90] These public and professional attitudes resulted in widespread institutionalisation of the intellectual disabled in England throughout the 1800s.[91] While there is a strong need for further research in both England and Ireland, it seems highly likely that individuals with intellectual disability who engaged in offending behaviour presented similar kinds of challenges to medical and judicial services in both jurisdictions. These were most likely problems with judicial and diagnostic procedures, lengthy durations of detention, and difficulties with community provision of appropriate discharge facilities.

Today, over a century later, many of these challenges remain highly relevant, urgent and important. It is in this context that the Irish College of Psychiatrists re-emphasised the need for dedicated service provision for this group and recommended that Ireland's Health Service Executive should 'make the development of a national forensic learning disability service a strategic priority'.[92] The proposals of the Irish College of Psychiatrists, along with the recommendations in A Vision for Change,[93] provide a set of clear, reasonable and achievable measures that would greatly improve the medical and judicial experiences of individuals with intellectual disability who offend. Although the identification of these measures has come too late for Patrick and thousands of unknown others, the implementation of these measures in a timely fashion today would undoubtedly transform the lives of thousands more in the decades to come.

SYPHILIS

The protean clinical syndromes associated with syphilis (an infection generally acquired through sexual contact) have lengthy, complex histories in medicine and psychiatry.[94] In the nineteenth century, syphilis and neuro-syphilis (which affects the brain) presented substantial challenges to medical and psychiatric services in Ireland and many other countries.

At the Sainte-Anne Asylum in Paris, for example, 'general paralysis of the insane' (a form of neurosyphilis) accounted for 30.5 per cent of voluntary and 17.4 per cent of involuntary male admissions between 1876 and 1914.[95] In Germany, syphilis-related disorders were similarly problematic and later formed one of the three categories in the Würzburger Schlüssel classification of psychological disorders (1930). The other two categories were alcohol-related disorders and the psychopathies (i.e. personality disorders).[96]

In Ireland, too, venereal (or sexually transmitted) diseases represented a significant public health problem throughout the eighteenth and nine-teenth centuries. In Dublin, Dr Steevens Hospital was opened in 1733 and treated patients with veneral disease with mercurial and arsenical compounds.[97] Several other hospitals dedicated to the treatment of veneral diseases were later established, including one at Rainsfort Street, Dublin (1755) and a private facility at King Street, Dublin (1758). 'Lock Hospitals' were also established in Limerick and Cork, although the former was closed in 1849.

Syphilis also presented challenges to the Irish asylum system, although the extent of the problem is unclear. The first systematic study of the psychi-atric implications of syphilis in nineteenth-century Ireland was performed by Hallaran in Cork,[98] and published in the second edition of his celebrated textbook, *Practical Observations on the Causes and Cures of Insanity*.[99] Hallaran attempted to identify the causes of insanity in 1,431 individuals admitted to Cork Lunatic Asylum between 1798 and 1818. Of the 351 in whom he identified a 'cause', however, only 13 (3.7 per cent) were categorised as having venereal disease.

While it is possible that Hallaran unwittingly placed individuals with neurosyphilis in other diagnostic categories (e.g. 'religious zeal', 'fever', 'heredity'), these data are consistent with the suggestion that syphilis, while problematic, was possibly not as prevalent in Irish asylums as it was in other jurisdictions (e.g. England, France). This impression is supported by mortality data from 1905, which shows that general paralysis of the insane accounted for 26.4 per cent of male and 7 per cent of female public asylum deaths in England, but only 5.3 per cent of male and 1.1 per cent of female public asylum deaths in Ireland.[100]

Notwithstanding the apparently low incidence of neurosyphilis in Ireland, individuals with neurosyphilis who were admitted to asylums in Ireland and elsewhere often presented significant challenges to asylum physicians and managers.[101] As the below studies show, examination of archival case records provides clear demonstrations of the clinical course (Richard) and diagnostic challenges (John) associated with neurosyphilis[102] in the Central Criminal Lunatic Asylum in the late 1800s and early 1900s.[103]

Richard: 'General Paralysis of the Insane' with 'Exalted Delusions'

Richard was a 34-year-old baker who was charged with 'felonious entry' but declared 'insane on arraignment' in the mid-1890s. Richard was sentenced to be detained in the Central Criminal Lunatic Asylum in Dundrum 'at the Lord Lieutenant's pleasure'. On admission, Richard was diagnosed with 'general paralysis of the insane' (i.e. neurosyphilis) with 'exalted delusions about doings in the army' and 'the campaigns he has been through with Lord Wolseley'. (The Field Marshal Garnet Joseph Wolseley (1833–1913) was a celebrated British Army officer who served in Burma, the Crimea, India, China, Canada and Africa.)

According to medical notes, Richard displayed 'loss of attention [and] impairment of memory'. He had 'an expression of apathy, melancholy and lack of ideas'. Richard's 'skin [was] muddy and greasy; nose spread out, flattened; putty faced'. His 'pupils [were] unequal' and 'eyes wide open' in a 'vacant stare'. There was 'twitching of the muscles of face, especially during speech', which was 'slow' with Richard 'searching for words, incoherent, stuttering'. His tongue was 'large, pale, flabby [and had] tremor on protrusion'. Richard was 'awkward with the use of his hands' and his gait was 'awkward and uncertain'. He had 'heart palpitation' and his 'reflexes

[were] exaggerated'. Richard also had 'seizures at night, epileptiform in character'. After such seizures, Richard was 'dull and stupid in the morning'. Throughout this time, Richard also had 'hallucinations and delusions' which persisted with varying levels of intensity.

One year after admission, Richard's 'general paralysis' had 'run a normal course. He is now feeble and paralytic, dirty in habits, demented, and is unable to swallow any food that is not minced and moist. He cannot live more than a few months.' Soon, Richard had to be 'fed, washed and dressed' and was in a 'very feeble state'. Five months later, Richard had a severe 'apoplectic seizure' with the 'muscles of left side of face and left upper extremity twitching and rigid at times'. His 'pupils were irregular and reacting badly to light' (i.e. the pupils of his eyes did not constrict as they should when light was shone upon them). Patellar reflexes were 'exaggerated on left side and absent on right'. Soon, Richard was confined to bed, 'unconscious [and] breathing heavily'. Early the following morning, Richard died, at the age of 35 years, less than two years after admission to the Central Criminal Lunatic Asylum.

Diagnosing Syphilis in the Nineteenth Century

Richard was diagnosed with 'general paralysis of the insane' which is a form of neurosyphilis. Syphilis results from infection with *Treponema pallidum*, a spiro-chete (infection) that can be acquired transplacentally (i.e. in the womb) or, most commonly, through close sexual contact. Congenital syphilis is associ-ated with stillbirth, failure to thrive and nasal infections. The later stages are associated with abnormalities of long bones, sabre tibia (malformation of the tibia bone in the lower leg), Hutchinson's teeth (small, widely spaced teeth with notches on biting surfaces), inflammation in the eye, skin lesions and nervous system abnormalities.[104]

'General paralysis of the insane' is a form of acquired neurosyphilis char-acterised by progressive dementia, tremor, altered nerve function, abnormal function of the pupils in the eye (Argyll Robertson pupils) and, in some cases, seizures.[105] Neurospyhilis is also associated with a range of psychiatric symptoms including personality change, impaired judgement, delusions of grandeur (10 per cent–20 per cent), decreased self-care and dementia.[106] Clinically, the later stages of acquired syphilis can have many features in common with late manifestations of congenital syphilis[107] although patients with late-stage neurosyphilis have a notably high mortality rate and many die within three years of diagnosis.[108]

In Richard's case, the diagnosis of 'general paralysis of the insane' was based on both psychiatric symptoms (e.g. delusions, hallucinations) and neurological symptoms (e.g. impairment of memory, unequal pupils, involuntary movements, seizures). Other possible diagnoses in Richard's case might include motor neuron disease, cerebrovascular disease or other forms of dementia. From the perspective of the nineteenth-century physician, however, the clinical features were consistent with, and highly suggestive of, general paralysis of the insane or neurosyphilis.

At the time of Richard's admission to the Central Criminal Lunatic Asylum, the diagnosis of neurosyphilis was based solely on symptoms: the complement-fixation test for syphilis by August Paul von Wasserman (a German bacteriologist, 1866–1925) was not developed until 1906. While medical notes reflect confidence in the diagnosis, that it was entirely reliant on the interpretation of clinical signs and symptoms made it a more difficult task in some other, more complicated cases. Some of these diagnostic challenges are illustrated by the case of John.

John: 'General Paralysis of the Insane' or Simply 'A Scrofulous Diathesis'?

John was a 38-year-old gamekeeper charged with 'attempting to upset trains' and sentenced to seven years in prison in the mid-1890s. After six months in prison, John was transferred to the Central Criminal Lunatic Asylum with a diagnosis of 'general paralysis of the insane'. On admission he was described as 'intemperate', 'weak-minded' and 'scrofulous', which refers to a form of tuberculosis affecting the lymph nodes (a bodily drainage system), most characteristically in the neck.

Medical notes record that John was 'well-conducted [and] is employed working on the farm. His speech is thick; has tongue tremors; reflexes are exaggerated; pupils irregular and dilated; [and he] is of a scrofulous diathesis.' Eight months after admission, the medical officer noted that John presented only 'some of the lesser diagnostic signs of general paralysis of the insane. Mentally is facile and demented. On the whole I should be inclined to think that the diagnosis is doubtful.'

Two years after admission, John was 'weak-minded and demented' but in 'robust bodily health'. He was a 'good worker' and 'the diagnosis made on admission of GPI was undoubtedly a mistake. He suffers from dementia.' Six years after admission, John was 'in good bodily health' and 'plays cricket'.

The following year, he was transferred to his local district asylum and there is no further record of his clinical outcome, although it is likely he spent many years in the district asylum and may well have died there.[109]

Syphilis in the Nineteenth Century and Beyond

In John's case, there were some features suggestive of syphilis in the form of general paralysis of the insane (e.g. 'tongue tremors', 'reflexes … exaggerated', 'pupils irregular and dilated') but medical notes place greater emphases on the diagnosis of 'dementia' and the observation that John was 'of a scrofulous diathesis' (tuberculosis). In the nineteenth century, the term 'dementia' was used to describe any severe, chronic or recurrent mental disorder; contemporary diagnostic equivalents include bipolar affective disorder and schizophrenia, especially chronic schizophrenia.[110] The observation that John was 'of a scrofulous diatheses' raised the possibility of tuberculosis, which was a substantial problem in both the general[111] and asylum populations at this time.[112]

Syphilis, however, also presented substantial challenges to physicians and psychiatrists throughout the nineteenth century, not only owing to its myriad clinical forms but also the absence of effective treatments. Mercury was commonly used and it was believed that the efficacy of mercury treatment depended on the amount of salivation it stimulated.[113] In addition, the administration of mercury was often preceded by purgation and bloodletting, resulting in a treatment that would present a considerable challenge to the constitution of a healthy individual, let alone an individual with advanced syphilis.[114] Later in the nineteenth century, potassium iodide replaced mercury as the treatment of choice. Although there is no record of either treatment being used for Richard or John, medical records for other patients indicate that these treatments were used in the Central Criminal Lunatic Asylum during the nineteenth century. However, there is no systematic record of their effectiveness.[115]

Notwithstanding the absence of effective treatments – or, perhaps, because of it – syphilis began to feature strongly in the Irish literary world throughout the eighteenth, nineteenth and twentieth centuries. There were, for example, suggestions that Jonathan Swift (1667–1745), author and founder of St Patrick's Hospital in Dublin,[116] may have been afflicted with a form of syphilis,[117] although Menière's disease (a disorder of the inner ear) now appears equally likely.[118] There was also considerable speculation about whether or not James Joyce (1882–1941), author of *Ulysses*, might have had syphilis.[119] He makes a powerful reference to the disease in the opening pages of *Ulysses*, and there is symbolic use of syphilis in 'The Sisters', the opening story in *Dubliners*.[120]

Notwithstanding professional concern, governmental alarm and burgeoning literary interest, the clinical course of neurosyphilis in nineteenth-century Ireland was generally one of progressive deterioration, often resulting in death (as in the case of Richard). This was also the case in other countries: while men with 'general paralysis of the insane' accounted for 30.5 per cent of voluntary and 17.4 per cent of involuntary male admissions to the Sainte-Anne Asylum in Paris between 1876 and 1914, they accounted for only 18.2 per cent of voluntary and 14.3 per cent of involuntary patient discharges.[121]

Today, over a century later, syphilis continues to present significant diagnostic and therapeutic challenges. Despite considerable advances in techniques, definitive diagnosis can still be challenging, especially in individuals with suspected neurosyphilis.[122] Treatment can also prove difficult, especially in relation to clinical follow up, monitoring and co-ordination of national guidelines between countries.[123] Whilst antibiotics have assisted greatly with treatment of syphilis (and prevention of progression to tertiary syphilis), there are now reports of both treatment failures and genetic mutation of the infection resulting in antibiotic resistance.[124]

Additionally, there is growing epidemiological concern about recent increases in the incidence of infectious syphilis in many countries, including England[125] and, between 2001 and 2003, Ireland.[126] At a global level, these increases have drawn attention to the substantial illness burden attributable to sexually transmitted diseases in general, in both developed and developing countries.[127] Increased attention has also been devoted to the identification of risk factors for sexually transmitted diseases, with a view to targeting interventions.[128]

Increases in the rates of acquired syphilis also have implications in terms of congenital syphilis (i.e. acquired in the womb). In Alberta, Canada, an increase in acquired syphilis in 2000 was followed, two years later, by the first reported case of congenital syphilis in over ten years.[129] In the Russian Federation, reported cases of acquired syphilis increased twenty-six fold between 1991 and 1999.[130] If the compelling case history of Richard serves to highlight the devastating clinical effects of tertiary neurosyphilis, then these recent epidemiological reports of acquired and congenital syphilis highlight a compelling and complementary need for ongoing epidemiological and clinical vigilance. Careful, coordinated approaches are urgently required if syphilis is to become a truly rare disorder that is not allowed to progress to the advanced and often fatal stages so regrettably common in the asylums of nineteenth-century Ireland.

5

Reformation and Renewal:
Into the Twentieth Century

This book is primarily concerned with the fate of the mentally ill, especially the 'criminally insane', in nineteenth- and early twentieth-century Ireland . However, this chapter concludes the book by examining the process of reform of Ireland's mental health laws, practices and institutions, in the early to mid-twentieth century.[1] This reform movement found its first clear expression in the Mental Treatment Act 1945, which coincided with new enthusiasm for increasingly scientific approaches to the treatment of mental disorder in Ireland and elsewhere. These important and ongoing developments are considered next.

THE MENTAL TREATMENT ACT 1945

The Mental Treatment Act 1945 had a decisive influence on the provision and development of psychiatric services in Ireland throughout the twentieth century. The background to the legislation is complex and relates not only to the state of mental health services in early twentieth-century Ireland, but also the fraught political situation that pertained in Ireland at that time.[2]

The Political Context of the Mental Treatment Act 1945

The start of the twentieth century was a period of considerable political and social change in Ireland. During the first decade of the century, Sinn

Féin was established as a political party with the aim of achieving self-government in Ireland, and the Irish Socialist Republican Party began to advance reformist socialist analysis of Ireland's situation. In 1911 the British Government declared its intention to pass another Home Rule Bill, prompting renewed Unionist resistance in the north and the establishment of the Ulster Volunteers. In 1916 the Easter Rising took place in Dublin and the subsequent execution of its republican leaders generated increased sympathy for Ireland's Republican cause.

Following the victory of Sinn Féin in the 1918 election, Dáil Éireann (the Irish parliament) met in Dublin and declared Irish independence. This was followed by the War of Independence with Great Britain (1919–21), the Anglo-Irish Treaty (a negotiated compromise settlement) (1921) and Irish Civil War (1922–23).[3] In 1922, the Irish Free State came into being. The subsequent post-war reconstruction of Ireland's economy was an especially challenging task, owing not only to the effects of sustained conflict and the recession of the 1930s, but also the development of a 'trade war' with Britain in the 1930s. In 1937, a new constitution was passed by referendum, but it was not until 1949 that the Republic of Ireland came into being. The Republic comprised twenty-six counties in the 'South' of Ireland and excluded six counties in 'Northern' Ireland.

These political and economic developments, and especially the movement towards Home Rule, had a substantial influence on the development of medical and psychiatric services in Ireland throughout this period.[4] On the one hand, Irish politicians were generally wary of expanding services and increasing the financial challenges they would face in the event of self-government,[5] while on the other hand the English were hesitant about any trade off on Home Rule they might have to make in order to ensure Irish support for reform.[6] Notwithstanding these tensions, there were several significant changes in medical services during this period, including two major reviews of the Poor Law and medical relief system in Ireland, performed by the Viceregal Commission on Poor Law Reform (1906) and the Royal Commission on the Poor Laws and Relief of Distress (1910). The National Health Insurance Act was introduced in 1911, aiming to provide widespread health cover underwritten by the State, and a system of benefits to cover care in sanatoria (for tuberculosis, a particular problem).[7]

As in many other countries, the First World War presented considerable challenges to health services in Ireland, and government involvement in this sector continued to grow in the 1920s. The Dáil Department of Local Government was central to public service reforms during this period, and the passing of the Public Charitable Hospitals Act of 1930 permitted the establishment of the Hospitals Sweepstakes, enhancing financial support for voluntary hospitals.[8] The 1930s saw the development of an improved network of hospitals throughout Ireland, followed, in the 1940s, by renewed debate about the broader direction of Irish health services, a debate that was informed by both Catholic social teaching and Britain's movement towards a National Health Service. In 1945, the Report of the Departmental Committee on Health Services, submitted to the Minister for Local Government and Public Health, presented a series of radical proposals for the Irish Health Service. It suggested that Ireland should double its spending on health services and aim to provide a free national health service for all.[9] The same year also saw a landmark development in Irish mental health services with the Mental Treatment Act of 1945.

'INSANITY IN IRELAND' (1944)

In 1944, the year when the Mental Treatment Bill was presented to Dáil Éireann for its second reading, an anonymous psychiatrist wrote an article on 'Insanity in Ireland' in *The Bell*, a prominent Irish literary journal.[10] The author summarised the history of mental health care in Ireland, from the perspective of the 1940s:

> The history of insanity in this country does not differ from that in others. Its incidence was about the same; its causes were similar; the attitude of the public towards it was equally callous and the absence of any attempt at scientific treatment equally noticeable. In the early decades of the 19th century some differences became apparent. Neighbouring countries began to do something about it and their Governments took active steps in providing 'Asylums' for the mentally afflicted, but the Irish Government lagged behind and, even though many years have passed, that lag is still apparent.

There were, however, signs of change:

> First had to come the knowledge that insanity was not due to possession by evil spirits. It gradually oozed into the minds of the public that insanity

was a disease. So, in time, the gaoler with the whip was replaced by the doctor … Today the treatment of mental disease is in its infancy and it is no wild hope to say that the mental experts of 2000 ad will write of 'the crude, unscientific treatment of mental disease in 1943'. In the two decades before the outbreak of the present war, Ireland began to gain lost ground in hospitalization generally, and a great impetus to the provision of modern buildings was given by the Government in sponsoring and controlling the Irish Hospital Sweepstakes. Not alone were many suitable additions made to existing Mental Hospitals, but the general public became aware that something could be done towards the treatment of mental disease.

The anonymous psychiatrist went on to outline the principles of treatment in the early 1940s:

There are many types of mental disease and it is to be understood that each type has to be treated in its own way. Nevertheless there are certain principles which govern the treatment of all cases. These in the main are: removal from home and relatives; rest; adequate diet; sleep. These can be achieved only in an Institution with a trained staff, and the sooner these can be had the more likelihood of speedy recovery. Modern special methods of treatment have from time to time received a lot of publicity in both the medical and lay Press. So much so that almost everyone has heard of Insulin treatment and Convulsive or 'shock' treatment, either medical or electrical. One with experience of these different methods can safely say this: 'In selected cases one or other of these methods of treatment may give excellent results. They are not cure-alls, and if used indiscriminately will do harm by lessening the enthusiasm of the workers and by killing the faith of the relatives of patients on whom they have been tried.' Most early cases will, however, respond favourably to one or other modern method.

As the anonymous psychiatrist points out, Irish mental health care had undergone considerable changes in the century preceding the Mental Treatment Act of 1945. A brief, interesting overview of the evolution of early Irish mental health services was given to the Dáil on 29 November 1944, by Dr Ward, Parliamentary Secretary to the Minister for Local Government and Public Health, who presented the Mental Treatment Bill 1944 for its second reading:

It is stated that in medieval times lunatics were treated in monastic hospitals, but to what extent those hospitals dealt with the problem of lunacy it would now be impossible to say. Subsequent to the suppression of the monasteries, the earliest provision for the institutional accommodation of the insane took the form of cells in workhouses or houses of industry. The first of these were provided in the Dublin House of Industry about the year 1728. Cells had been provided in the year 1711 in the Royal Hospital, Kilmainham, for soldiers who were mentally deranged. During the course of the next century the authorities of houses of industry continued to provide cells or wards for the insane. In some few cases asylums were provided at the houses of industry. In connection with the Cork House of Industry, an asylum was erected in 1787 which subsequently became the Cork District Lunatic Asylum. In that year, also, a Prisons Act was passed containing a section which empowered grand juries to raise moneys for the support of wards for destitute insane persons in houses of industry. In 1815 there was established in Dublin an asylum which subsequently became the Richmond Asylum, and many of the insane persons in the house of industry were transferred to it.

Ward also outlined the legislative background to the new bill:

Acts were passed in the years 1817 and 1820 providing for the establishment of asylums for lunatics. These were superseded by the Lunacy (Ireland) Act, 1821, which provided for the formation of asylum districts and the establishment of district asylums. This Act formed the basis of the legal code under which lunatic asylums were established and maintained.

An Act passed in 1845 provided for the removal of all lunatics from the houses of industry to the lunatic asylums. Section 15 of that Act gave power for the establishment of an asylum for each of the provinces to be appropriated to any particular class or classes of lunatics. The object was to permit the establishment of asylums for chronic and harmless patients. Section 9 of the Lunatic Asylums (Ireland) Act, 1875, authorised the reception into workhouses of such chronic lunatics as were not dangerous and might be transferred thereto from lunatic asylums.

No advantage was taken of Section 15 of the Act of 1845. It was repealed by the Local Government (Ireland) Act, 1898, Section 76 of which gave power to asylum authorities to establish auxiliary asylums for the reception of chronic lunatics who, not being dangerous to themselves or others, were certified not to require special care and treatment in a fully equipped lunatic asylum. Where an auxiliary asylum was so provided Section 9 of the Act of 1875, relating to the accommodation of chronic lunatics in workhouses, ceased to apply. The Act of 1898 also imposed a duty on the county councils to provide and maintain sufficient accommodation for the lunatic poor.

The provision of psychiatric care to prisoners, offenders and the violent mentally ill presented particular cause for concern at this time:

> Towards the end of the eighteenth century a large number of violent lunatics and wandering idiots were committed to the county prisons, a separate portion of each prison being set apart for them. By direction of the Government of the day, given in the year 1816, admission to lunatic cells or wards in the Dublin House of Industry was restricted to such patients as were deemed incurable and had previously been received into the lunatic asylum. Although the Act of 1821, to which I have already referred, provided that all the lunatic poor within an asylum district were to be maintained and taken care of in the asylum for the district, the only provision it contained governing admission to those asylums was one providing for the admission of prisoners found insane.
>
> Dangerous lunatics were dealt with by an Act passed in 1838 for the prevention of offences by insane persons. It empowered two justices of the peace to commit a person to gaol on his being found to be a dangerous lunatic or a dangerous idiot. The Lord Lieutenant could at his discretion order the removal of any such person from the gaol to the district lunatic asylum. Committal of dangerous lunatics to gaols was prohibited by the Lunacy (Ireland) Act, 1867, Section 10 of which empowered any two justices of the peace to commit to the district lunatic asylum any person apprehended or discovered under circumstances denoting derangement of mind and a purpose of committing an indictable crime. The purpose of the section was to provide a substitute for the committal of dangerous lunatics to gaol, but the provisions of the section have been very widely availed of and by far the greater number of poor persons admitted to public institutions are committed in pursuance of that section.

Overall, the nineteenth century had seen a relatively large amount of mental health legislation implemented in Ireland, including the Lunacy (Ireland) Act 1821, the Criminal Lunatics (Ireland) Act 1838 and the Private Lunatic Asylums (Amendment) Act 1842. Owing to widespread abuse of the Criminal Lunatics (Ireland) Act 1838, which based committals on information provided while not under oath, the Central Criminal Lunatics Asylum Act 1845 was subsequently passed, requiring that evidence be given under oath prior to committing an individual to an asylum.[11] Nonetheless, committal abuses persisted throughout the nineteenth century[12] and, as a result, the Lunacy Act 1867 was passed, allowing two magistrates to commit an individual to an asylum under specified conditions only if they obtained a certificate from a dispensary medical officer.

Introducing the Mental Health Bill to the Dáil in 1944, Ward summarised the (still prevalent) process of 'committal in pursuance of Section 10 of the Lunacy (Ireland) Act, 1867' as follows:

> The committal order was made by two peace commissioners or a district justice after the person concerned had been certified as a dangerous lunatic by a dispensary medical officer. The expenses connected with the committal, including the payment to the medical officer for his services, were defrayed by the local public assistance authority.[13]

In addition, the Lunacy (Ireland) Act of 1867 permitted medical staff to discharge patients without recourse to higher authorities following their course of treatment at the asylum.[14] While the Act brought further reform by permitting the admission of private patients to district asylums, a three-person commission established by the lord lieutenant in 1891 still identified a clear need for reform in this area and recommended, among other measures, the introduction of a voluntary admission status.

THE NEED FOR REFORM IN THE 1940S

The need for broad reform of Ireland's asylum system was very evident by the 1940s. In 1893 the Inspector of Lunatics (Ireland) reported that:

> The accommodation in District Asylums in this country continues quite inadequate to supply the wants of the insane population. We have again to repeat the statement made in former reports that the overcrowding is rapidly increasing, and that the necessity for further accommodation is becoming more and more urgent.[15]

Even then, the inspector was also concerned about the number of 'pauper lunatics and imbeciles residing in Workhouses' who:

> ... have not always received that attention which their helpless condition requires ... Their condition in many of these establishments continues to be far from satisfactory, notwithstanding the interest as regards this class which the Local Government Board and its Inspectors have shown. In many workhouses they continue to be practically untended, their only attendants being pauper inmates, while the accommodation provided is inadequate to meet their requirements, and, as a result, proper attention is not in all cases given to personal cleanliness.

The inspector's general observations about the level of mental healthcare in workhouses are confirmed by contemporaneous historical records. This includes, for example, the records and minutes of Ballinrobe Poor Law Union, County Mayo, which demonstrate substantial deficiencies in the provision of medical, psychiatric and social care (Chapter 1).[16] Little was recorded about the outcome of mental or medical illness in Ballinrobe workhouse; this is consistent with the observation of the Inspector of Lunatics (1893) that 'as regards the remaining inmates of unsound mind in Irish workhouses, we have no returns showing admissions, discharges and deaths'.

There is strong evidence that the plight of the destitute mentally ill in other parts of the United Kingdom was similarly determined by inadequate or inappropriate statutory and administrative responses to their situation at this time.[17] In Ireland, the Inspector of Lunatics (1893) highlighted the particular absence of adequate legislative provision for the destitute mentally ill:

> These results are due as much to the want of proper legislative enact-ments for the protection of these persons as to the fault of local authorities, who have not the requisite knowledge of the requirements now demanded for the proper care of the insane poor, while, owing to the same deficiency of law regarding the status and recognition of lunatics in workhouses, the Local Government Board possess very insufficient powers to compel Boards of Guardians to make adequate provision for the care and treatment of the insane and imbecile inmates under their charge.[18]

In the following year, Tuke added to the scale of concern about these problems by arguing, in the *Journal of Mental Science*, that there was a substantial increase in the number of individuals with mental disorder in Ireland.[19] Having examined statistics from 1875 to 1893, Tuke concluded that the number of 'certified lunatics' in Ireland had increased by 60 per cent over this period, compared with an increase of not more than 22 per cent in England and Wales. This apparent increase in the levels of insanity in Ireland was a cause of considerable concern, not only in other professional journals such as the *American Journal of Insanity*,[20] but also in the reports of the Irish Inspectors of Lunatics, who were worried about worsening overcrowding and understaffing.[21]

Concerns about standards of accommodation and care were to persist well into the twentieth century: in 1924, for example, E. Boyd Barrett, SJ, painted a very similar picture of public psychiatric care in an article published in *Studies: An Irish Quarterly Review*. He wrote:

> Thanks to the indifference of the public, our asylums are in a bad way. They are over-crowded. They are both understaffed and inefficiently staffed. Curable and incurable cases are herded together. There is practically no treatment. The percentage of cures remains at a very low figure. Public money is wasted. The asylums are unsuited for their purpose in almost every respect. The rate of committals to asylums goes on increasing, and there exists no means of treating cases of incipient insanity. Curable nerve cases are allowed to develop into incurable cases. The public, ignorant and indifferent as regards mental disease, gives no encouragement to the setting up of nerve clinics or to the practice of the new methods of psychotherapy ...
>
> The most lamentable feature of the present asylum system is the absence of treatment. Apart from the many hardships that the unfortunate patients have to put up with – the poor and monotonous diet, the repulsive prison-like surroundings, the dreary exercise yards, the hideous clothing, the punishments for refractory patients, the uncongenial associates, the nerve-racking cries, the dirt and general gloom, the almost total absence of amusement and recreation – there is this appalling difference between the mental hospital (as an asylum should be) and the ordinary hospital, that in the latter each kind of disease is carefully treated by the best modern methods, whereas in the former no type of mental disease is fully treated ... To put it bluntly, the patients committed to asylums are condemned to a degrading and miserable imprisonment for life.[22]

The association between imprisonment and psychiatric admission was perpetuated by the absence of any clear legislative provision for voluntary admission, prior to the Mental Treatment Act of 1945. In 1944, the anonymous psychiatrist writing in *The Bell* paid particular attention to the need for a voluntary admission status in public psychiatric institutions.[23] The need for voluntary admission status had been previously emphasised in 1927 by the 'Report of the Commission on the Relief of the Sick and Destitute Poor including the Insane Poor', which recommended the establishment of a system of auxiliary mental hospitals in old workhouses, the development of outpatient clinics and the introduction of a voluntary admission status.[24] These recommendations, along with legislative developments in other countries, had a significant influence on the drafting of the Mental Treatment Bill in 1944.

Interestingly, the 1944 Bill was ultimately tabled without significant consultation with interested parties, although some of the reforms discussed at the Conference of the Irish Asylums Committee in 1903, especially those related to community care, were advanced by the new Act.[25] In addition, the government had sanctioned a Committee of Investigation in 1933 to examine mental health services internationally, and many of this committee's recommendations (e.g. outpatient services, voluntary admissions, research facilities) were also reflected in the Act.[26] Finally, the Act also reflected some of the reforms that certain psychiatrists had recommended repeatedly over many years previously; for example, Norman at Grangegorman Mental Hospital had repeatedly promoted the idea of 'boarding out' for patients with mental disorder[27] and this measure was ultimately addressed in some detail in the Act.

In any case, by 1945 it was clear that the problem of the increasing numbers of involuntary psychiatric inpatients was reaching crisis level. In 1804 a parliamentary committee had recommended the establishment of asylums throughout Ireland and within thirty years asylums had been built in Dublin, Derry, Belfast, Limerick and Armagh;[28] further asylums were soon opened at Killarney in 1852, Kilkenny in 1852, Omagh in 1853, Mullingar in 1855 and Sligo in 1855.[29] In parallel with this structural expansion, the number of inpatients also increased substantially throughout the latter half of the nineteenth century and first half of the twentieth century, interrupted only by two short-lived declines during the world wars.[30] By 1945, there were some 17,708 individuals resident in asylums in the southern part of Ireland, including the Central Criminal Lunatic Asylum in Dundrum. Reform was clearly needed.

MAIN PROVISIONS OF THE MENTAL TREATMENT ACT 1945

The Mental Treatment Act of 1945 aimed to address legislative deficiencies in Irish mental health law and strengthen the delivery of appropriate care to individuals with mental disorder. Introducing the 1944 Mental Treatment Bill for a second reading in the Dáil, Ward noted that some of the legislation governing mental disorder dated 'back as far as the year 1821. The general consensus of opinion with persons engaged in administration favours the replacement of those Acts by one complete measure.' Ward went on to note that:

> The Commission on the Relief of the Sick and Destitute Poor, including the insane poor, in their report, which was published in 1927, said: 'The law governing lunacy is as we have shown, to be found in numerous statutes passed in the course of a century. These statutes do not form one consistent whole; they are in some respects obsolete, defective, and even contradictory. We, therefore, recommend that all the existing lunacy Acts be repealed and that new legislation take the form of an amending and consolidating Act'.
>
> That commission made other suggestions for the amendment of the law, particularly in regard to the procedure by which admission to mental institutions was obtained and to the question of provision for early treatment of incipient mental disease. Their views in these matters are endorsed by medical practitioners engaged in the treatment of mental disease. They support the opinion that the law on the subject requires radical reform. There is no provision in the law to enable a poor person to submit himself voluntarily for mental treatment, nor is it possible for a patient to be admitted to an institution for treatment for temporary mental disorder. Furthermore, very little latitude is given as to the nature and kind of mental institutions which may be provided by mental hospital authorities.
>
> In the Bill before the House it is proposed to remedy these defects and to make other amendments in the law to secure for mental patients the benefits of the advances made in medical science and treatment in the present century. It is proposed in the Bill to substitute for the law at present in force relating to the prevention and treatment of mental disorders a new code in harmony with modern views on the treatment of mental illness.

Definitions, Inspector of Mental Hospitals, Mental Hospital Authorities

The formal preamble to the Mental Treatment Act of 1945 stated that the Act aimed 'to provide for the prevention and treatment of mental disorders and the care of persons suffering therefrom and to provide for other matters connected with the matters aforesaid'. Part 1 was concerned with 'preliminary and general matters' including definitions of terms used throughout the Act. For example, Section 3 defined a 'temporary patient' (i.e. a detained patient) as:

> a patient either (a) who is (i) suffering from mental illness, and (ii) is believed to require, for his recovery, not more than six months suitable treatment, and (iii) is unfit on account of his mental state for treatment as a voluntary patient, or (b) who is (i) an addict, and (ii) is believed to require, for his recovery, at least six months preventive and curative treatment.

Most importantly, a voluntary patient was defined as 'a person who, acting by himself or, in the case of a person less than sixteen years of age, by his parent of guardian, submits himself voluntarily for treatment for illness of a mental or kindred nature'. This was an important and clear, albeit belated, recognition of the legal status of a voluntary patient in Ireland.

Part 3 of the Act divided the country into 'mental hospital districts', each with a defined 'local administrative authority' (i.e., county council, county borough corporation or a specially appointed 'joint board'). Part 4 outlined the duty of the 'mental hospital authority to provide treatment, maintenance, advice and services' to individuals living in the 'mental hospital district' who developed mental disorder and could not otherwise afford treatment (i.e. it provided public mental health care for the poor). Part 5 of the Act outlined the obligation of the 'mental hospital authority' to 'provide and maintain proper and sufficient accommodation for carrying out their functions' and permitted mental hospital authorities to establish 'consulting rooms or clinics for affording advice and preventive and curative treatment' (i.e. outpatient clinics).

Part 10 of the Act concerned 'private institutions' which were institutions or premises 'in which one or more than one person of unsound mind is or are taken care of for profit'. This part of the Act directed that the Minister for Local Government and Public Health keep a register of private institutions and outlined a range of detailed regulations governing private institutions.

Part 11 concerned 'private charitable institutions' which were institutions 'for the care of persons of unsound mind' which were 'supported wholly or in part by voluntary contributions' and 'not kept for profit by any private individual'. These measures increased regulation and oversight of asylum facilities operated by private and charitable organisations rather than the State.

Involuntary Admission Procedures for 'Persons of Unsound Mind'

Part 14 of the Act concerned 'reception orders' governing admission to psychiatric hospitals. Chapter 1 of this part concerned 'chargeable patient reception orders' where 'it is desired to have a person received and detained as a person of unsound mind and as a chargeable patient'. In essence, this 'person of unsound mind' status permitted involuntary detention and treatment for an indefinite period without automatic review of status. An application for such admission could be made '(a) by the husband or wife or a relative of the person to whom the application relates, or (b) at the request of the husband or wife or a relative of such person, by the appropriate assistance officer, or (c) subject to the provisions of the next following sub-section, by any other person'.

The next step involved the 'authorized medical officer' who:

> shall within twenty-four hours after receipt of the application (a) visit and examine the person to whom the application relates, and (b) after such examination, either (i) if he is satisfied that it is proper to make the recommendation and is of the opinion that the person to whom the application relates will, if received, be a chargeable patient, make the recommendation in the prescribed form, or (ii) in any other case, refuse the application.

Within 'seven clear days' of the making of the 'recommendation for reception' the 'applicant for the recommendation or any person authorized by him or ... any member of the Gárda Síochána [Irish police force] ... may ... take the person to whom the recommendation relates and convey him to the district mental hospital'. At the hospital:

> the resident medical superintendent of the hospital or another medical officer of the hospital acting on his behalf shall, on the arrival of the

person at the hospital and on presentation of the recommendation, examine the person, and shall thereupon either (a) if he is satisfied that the person is a person of unsound mind and is a proper person to be taken charge of and detained under care and treatment, forthwith make in the prescribed form an order ... for the reception and detention of the person as a person of unsound mind in the hospital, or (b) in any other case refuse to make such an order.

When the chargeable patient reception order was made, the mental hospital authority, resident medical superintendent or 'the other officers and the servants of such hospital' may 'receive and take charge of the person to whom the order relates and detain him until his removal or discharge by proper authority or his death'. Interestingly, 'private patient reception orders' required 'two separate examinations' by registered medical practitioners. In all cases, the 'person of unsound mind' procedure resulted in detention of indefinite duration without automatic review.

Involuntary Admission Procedures for 'Temporary Chargeable Patients'

Chapter 3 of Part 14 of the Act concerned 'temporary chargeable patient reception orders and temporary private patient reception orders'. In essence, 'temporary chargeable' status permitted involuntary detention and treatment for up to six months. Again, an application had to be made (e.g. by a relative) and be accompanied by a:

> certificate in the prescribed form of the authorized medical officer certifying that he has examined the person to whom the application relates on a specified date not earlier than seven days before the date of the application and is of the opinion either (a) that such person (i) is suffering from mental illness, and (ii) requires, for his recovery, not more than six months suitable treatment, and (iii) is unfit on account of his mental state for treatment as a voluntary patient, or (b) that such person (i) is an addict, and (ii) requires, for his recovery, at least six months preventive and curative treatment.

In the case of a private patient reception order, the certificate had to be 'signed by two registered medical practitioners'. Following completion of the certificate, 'the applicant for the order or any person authorized by him may, not later than seven days after the date on which the order is made, take the person to whom the order relates and convey him to the approved institution'. At the hospital, the person in charge, or 'his officers, assistants, and servants and any medical officer of such institution' may 'receive and take charge of the person to whom the order relates and detain him until the expiration of a period of six months'. The period of detention could be extended 'by a further period not exceeding six months or by a series of orders … by further periods none of which shall exceed six months and the aggregate of which shall not exceed eighteen months'.

Transfer to the Central Criminal Lunatic Asylum

The 1945 Act revised certain admission procedures for the Central Criminal Lunatic Asylum.[31] Section 207 provided that if a detained person 'is charged with an indictable offence' and 'evidence is given which, in the opinion of the justice, constitutes *prima facie* evidence (i) that such person committed the offence, and (ii) that he would … be unfit to plead, the justice shall by order certify that such person is suitable for transfer to the Dundrum Central Criminal Lunatic Asylum'. Following a period of detention at the hospital, and 'where the resident governor and physician of the Dundrum Central Criminal Lunatic Asylum and the Inspector of Mental Hospitals agree and certify that [the person] has ceased to be of unsound mind, the said governor and physician shall discharge such person'.

Section 208 stated that where a mental hospital authority was of the opinion that a detained person 'requires treatment (including surgical treatment) not available save pursuant to this section, the authority may direct and authorise the removal of such person to any hospital or other place where the treatment is obtainable'. This section could also be used to mandate transfer from the district mental hospital to the Central Criminal Lunatic Asylum, under certain circumstances.

The remainder of the 1945 Act concerned a range of issues pertaining to detained patients, including arrangements for 'boarding-out in a private dwelling' and for discharge of a detained person who 'becomes capable of expressing himself, and does express himself, as desirous of being received as a voluntary patient in an approved institution'. Other regulations related to orders for independent examinations of detained patients; visiting discharged persons so as to provide 'advice as to any mental treatment'; and the role of the Inspector of Mental Hospitals in relation to detained persons. There were also provisions regarding the precise 'powers and duties of the Inspector of Mental Hospital' and the establishment of inquiries into complaints. Part 19 also contained the important stipulation that 'where mechanical means of bodily restraint are applied … full particulars of the application shall be entered forthwith in a book to be kept for that purpose'.

The Effects of the Mental Treatment Act, 1945 on Admission Rates

Ireland's Mental Treatment Act 1945 was introduced at a time of considerable change and reform in mental health services, both in Europe and elsewhere. As discussed in previous chapters, the nineteenth century had seen a considerable rise in the number of individuals confined to psychiatric institutions in many countries. In England in 1800, for example, there were relatively low numbers of individuals in asylums, with well-known asylums such Bedlam in London housing hundreds rather than thousands of patients.[32] By the end of the 1800s, however, the London region alone had sixteen asylums, some with more than 2,000 patients. By 1891, France had 108 asylums. In 1904 there were some 150,000 patients in asylums in the United States, accounting for two individuals for every 1,000 population.[33] A similar pattern was clearly evident in Ireland (Chapter 2).

There were myriad reasons for the increasing confinement of the mentally ill over this period, including better recognition of mental disorder, evolving concepts of the mind and various other interrelated societal, political and demographic factors (Chapter 2).[34] One of the aims of Ireland's Mental Treatment Act 1945 was to reduce the numbers in asylums. Ward made this clear when he presented the Bill in the Dáil in 1944, and linked it with the establishment of outpatient clinics:

It is the considered opinion of specialists engaged in the treatment of mental disease that to reduce the numbers in the mental institutions attention should be focused on the treatment of early cases of mental disorder and that failure to make provision for the treatment of such cases must result in an increase of the numbers suffering from mental afflictions and requiring prolonged or permanent treatment in mental institutions.

The arguments already put forward in favour of the establishment of consulting rooms and clinics apply with equal force to the provision of facilities for the treatment of voluntary patients. Persons suspecting symptoms of mental or nervous disease should be encouraged to seek advice and treatment in the early stages before the disease is too far developed. It is essential, therefore, to remove all formalities such as certification and formal committal to mental institutions which are likely to deter or discourage patients from seeking treatment of their own accord.

The Mental Treatment Act 1945 did not prove immediately effective in reducing inpatient numbers: by 1960 the number of individuals in Irish mental hospitals had actually risen to 20,506. In some towns, the asylum continued to dominate the local economy: in 1951, for example, the town of Ballinasloe had a total population of 5,596 of whom 2,078 were patients in the mental hospital.[35] Presumably, most of the others either worked in the mental hospital, helped supply it with goods and services, or were dependents of those who did.

A similar trend of increasing admissions was evident at the Central Criminal Lunatic Asylum, where admissions of women rose significantly following the introduction of the 1945 Act. Prior to its introduction, between 1910 and 1945, female committal rates had actually decreased steadily in the asylum: in the five-year period commencing in 1910 there were twelve female committals while in the five-year period commencing in 1940 there was one female committal (Chapter 3).[36] Female committal rates rose again, however, with the introduction of the Mental Treatment Act 1945; in the three years following 1945, there were seven female committals, chiefly owing to transfers from district mental hospitals (Section 208).

This trend was echoed nationally and continued for many years following introduction of the 1945 legislation. By 1961, one in every seventy Irish people above the age of 24 was in a psychiatric hospital bed.[37] In October 1968, *The Irish Times* published an influential series of articles by Michael Viney highlighting the broad range of problems related to mental health care and, in particular, this strikingly large number of individuals still resident in Irish asylums at that time.[38]

One area in which the Mental Treatment Act 1945 was arguably more successful, and which may help to account for its failure to reduce inpatient numbers, was its efforts to reduce the stigma associated with mental disorder. In particular, the new Act saw the removal of the term 'lunatic' and its replacement with terms such as 'person of unsound mind', which were less stigmatising at that time. The reduction of stigma was one of the express aims of the new Act: in the Dáil, Ward had pointed out that 'it is proposed to depart entirely from the term "district lunatic asylum" and to continue the use of the term "mental hospital" provided for in Section 79 of the Local Government Act, 1925. It is proposed also to use the term "person of unsound mind" instead of the term "lunatic".' In addition, the introduction of a new voluntary admission status and the centrality of medical rather than judicial personnel in the detention process may have further helped reduce stigma and increase patient numbers, as may have the simultaneous introduction of various 'modern physical methods of treatment' (e.g., convulsive treatment, insulin coma treatment and psychosurgery).[39]

The International Legislative Context

In the decades leading up to Ireland's Mental Treatment Act 1945, both the United Kingdom (1930) and Northern Ireland (1932) had introduced relatively liberal mental health legislation which included, among other measures, voluntary admission status.[40] This trend towards substantial reform of mental health legislation was also apparent in many other jurisdictions: in 1936 and 1939, Switzerland passed laws that drew a clearer distinction between *admissions libres* which were requested by the patient and other admissions which were requested by third parties, such as parents, authorities, etc.[41] Some twenty years earlier, Japan had started to reform its system of psychiatric care, replacing its Mental Patients' Custody Act 1900 with a Mental Hospitals Act 1919 which heralded a substantial expansion of hospital-based care for individuals with psychiatric illness.[42] In India, a division of the Royal Medical Psychological Association was formed in the mid-1930s, and in 1946 the Health Survey and Development Committee performed a survey of psychiatric services, also recommending substantial reform in the provision and administration of care in India.[43]

The 1940s also saw considerable legislative change in the United States with the introduction of the National Mental Health Act of 1946. The aims of this Act were to: (a) support research into the aetiology and treatment of neuropsychiatric disorders; (b) support training of mental health workers by awarding fellowships to individuals and institutions; and (c) provide grants and assistance to States in order to establish treatment centres for neuropsychiatric disorders.[44] This Act stemmed in part from the particular emphasis placed on neuropsychiatric disorders by Vannevar Bush, director of the United States Office of Scientific Research and Development, who advised the US president, Franklin D. Roosevelt, that there were approximately 7 million persons in the USA with mental disorder, resulting in considerable costs to the public purse.[45]

Bush's report coincided with growing public interest in mental disorder, which was attributable to a number of factors, including the publication of Clifford Beers' autobiography *A Mind That Found Itself* in 1908[46] and increased recognition of the prevalence of mental disorder, as a result of the systematic medical inspection of immigrants in New York.[47] The Second World War also generated interest in mental disorder as some 1.1 million men were rejected for military duty owing to neurological or mental disorder; the practice of military psychiatry also later demonstrated the effectiveness of multidisciplinary treatment involving psychiatric nurses, psychologists and social workers.[48]

The US National Mental Health Act of 1946 was also consistent with the legislative trend demonstrated in the US Public Health Service Act of 1944, which increased health assistance to States and broadened the remit of the Public Health Services.[49] Ultimately, the 1946 Act not only authorised a broad Federal programme to treat mental disorder and promote mental health, but also provided for the creation of a National Neuropsychiatric Institute, which was established as the National Institute of Mental Health in 1949.

Like the US National Mental Health Act of 1946, Ireland's Mental Treatment Act 1945 aimed 'to provide for the prevention and treatment of mental disorders and the care of persons suffering therefrom and to provide for other matters connected with the matters aforesaid'. The Irish legislation also made clear reference to the importance of research, stating, for example, that 'a mental hospital authority may, with the consent of the Minister, and shall, if the Minister so directs, provide and maintain a laboratory for research in connection with mental and nervous diseases'. The Irish legislation, however, failed to provide for the establishment of a national 'Institute of Psychiatry' to promote research into the causes and treatment of mental disorder, despite occasional considerations of the idea since then within Irish psychiatry.[50]

CHANGES IN PSYCHIATRIC PRACTICE SINCE THE MENTAL TREATMENT ACT 1945

In the decades following the introduction of the Mental Treatment Act 1945, the international legislative environment changed considerably in response to myriad factors, including increased recognition of human rights in general[51] and the human rights of the mentally ill in particular, especially through United Nations' Principles for the Protection of Persons with Mental Illness and the Improvement of Mental Health Care (1991).[52] By this time, almost fifty years after the 1945 Act was introduced, it was apparent that there were significant problems with the legislation from a human rights perspective, not least because it permitted indefinite involuntary detention and treatment without automatic review, and detention of individuals who were not alleged to be dangerous to self or others.[53]

In addition, in 2008, two years after the Mental Treatment Act 1945 had been fully replaced by the Mental Health Act 2001,[54] the Irish Supreme Court actually found that part of the 1945 Act had been unconstitutional all along, as it restricted grounds for challenging detention to two specific grounds (that the hospital had acted in 'bad faith' or proceeded 'without reasonable care').[55] The Court found that this was a disproportionate restriction on the detained patient's right to access the courts where a fundamental right, liberty, had been restricted, and was, thus, contrary to the Constitution of Ireland.

At the time of its introduction, however, the Mental Treatment Act 1945 was an important, albeit belated, recognition of the need to reform Ireland's asylum system. It also coincided with a period of considerable optimism in clinical psychiatry, as new treatments were being introduced and tested, and psychiatrists in Ireland and elsewhere found renewed enthusiasm for the prospects of recovery from mental disorder. These clinical developments are considered next, with particular reference to Ireland's largest asylum, Grangegorman Mental Hospital in Dublin, and to the work and words of Professor John Dunne, who worked there for almost three decades, from 1937 until 1965.

THE 'CONTRIBUTION OF THE PHYSICAL SCIENCES TO PSYCHOLOGICAL MEDICINE'

In 1955, Professor John Dunne of Grangegorman Mental Hospital and University College Dublin became president of the Royal Medico-Psychological Association (RMPA), forerunner of the present-day Royal College of Psychiatrists.[56] The organisation aimed to facilitate communication between doctors working in asylums, with a view to improving quality of care for the mentally ill.[57] In 1894, the organisation had admitted its first female member, Dr Eleonora Fleury (1867–1960), from the Richmond

Lunatic Asylum in Dublin (later renamed Grangegorman Mental Hospital) where Dunne worked.[58]

Dunne was the sixth Irish president of the RMPA. The previous Irish presidents were Dr Lalor of the Richmond Lunatic Asylum (1861), Dr J.E. Duncan (1875), Dr Conolly Norman of Grangegorman Mental Hospital (1894), Dr W.R. Dawson (1911), Dr M.J. Nolan of Downpatrick (1924) and Dr R. Leper (1931). Dunne's appointment as president was an important recognition of work being done in Irish psychiatry and, on 13 July 1955, Dunne duly delivered a commanding presidential address at the annual meeting of the RMPA in Dublin. The following year, his address was published in the *Journal of Mental Science*, forerunner of the present-day *British Journal of Psychiatry*.[59]

Dunne is one of the most significant figures in Irish psychiatric history. His address to the RMPA in 1955 highlights many of the major themes of his life's work. It also provides an important insight into the clinical enthusiasms of Irish psychiatry as reform commenced in earnest in the 1940s and 1950s. Dunne had taken up the post of chief RMS at Grangegorman Mental Hospital on 10 September 1937.[60] Twelve years earlier, he had worked there as an assistant medical officer and had introduced malarial treatment for general paralysis of the insane. This novel physical treatment was pioneered by Julius von Wagner-Jauregg, a professor of psychiatry at the Vienna Asylum in Austria, who received a Nobel prize for his work in 1927.[61]

Following his appointment as RMS in 1937, Dunne went on to introduce several new forms of physical treatment for mental disorders,[62] and was the first medical superintendent in Ireland to use insulin therapy for the treatment of schizophrenia.[63] While there had been early work with administration of insulin for the treatment of mental disorder at the Psychopathic Hospital at Ann Arbour in the 1920s, most of the pioneering work on insulin treatment for schizophrenia had been performed by Dr Manfred Sakel in Vienna in the early 1930s.[64] Following Sakel's positive reports, insulin therapy was soon introduced at several centres throughout the United States and Europe, including the Maudsley Hospital in London. In 1938, Dunne reported positive results with insulin therapy at Grangegorman Mental Hospital.[65] Four years later, electroconvulsive therapy (ECT) was also introduced to Grangegorman Mental Hospital, demonstrating Dunne's ongoing interest in delivering novel forms of treatment to patients who were often suffering from severe and prolonged psychiatric illness, as well as the effects of long-term institutionalisation.[66]

While many of these physical treatments are no longer in use today, it is worth noting that they were all viewed as the progressive treatments in their time. In addition to pioneering physical treatments, Dunne's arrival also heralded a range of other reforms at Grangegorman, including the following measures:

- Benches that were used to hem in challenging patients were removed and extra attendants were employed so as to give patients more liberty
- Old box beds were replaced by cast-iron bedsteads
- A medical library was established to keep staff in touch with scientific developments
- A separate unit for the disturbed elderly and a separate ward for children were sought.[67]

Therefore, while many problems certainly persisted at the hospital during Dunne's time there, as highlighted by inspectors' reports, there were also real attempts to remedy many of the deficiencies. This even included the development of a 'ladies after-care committee' dedicated to assisting recently discharged patients to settle down and find employment. Despite many such reforms throughout the 1940s and 1950s, however, and despite the introduction of the Mental Treatment Act in 1945, there remained a large custodial element to most psychiatric institutions, and there were significant problems with overcrowding at Grangegorman, concerning Dunne greatly.

PRESIDENT OF THE ROYAL MEDICO-PSYCHOLOGICAL ASSOCIATION

In 1955, Dunne commenced his first address as president of the RMPA by noting the honour of being appointed and offering his thanks to the RMPA:

The honour which the RMPA has bestowed on me fills me with a mixture of pride and apprehension; pride that I occupy the Chair where have sat so many distinguished psychiatrists and apprehension lest I might be unequal to the task of upholding the noble traditions of my prede-cessors ... The first Irish President was Dr Lalor, who was the Medical Superintendent of this Hospital [Grangegorman Mental Hospital], in 1861. He was an outstanding figure in the psychiatric world at that time. Under the direction of Dr Lalor, the Richmond Lunatic Asylum, as this hospital was then known, had achieved a very high reputation for the manner in which the mentally ill were treated. Dr Lalor was in fact renowned for having initiated and developed a system of education of the patients as a front line of treatment in this hospital.[68]

Having next paid a warm tribute to the previous president of the RMPA, Dr Noel Harris, Dunne turned his attention to 'more serious topics':

> It is a tradition of the Association that the newly-installed President begins his term of office by delivering a Presidential Address on some topic of his own choice. Like the newly-born infant, whose first cry is hailed with delight by the mother, the new President must give tongue so that his subjects may have audible proof of his vigour. I found great difficulty in selecting a theme for my Address. Many headings occurred to me, such as 'The Scottish Influence on Psychological Medicine in England' or 'Eccentricities and Idiosyncrasies of Psychiatrists'. My muse, however, rejected these titles and decided that I should attempt to present my impressions of the effect of modern scientific advances on psychological concepts ....
>
> Medicine today has progressed far beyond its conception as an art and has become a vast field of scientific knowledge which derives from a combination of research in practically all other branches of science. The isolation of pathogenic organisms, the discovery of antibiotics, sulphonamides and other bactericidal substances, the advances in anaesthesia and surgical technique, are only some of the bewildering series of successes which have yielded to research in recent times. It must be admitted, however, that progress in psychological medicine has not kept pace with that of somatic medicine. Scientific explanation of the aetiology of mental illness still remains obscure, and treatment is largely based on empiricism.

From this point onwards, Dunne focused on the specific contributions of 'the physical sciences to psychological medicine'. In particular, he explored (a) the principle of conditioning and the work of Hans Selye, especially in relation to 'General Adaptation Syndrome' and the role of stress in producing psychosomatic or physical symptoms; (b) cybernetics and the generation of partial models of cerebral functioning, such as Grey Walter's Conditioned Reflex Analogue and the Electronic Delayed Storage Automatic Computer of Cambridge; and (c) the development of integrated, holistic models of cerebral functioning, that took account of advances in both physical medicine and psychoanalytic thought.

THE PRINCIPLE OF CONDITIONING, THE ROLE OF STRESS, AND THE WORK OF HANS SELYE

Turning his attention firstly to the science of the nervous system, Dunne noted that 'three hundred years ago, Descartes first propounded that nervous and mental activity depended on mechanisms which had an anatomy and physiology; that nervous and mental activity was a response to external or internal stimuli; that the responses to stimuli were automatic, whether as a result of inherent or acquired influence'. The animal experiments of Pavlov had 'successfully shown that reflexes may be conditioned and altered by the effects of environmental influence ... The discovery of the manner in which reflexes can be conditioned opened a new path towards the understanding of psychological processes ... The modern psychoanalytical and therapeutic approach to mental abnormality, whether of the major or minor variety, is largely based on the principle of conditioning, even though such may not be admitted by psychological purists'.

Dunne devoted particular attention to the idea of 'conditioning', a form of learning that involves associating specific behaviours with certain stimuli or rewards:

> The principle underlying the conditioning of reflexes would seem to be the underlying basis of well-known aetiological concepts, including those of Hans Selye, whose contributions to the science of medicine are held in such high esteem today ... His exposition of the General Adaptation Syndrome (specific and non-specific) and diseases of adaptation marks a highlight in medical science. His concepts of stress as a disease-producing agent and of the manner in which it produces disease, is an example of the application of careful study of mechanism as an essential part of the holistic approach.

Hans Selye (1907–82) was an Austrian physician and endocrinologist who served as a professor and director of the Institute of Experimental Medicine and Surgery at the University of Montreal, Canada. Selye's chief research interest was stress and its relationship with physical and mental disorder. As Dunne noted, Selye recognised:

the important part which conditioning plays in psychological and psychiatric problems and relates the phenomenon to physiological mechanisms. He emphasizes particularly the influence of steroid hormones which are released by stress, and refers to the manner in which the action of those hormones can be inhibited or accentuated by metabolic processes ... Selye has shown that mental stress is responsible for the production of psychic or psycho-somatic symptoms and that stress is always associated with the production of ACTH [adreno-cortico-trophic hormone] and adreno-steroids.

Selye was right: it is now well recognised that hormones such as those mentioned by Selye and Dunne are indeed central to the genesis of certain mental disorders, with particular attention now devoted to corticotropin-releasing hormone (CRH) in the reaction and adaptation to stress.[69] This approach finds further support in recent work in the related field of psycho-neuro-immunology, which further clarifies the roles of endocrinology, immunology and adaptation to stress in the genesis of mental disorders.[70]

In his 1955 presidential address, Dunne went on to discuss the role of the electroencephalogram (EEG) in elucidating the physical underpinnings of mental disorder. The EEG is a recording of electrical activity in the brain (i.e. brainwaves) which can help demonstrate levels and patterns of brain activity. Dunne noted that this technique 'has made great strides in the short time that has elapsed since Berger's first observation. It has become one of the most valuable aids in the diagnosis of brain disturbances such as epilepsy, brain tumour and brain damage.'

In the decades since Dunne's comments, some of the diagnostic roles of the EEG have been supplanted by brain imaging, owing in part to the development of techniques such as computed tomography and magnetic resonance imaging, and also owing to the limitations of the EEG in terms of specificity and sensitivity. Even in 1955, however, Dunne was aware of the limits of EEG and that, for many EEG abnormalities, 'the electroencephalographic expert was unable to ascribe any typicality to these abnormalities and even regarded them as somewhat equivocal'. Nonetheless, Dunne concluded that 'many, if not all, functional disturbances of the brain, such as encephalopathies, psychotic depression, types of schizophrenia, are associated with a breakdown or disturbance of the electrical mechanism'. Today, several decades later, the EEG is still used as one element in an increasingly complex diagnostic process for a range of conditions, including, as Dunne noted, 'brain disturbance such as epilepsy, brain tumour and brain damage'.

CYBERNETICS AND THE GENERATION OF PARTIAL MODELS OF CEREBRAL FUNCTIONING

Dunne next examined the development of models or partial models of brain function, which was a popular and exciting field of endeavour in the 1950s:

> The amazing developments in the sciences of physics, chemistry, electronics and mathematics has resulted in the construction of complex machines which can perform functions that hitherto seemed to be the monopoly of the human brain. Grey Walter's Conditioned Reflex Analogue and the Electronic Delayed Storage Automatic Computer of Cambridge, are instruments in which reflex responses can be conditioned to substituted stimuli similar to the conditioned reflexes of Pavlov. These achievements have led to a comparison between the mechanisms of these man-made machines and the mechanism of the brain ...
>
> The analogy has stimulated the application of a new method of study to the mechanism of the brain, the science of Cybernetics ... The works of Wiener, Ashby, Grey Walter, McCulloch and others, are convincing masterpieces of logical, mathematical, scientific, deduction. There can be no doubt of the soundness of their demonstration of similarities in the mechanism of the nervous system and man-made machines and that the principles underlying one can apply to the other. They have shown that there is a basic principle, the feed-back, which is common to all mechanisms no matter how complex ...
>
> The principle of the feed-back of the cyberneticist and the reflex of the physiologist are one and the same ... On the higher scale of thought, the same principle exists, but the communication between cells is very much more complex, depending not only on associated nerve pathways, but also on direct influences from cell to cell by means of chemical and electrical interchanges, and on the influences of distant metabolic and glandular products, the result of nervous activity. The final response to stimuli then on a higher plane, may be regarded as the end solution of a problem presented by the stimulus ... The application of the cybernetic approach to the mechanism of cerebral functioning, including

psychological processes, suggests the presence of compartments or areas in which stimuli are subjected to various processes before the nature of the response is decided. Such compartments or areas are not meant to signify separate anatomical areas, such as Broca's area, but a separate mechanism ...

The notion of developing models or partial models of cerebral function is one which has long held attraction for scientists and psychiatrists alike, and which persists today.[71] The idea of 'cybernetics' was, perhaps, most clearly enunciated by Norbert Weiner (1894–1964), who focused on the relationships and similarities between feedback mechanisms, computing machines and the human nervous system.[72] Using a cybernetic paradigm, Weiner suggested that many mental disorders may be due to disorders of information circulation, owing to altered synaptic thresholds (i.e. altered patterns of communication between brain cells). Dunne's account of the 'cybernetic approach to the mechanism of cerebral functioning', as outlined in his 1955 address, is presented in Figure 3.

The development of computers in the 1950s and the emergence, in subsequent years, of 'neural network' theories regarding the brain transformed many aspects of this school of thought, especially in relation to the field of cybernetics which so interested Dunne. Neural network modelling remains a subject of considerable scientific interest today, especially in relation to the development of models to better explain how information is represented by large numbers of interconnected units, such as brain cells.[73] As in Dunne's presidential address, there is still considerable interest in the relevance of neural networks and remodelling in relation to auditory, visual and linguistic processing,[74] learning processes,[75] autism,[76] recovery after stroke[77] and borderline personality disorder.[78]

THE DEVELOPMENT OF INTEGRATED, HOLISTIC MODELS OF CEREBRAL FUNCTIONING

One of the recurring themes of Dunne's 1955 address was that of holism, and this is especially evident in his attempts to link various scientific, psychoanalytic and spiritual theories with each other so as to form an overall, integrated model of mental functioning. In the interests of developing more unified theories about mental functioning, Dunne stated:

FIGURE 3

Professor John Dunne's account of 'the cybernetic approach to the mechanism of cerebral functioning'.

In his presidential address, Dunne stated that:

the application of the cybernetic approach to the mechanism of cerebral functioning, including psychological processes, suggests the presence of compartments or areas in which stimuli are subjected to various processes before the nature of a response is decided ... These compartments may be approximately represented in the following rough schema:

- Impressions are first received
- Selected, namely priority of attention is given to selected stimuli such as visual over olfactory stimuli
- Analysed, namely important data are distinguished from less important data
- Synthesised, namely different important data are related to one another
- Computed, for example the speed of an oncoming car, the speed of a person crossing, and of distance, are computed so that an appropriate decision may be made
- Referred to problem-solving area of selected, analysed and computed data where:

a) The problem is solved.
b) The incomplete solution is stored for future reference, for example, learning by mistakes.
c) The solutions of solved problems are stored, which represents having learned to do something.
d) Data without any problems are stored, for example, learning a poem.

Note to Figure 3

Quotation is taken, with permission, from: Dunne J. 'The Contribution of the Physical Sciences to Psychological Medicine' in *Journal of Mental Science* (1956; 102: 209–20). See Acknowledgements for further details.

To summarize briefly, it is suggested that the successful functioning of mind depends on the integrity of the following mechanisms:

(1) A complex combination of reflex arcs, consisting of nerve cells and fibres, intimately associated with, and depending upon one another.

(2) A system of production of various substances which affect the integrity of this nervous mechanism, namely ACTH, Corticoids, Minerals, etc.

(3) The generation of electrical potential.

(4) A complicated electrical mechanism which is essential to preserve the communications between the various areas through which the products stimuli must pass before a problem is solved and effect given to the solution.

(5) The existence of special compartments within this mechanism for reception of data, selection, analysis, synthesis, computing and solving of data; of storage areas for unsolved and solved problems; for automats, which are the compartments which govern ordinary behaviour.

Dunne went on to explore specific relationships between a number of different areas within psychology and related fields, including the relationship between cybernetics and psychoanalysis, and between psychoanalysis and spirituality. Regarding cybernetics and psychoanalysis, Dunne stated:

The difference between the language of the cyberneticist and the psychoanalyst would … seem to be no more than exists between the spoken tongue of two different countries … It is a source of wonder that the language invented by Freud when the physiology of the brain was practically unknown, should so closely conform to the mechanisms later uncovered by physiological research … The following few examples give an indication of the unity of meaning between the language of Psychologists and Cyberneticists – censoring, involving repression, appears to be identical with the process of selection and storage of data; reasoning and judgement are identical with computing and problem solving; the unconscious, with the storage of data and solved and unsolved problems.

Regarding psychoanalysis and spirituality, Dunne stated that 'a stage has been reached in which different scientific discoveries form a compatible relationship with one another and conform to the requirements of scientific and spiritual concepts'. In particular, he noted that:

> Freud's greatest achievement ... was his structural delineation of mental processes. His exposition of the manner in which personality and character are developed and moulded, his demonstration of the effect of environmental influences on the shaping of personality, his schematic representation of mental mechanisms, are concepts which form the basis of all modern psychology.

He went on to clarify that:

> The Id [described by Freud as that part of the mind concerned with primitive drives, such as hunger and sex], being the seat of Instincts, may be regarded as containing pre-setting influences which guide behaviour. While the Instincts are the main pre-setting influences in lower animals, they should only be regarded in man as subordinate to an overall pre-setting direction of what may be termed the spiritual instinct. This spiritual instinct is contained in the religious concept of the desire for good in the human ... While the standards of good may vary in different races it cannot be denied that the overall aspirations of the human mind are towards good ... Conscience may, therefore, be regarded as an essential part of human mental equipment, embryonic at birth, but later to reach its full development in what Freud called the Super-Ego ... Freud defines the Super-Ego as activities of self-observation, conscience and the holding-up of ideals; the representation of all moral restrictions; the advocate of the impulse towards perfection. These concepts from such varying schools of thought would seem to establish that the most important aspect of mental mechanisms, namely the pre-setting, depends on a spiritual instinct.

Through these syntheses of cybernetics with psychoanalysis, and psychoanalysis with spirituality, Dunne sought to present a progressive and unified model of mind, drawing on myriad fields within and related to psychiatry, in order to better understand the human mind and guide the treatment of the mentally ill. Similar efforts continue today.[79]

The Search for Integrated Theories of Brain Function

The recurring themes in Dunne's presidential address to the RMPA include, as its title suggests, the 'contribution of the physical sciences to psychological medicine', as well as the search for integrated theories of brain function, and the need to re-evaluate the theories of the past in light of more recent developments and discoveries. These themes were timely, as the 1940s and 1950s were decades of considerable change in psychiatry, with the theories of Freud being substantially re-evaluated in light of developments in psychology and the physical sciences.[80] In his address, Dunne referred openly to these controversies and discussions:

> The fact that different schools of psycho-analysts and psycho-therapists disagree with Freudian analysis because of his emphasis on the dominance of the sexual instinct in the shaping of the personality should not blind us to the wonderful advances in knowledge of the mind which were the result of the researches of Freud, his contemporaries, Adler and Jung, and of his numerous successors in the field … The importance which is attached to psychology today in all forms of disease, individual, collective, social, industrial and international mal-adjustments, owes its position to psycho-analytical research.

Throughout his 1955 address, however, Dunne placed his greatest emphasis on the development of comprehensive, scientific models of brain function. His words captured the optimism of the era clearly, as he stated that 'the various scientific approaches to the explanation of mental functioning by physiologists, neurologists, bio-chemists, electrologists, cyberneticists, not only appear to harmonize, even synchronize, in the elucidation of mental mechanistics, but also appear to harmonize very closely with the concepts of the psychological purist'.

These attempts to integrate various areas of physical, psychological and spiritual thought belong firmly within the long-standing tradition of efforts to develop comprehensive, integrated models of the human mind.[81] In the decades since Dunne's address, much of this type of integrated theorising has focused on understanding the mind by exploring the phenomenon of human consciousness and embarking on a similar integration of research findings from various fields of neuroscience, including neurology, brain imaging, psychiatry, psychology and evolutionary biology.[82]

In similar fashion, there is continuous and increasing interest in the development and improvement of comprehensive, scientifically based models of psychiatric care that integrate biological, psychological and social perspectives on mental disorder.[83] This point was especially emphasised by Dunne in 1955: 'The urgent pleas by Gladstone, Henderson et al., for a holistic approach to sickness can only be effected by a realization of the inseparability of psychological concepts and mechanistic concepts. The barriers between the two concepts are only figments which do not exist in reality. Each is essential to the other'.

Many of the innovations that Dunne introduced at Grangegorman Mental Hospital (reduced use of restraint, better bedding, the aftercare committee, the medical library)[84] were to contribute significantly to the development of more integrated models of psychiatric care there and elsewhere. Dunne was also outspoken in condemning the overcrowding of Grangegorman Mental Hospital and in campaigning for generally better conditions for the institutionalised mentally ill.

All of these concerns are well reflected in Dunne's presidential address. His remarks reflect a passionate concern, not only with the scientific basis of contemporary psychiatric practice, but also with the mechanisms by which such practice is determined; that is, the roles of medical education and scientific research in shaping psychiatric practice. This was a progressive, positive approach which held out considerable hope for the tens of thousands detained within Ireland's asylum system at that time. In his own practice, Dunne combined this scientific approach with a pragmatic and patient-centred attitude to the reform of psychiatric care, within the context and limitations of the existing laws and social setting.

The occasion of the RMPA presidential address gave Dunne the opportunity to explore in some depth many of the themes that had informed his career in psychiatry up to that point. It was traditional for new presidents of the RMPA to use the presidential address to set out their vision of psychiatry for the future, too, and to provide an overview of their ambitions in relation to key issues.[85] In 1899, for example, Dr Beveridge Spence was elected president and took the opportunity to review progress in nursing education and highlight that educational initiatives were leading to improvements in the position of nurses in asylums.[86] In 1933, Dr F.D. Turner devoted much of that year's presidential address to 'mental deficiency', focusing on training and re-socialisation as key elements of care.[87] In 1947, Dr W.G. Masefield used his presidential address to appeal for a broader acceptance of varied forms of therapy and improvements in mental health laws.[88] Placed in the context of these other presidential addresses, Dunne's address was notable for the breadth of its vision and emphasis on the scientific basis of treatment.

Prior to Dunne assuming the presidency of the RMPA, there had been several earlier Irish presidents who had made their marks on the organisation in various different ways.[89] Dunne continued this tradition and was notable not only for his emphasis on the need for a scientific basis for psychiatric practice, but also his rational and pragmatic approach to the limitations of present knowledge. Indeed, as he concluded his address, Dunne acknowledged that his attempt to present a complete and integrated model of brain function was, of course, incomplete. As ever, more work needed to be done, and, as ever, Dunne believed the key to progress lay in understanding disparate fields of research and integrating the findings into a unified whole:

> I have attempted to make a digest of the scientific aspects of psychological medicine and to compress them into a cohesive whole. I fear that my achievement has fallen far short of what I set out to do. I hope, however, that in bringing the physical sciences and psychological and spiritual concepts into a compressed relationship, my address will help to clarify in a very small way the confusion that so many different approaches might well inspire in the student of Psychiatry. I would also express the hope that the broad perspective I have outlined may perhaps help the pioneers in different schools of thought to realise that in each approach is contained values not always conceded.

Reforming Ireland's Asylum System

Given these reforms in mental health law, as evidenced by the Mental Treatment Act 1945, and renewed optimism within Irish psychiatry, as evidenced by Dunne's presidential address to the RMPA in 1955, did the position of the mentally ill in Ireland's mental hospitals truly improve during the 1940s and 1950s?[90] Did these developments in legal and clinical approaches truly impact on the lives and institutional experiences of men and women in mental hospitals and the Central Criminal Lunatic Asylum in Dundrum?

The most important point to note is that, despite these apparently positive changes, the number of individuals in Irish psychiatric institutions did not peak until 1958 and was notably slow to decline even after that; even in 1961, one in every seventy Irish people above the age of 24 was in a psychiatric hospital.[91] The decline in numbers only commenced in earnest in the early 1960s, when the number of individuals in Irish psychiatric units and hospitals finally decreased from 19,801 in 1963 to 3,658 in 2003 — a decrease of some 16,143 individuals (or 81.5 per cent) over forty years.[92]

Prior to this decrease, however, Irish mental hospitals were still large, overcrowded institutions throughout the 1940s and 1950s, and clearly in need of reform. The reduction of the stigma associated with both mental hospitals and mental disorder was important for rallying public support for reform. As the anonymous psychiatrist noted in *The Bell* in 1944:

> When people learn that insanity is a disease and not a disgrace, and act on it, there will be a hope of getting a large percentage of cases early enough for a quick recovery.[93]

One of the key initiatives aimed at reducing stigma was the introduction of outpatient clinics, and the decades following the Mental Treatment Act 1945 saw significant progress in the promotion of outpatient rather than inpatient care. In 1967 and 1968, Dunne audited outpatient clinical activity at the Mercer's Hospital clinic in Dublin and reported 2,274 attendances by 413 patients over this period.[94] The most common diagnoses were depression (31 per cent), anxiety hysteria (16 per cent) and schizophrenia (9 per cent). This recognition of the importance of outpatient care as an alternative to admission was an important step in the reform of Ireland's mental health services.

The decades following the 1945 Act were also a time of significant interest in new physical or biological treatments for mental disorder and, in 1950, Dunne published a 'Survey of Modern Physical Methods of Treatment for Mental Disorder Carried Out in Grangegorman Mental Hospital', where he was RMS.[95] Dunne's paper focused chiefly on the physical treatments of the 1930s and 1940s and discussed, in some detail, results he observed with electroconvulsive therapy, insulin coma and psychosurgery. Dunne's interest in physical treatments for mental disorder was consistent with a broader renewal of enthusiasm for physical treatments in psychiatry, as reflected in Dunne's presidential address.[96] This enthusiasm reached a new peak in the early 1950s with the introduction of chlorpromazine, the first effective antipsychotic medication and, thus, the first effective medication for schizophrenia.[97]

Notwithstanding these legislative reforms, service developments and scientific enthusiasms, however, there were still substantial problems in Irish mental health services in the decades following the Mental Treatment Act of 1945. Most worryingly, by 1958 the number of individuals in psychiatric hospitals had risen to an all-time high of approximately 21,000, or 0.7 per cent of the entire population.[98] In 1968 Michael Viney painted a stark picture of psychiatric institutionalisation in *The Irish Times*:

> Seven in every thousand people in Ireland spent last night in a mental hospital bed. In no other country in Europe – nor, probably, in the world – did so large a fraction of the nation's population find themselves in such surroundings. Comparatively few of these 19,656 people spoke to a doctor yesterday or are likely to speak to one today. And in a more prosperous and progressive society, one third of them (at a rough but not a reckless guess) would have left hospital years ago or would never have been admitted.
>
> They may long since have recovered from the illness which brought them into hospital. But they have lost their place in the world outside: no home, no friends, no job. If they have an illness now, it is the one called 'institutional neurosis': a steady sapping of interest and initiative, an ever-growing dependence on the security, authority and routine of mental hospital life.[99]

In the 1960s, the Irish Government established a Commission of Enquiry on Mental Illness which attempted to examine the high rates of psychiatric institutionalisation in order to determine whether they truly reflected a raised incidence of mental disorder in Ireland.[100] While drawing much-needed attention to the state of mental health services in Ireland at this time,[101] however, the Commission was unable to reach definite conclusions about incidence of illness owing to a paucity of reliable data. The Commission recommended that the Medico-Social Research Board examine the matter. Subsequent data collection was more systematic and reliable, and data from the 1960s and 1970s showed a gradual, steady decline in the number of psychiatric inpatients.[102]

Notwithstanding this welcome reduction in inpatient numbers, there was little convincing evidence of the kind of comprehensive, system-level change that was required in order to reverse the strong legacy of institutional care. In 1984, however, the Department of Health published a comprehensive revision of mental health policy, entitled 'The Psychiatric Services – Planning for the Future', which recommended that mental health services should deliver comprehensive, co-ordinated, multi-disciplinary

care with a strong community orientation.[103] Services were to be organised
through consultant-led teams, each of which would be assigned a population 'sector' comprising 25,000 to 30,000 individuals. Day hospitals were
to be provided and a range of other services (e.g. child psychiatry services)
were to be strengthened and reformed.

'Planning for the Future' was a generally progressive and ambitious
document, aimed at transforming Irish mental health care and reori-
enting services towards the community. While some progress was made
in subsequent years, however, there were significant problems with full
implementation, especially in relation to levels of community provision.[104]
On foot of these concerns, as well as significant changes in Irish population and society over the previous twenty years, a new policy document
was published in 2006, titled 'A Vision for Change'.[105] 'A Vision for Change'
largely restated the principles of 'Planning for the Future', but contained
a renewed commitment to implementation.[106] One of the most pressing
needs by this time, however, was for the reform of Ireland's mental health
legislation, as the Mental Treatment Act of 1945 was increasingly inconsistent with the directions of Irish mental health policy and international
human rights declarations, such as United Nations' Principles for the
Protection of Persons with Mental Illness and the Improvement of Mental
Health Care and the European Convention on Human Rights.[107] These
concerns led to the emergence of new mental legislation in Ireland, in the
form of the Mental Health Act 2001.

THE MENTAL HEALTH ACT 2001

Ireland's Mental Health Act 2001, was formally enacted on 8 July 2001 and
implemented in full by 1 November 2006. This Act was chiefly concerned
with involuntary admission to 'approved centres' and mechanisms for
inspection and quality assurance in mental health services.[108] The Act uses
the term 'mental disorder' to include 'mental illness, severe dementia or
significant intellectual disability'. 'Mental illness' is defined as 'a state of
mind of a person which affects the person's thinking, perceiving, emotion
or judgment and which seriously impairs the mental function of the person
to the extent that he or she requires care or medical treatment in his or her
own interest or in the interest of other persons'.

Under the new legislation, an individual with 'mental disorder' can
be involuntarily admitted following (a) application by a spouse, relative,

'authorized officer', member of the Garda Síochána (Irish police force) or another person; (b) 'recommendation' by a registered medical practitioner (e.g. a general practitioner) 'within 24 hours of the receipt of the application'; and (c) completion of an 'admission order' by a consultant psychiatrist on the staff of the approved centre, if they are 'satisfied that the person is suffering from a mental disorder' and fulfils certain other criteria. The Act also provides regulations governing means of transport to the 'approved centre' and details the timescale involved in the various steps in this process. The 'admission order' may remain in force for twenty-one days, during which time the Mental Health Commission must appoint a Mental Health Tribunal to review the matter independently.

The Mental Health Act 2001 directed the establishment of a 'Mental Health Commission' in order 'to promote, encourage and foster the establishment and maintenance of high standards and good practices in the delivery of mental health services and to take all reasonable steps to protect the interests of persons detained in approved centres under this Act'. One of the roles of the Mental Health Commission is to appoint mental health tribunals to review involuntary admission orders. Each tribunal comprises one consultant psychiatrist, one barrister or solicitor and one lay person. Prior to the tribunal, an independent psychiatrist examines the detained patient, interviews the patient's consultant psychiatrist and reviews the records. The tribunal then reviews the detention of the patient and, 'if satisfied that the patient is suffering from a mental disorder' and correct procedure has been followed, affirms the detention order. If it is not satisfied, it shall 'revoke the order and direct that the patient be discharged from the approved centre concerned'. If the order is affirmed, it can be renewed by the consultant psychiatrist for defined periods, each renewal being subject to a further tribunal. Most importantly, there is no longer any provision for indefinite detention without automatic review, as there was under the Mental Treatment Act 1945.

In addition to reforming procedures governing involuntary admission, the Mental Health Act 2001 has also introduced a series of measures and regulations relating to child and adolescent psychiatry, consent to treatment (including psychosurgery), registration of 'approved centres', use of seclusion, appointment of clinical directors and instigation of civil proceedings in respect of the Act. The Act also outlines an extensive and expansive role for the Mental Health Commission, not only in appointing mental health tribunals but also in promoting high standards of care and regular inspection of all aspects mental health services. On this basis, the Mental

Health Commission is active in providing information and training to mental health service providers and service users, promoting research in mental health services and formulating regulations governing matters such as the use of seclusion and ECT.[109]

The introduction of the Mental Health Act 2001 was not without controversy.[110] While there was broad agreement on the need for new legislation, there was concern that it did not address several important areas, including the process of voluntary admission, involuntary treatment as an outpatient (which is still not permitted) and involuntary admission solely for assessment purposes (which is still not permitted).[111] There was particular concern about the resource implications of the new Act,[112] the timing and nature of tribunals,[113] and the Act's relationship with other legislative measures, such as the Criminal Law (Insanity) Bill 2002.[114]

Notwithstanding these concerns, the Act was implemented in full by 1 November 2006 and, in the first eleven months following implementation, 12 per cent of involuntary admission orders that were reviewed by mental health tribunals were revoked.[115] A review of the operation of the Act was published in 2007 and highlighted considerable progress, but also concerns, relating to involuntary admissions procedures (especially for children), timing of mental health tribunals, procedures for the detention of voluntary patients and matters related to treatment (e.g. ECT, medication).[116] In 2011, when a substantive review of the legislation was launched, the government emphasised the centrality of 'a human rights-based approach to mental health legislation'.[117] In 2012, the Interim Report of the Steering Group on the Review of the Mental Health Act 2001 duly confirmed that a 'rights-based approach to mental health law should be adopted' in any revisions to the legislation.[118]

CONCLUSIONS: THE FATE OF THE 'CRIMINALLY INSANE'

This book has taken the story of mental health services in Ireland from the early 1800s to the reforms of the early decades of the current millennium. This slow, painful evolution reflected myriad, diverse factors, including reform of mental health legislation, changes in asylum administrative practices, diagnostic and therapeutic advances, and, possibly, demographic and/or biological changes affecting the incidence of illness. All of these factors emerged and were interpreted within a specific societal context in Ireland, commonly involving social disadvantage or even famine, which had significant and arguably decisive effects on the experiences of the mentally ill and direction of change.

The apparent increase in incidence of mental disorder, in the late 1800s in particular, occurred in close temporal intimacy with a dramatic increase in availability of asylum beds which was, in turn, related to growing societal pressure on administrative authorities to increase resources for the mentally ill. This was related to both changes in psychiatric practice throughout Europe and a significant increase in general enthusiasm for social reform throughout the 1800s. It was then societal and political factors, such as decreased public tolerance for untreated mental disorder, which largely determined the direction of mental health service development in Ireland from the start of the nineteenth century onward. In the words of the nineteenth-century German pathologist, Rudolf Virchow: 'Medicine is a social science, and politics is nothing but medicine on a large scale.'[119]

Many of the reforms to mental health services over this period, however, centred on Ireland's district mental hospitals where the impact of changing committal laws and the therapeutic enthusiasms of psychiatrists were most notably apparent. How did these changes impact on individuals in the Central Criminal Lunatic Asylum? Did the institutional experiences of the 'criminally insane', such as those whose case histories feature in this book, improve significantly over this period?

The case histories presented here range from the 1800s to the early 1900s, and demonstrate the consistently high levels of psychiatric, medical, social, economic and legal challenges that the population faced over this time. Systematic reform of the broader asylum system, however, did provide an important context for reforms that saw the Central Criminal Lunatic Asylum transformed into today's Central Mental Hospital and National Forensic Psychiatry Service. The most dramatic legal change occurred with the Criminal Law (Insanity) Act 2006, which replaced the 'guilty but insane' verdict with 'not guilty by reason of insanity', and provided for the concept of 'diminished responsibility' in murder cases, among other reforms.[120] Today, the National Forensic Psychiatry Service is a deeply reformed service, highly progressive by national and international standards, with specialised, multi-disciplinary inpatient treatment, award-winning prison in-reach services,[121] and a comprehensive research programme.[122]

Despite such service-level reforms, however, certain society-level problems which were common in the 1800s and 1900s still persist today in relation to mentally ill offenders in Ireland and abroad. Both mental disorder and offending behaviour are still strongly associated with lower socioeconomic status and individuals in lower socioeconomic groups are still more likely to be incarcerated for offending behaviour.[123] Individuals with mental disorder remain more likely to be taken into custody following an offence, compared to individuals without mental disorder.[124] Most worryingly, rates of mental disorder in prison remain remarkably high, consistent with the clinical records of the 1800s and 1900s examined throughout this book: today, almost 4 per cent of prisoners have a psychotic mental disorder (i.e. serious mental illness) and over 10 per cent have major depression.[125] Finally, admission to forensic psychiatric facilities still shows a strong socioeconomic gradient,[126] just as it did in the 1800s and 1900s.

Resolving these concerns is likely to be a complex matter, as the history of mental health services over past centuries indicates that systemic reform is both challenging and slow. Against this background, the anonymous psychiatrist writing in *The Bell* in 1944 had words of advice that remain relevant for clinicians, administrators and reformers today, especially as they seek to balance the need for treatment and the public's expectation of safety, with the individual's right to liberty:

> If psychology has a great lesson for the average citizen – that of accepting necessary restrictions – it has also a very important one for the governors and reformers: for the one – Do not restrict more than is necessary; and for the other – Hasten slowly.[127]

In this important, complex area, reform is a continuous process that needs to meticulously planned and resolutely performed, in order to meet, as best as possible, the myriad needs of the troubled population.

Notes

Foreword

1   Hacking, Ian, *The Emergence of Probability* (Cambridge: Cambridge University Press, 1975); Hacking, Ian, *The Taming of Chance* (Cambridge: Cambridge University Press, 1990)

2   Finnane, M., *Insanity and the Insane in Post Famine Ireland* (London: Croom Helm, 1981) p 136; Walsh, D. & A. Daly, *Irish Psychiatric Hospitals and Units Census 2001*, (Dublin: Health Research Board, 2002); D. Brennan, 'A Theoretical Exploration of Institution-based Mental Health Care in Ireland' in Pauline M. Prior (ed), *Asylums, Mental Health Care and the Irish 1800-2010* (Dublin: Irish Academic Press, 2012)

3   Cannon M., P.B. Jones, R.M. Murray, 'Obstetric Complications and Schizophrenia: Historical and Meta-Analytical Review' *American Journal of Psychiatry* (2002; 159: 1080-1092)

4   Synge, John M., 'The People of the Glens' in *Wicklow and West Kerry* (Dublin and London: Maunsel & Company Ltd, 1912) pp 29-30.

5   Prunty, Jacinta, *Dublin Slums 1800-1925: A Study in Urban Geography* (Dublin: Irish Academic Press, 1998)

6   Clare Hickman, *Therapeutic Landscapes: A History of English Hospital Gardens since 1800* (Manchester: Manchester University Press, 2013)

7   Kirkbride, Thomas S., *On the Construction, Organization and General Arrangements of Hospitals for the Insane, with some Remarks on Insanity and its Treatment* (second edn) (Philadelphia: Lippincott & Co., 1880)

8   Bancroft, J.P., 'The Bearing of Hospital Adjustments Upon the Efficiency of Remedial and Ameliorating Treatment in Mental Diseases' in Henry C. Burdett, *Hospitals and Asylums of the World. Vol 2* (London: JA Churchill, 1891) pp 265-277

9 Kirkbride, *op cit.*

10 *The Irish Times* Obituary: Psychiatrist who revolutionised care of mentally ill (28 December 2013)

11 Walsh, Dermot, 'Mental Health Services in Ireland 1959-2010' pp 74-102 in Pauline M. Prior (ed), *Asylums, Mental Health Care and the Irish 1800-2010* (Dublin: Irish Academic Press, 2012)

12 Ministry of Health, *Special Hospitals: Report of a Working Party* (Emery Report) (London: HMSO, 1961)

13 Home Office & Department of Health and Social Security, *Report of the Committee on Mentally Abnormal Offenders* Cmnd. 6244 (London: HMSO, 1975)

14 Department of Health & Home Office, R*eview of Health and Social Services for Mentally Disordered Offenders and others Requiring Similar Services* Cmnd. 2088 (London: HMSO, 1995)

15 Fazel, S. & K. Seewald, 'Severe Mental Illness in 33,588 Prisoners Worldwide: Systematic Review and Meta-Regression Analysis' *British Journal of Psychiatry* (2012; 200: 364-373)

16 Kelly, B.D., 'Penrose's Law in Ireland: An Ecological Analysis of Psychiatric Inpatients and Prisoners' *Irish Medical Journal* (2007; 100: 373-4)

17 Curtin, K., S. Monks, B. Wright, D. Duffy, S. Linehan & H.G. Kennedy, 'Psychiatric Morbidity in 615 Male Remanded and Sentenced Committals to Irish Prisons' *Irish Journal of Psychological Medicine* (2009; 26: 169-173)

18 Commission on relief of the Sick and Destitute Poor, *Commission on Relief of the Sick and Destitute Poor including the Insane Poor, appointed on the 19ʰ March 1925* (Dublin: Stationery Office, 1926) www.lenus.ie/hse/ handle/10147/238535

19 Department of Health, *Report of the Commission of Inquiry on Mental Illness* (Dublin: Stationary Office, 1966)

20 Department of Health, *Planning for the Future* (Dublin: Stationary Office, 1984)

21 Department of Health, *Vision for Change* (Dublin: Stationary Office, 2006)

22 Brennan, D. 'A Theoretical Exploration of Institution-based Mental Health Care in Ireland' in Pauline M. Prior (ed), A*sylums, Mental Health Care and the Irish 1800-2010* (Dublin, Irish Academic Press 2012)

23 Winterwerp – v – The Netherlands, [1979-80] 2 EHRR 387; [1979] 6301/73; ECHR 4; [1981] ECHR 7; X – v – United Kingdom [1981] 7215 / 75 ECHR 6; [1982] ECHR 8

24 Walsh, D., E. O'Shea, 'Delivery of Psychiatric Care to those Mentally Ill in Ireland: Proposals for Change' *Journal for Statistical and Social Inquiry Society of Ireland* (1989; 25: 147-161). www.tara.tcd.ie/ bitstream/2262/7298/1/jssisiVolXXV147_161.pdf

25 O'Neill, C., H. Sinclair, A. Kelly, H.G. Kennedy, 'Interaction of Forensic and General Psychiatric Services in Ireland: Learning the Lessons or Repeating the Mistakes?' *Irish Journal of Psychological Medicine* (2002; 19(2): 48-54)

26 Morganroth, E., 'Buchanan Report' in B. Lalor (ed), *The Encyclopedia of Ireland* (Gill & MacMillan, Dublin 2003)

27 Department of Public Expenditure and Reform, *Third Report of the Organisational Review Programme* (Dublin: Stationary Office, January 2012). http://per.gov.ie/wp-content/uploads/ORP-Third-Report.pdf; RTÉ News, 'Decentralisation Damaged Civil Service: Report', www.rte.ie/news/2012/0126/311538-decentralisation/; RTÉ News, 'More Decentralised Offices to be Closed', 16 February 2012. www.rte.ie/news/2012/0215/312398-decentralisation/

28 Norris v. Ireland (Application no. 10581/83). European Court of Human Rights, 26 October 1988; *Norris v. A.G.* [1983] IESC 3, [1984] IR 36 (22 April 1983).

29 Criminal Law (Sexual Offences) Act, 1993 Irish Statute Book.

30 Garvin, T., *Preventing the Future: Why was Ireland so Poor for so Long?* (Gill & MacMillan Dublin 2004)

31 Croke – v – Ireland 33267/96 (2000) ECHR 680. www.bailii.org/eu/cases/ECHR/2000/680.html

32 Council of Europe Committee for the Prevention of Torture and Inhuman or Degrading Treatment or Punishment: visits to Ireland, www.cpt.coe.int/en/states/irl.htm

33 Commission on Relief of the Sick and Destitute Poor, *op cit.* at par. 411, p100.

34 European Commission Health and Consumer Protection Directorate-General, Green Paper: Improving the Mental Health of the Population: Towards a Strategy on Mental Health for the European Union. Brussels 14.10.2005. COM(2005)484 http://ec.europa.eu/health/archive/ph_determinants/life_style/mental/green_paper/mental_gp_en.pdf; http://ec.europa.eu/health/mental_health/policy/index_en.htm

35 Curtin et al, op cit

36 Giblin, Y., A. Kelly, E. Kelly, H.G. Kennedy, D.J. Mohan, Reducing the Use of Seclusion for Mental Disorder in a Prison: Implementing a High Support Unit in a Prison Using Participant Action Research' *International Journal of Mental Health Systems* (2012; 6:2. doi:10.1186/1752-4458-6-2)

37 McInerney, C., M. Davoren, G. Flynn, D. Mullins, M. Fitzpatrick, M. Caddow, F. Caddow, S. Quigley, F. Black, H.G. Kennedy & C. O'Neill, 'Implementing a Court Diversion and Liaison Scheme in a Remand Prison by Systematic Screening of New Receptions: a 6 Year Participatory Action Research Study of 20,084 Consecutive

Male Remands' *International Journal of Mental Health Systems* (2013; 7:18 doi:10.1186/1752-4458-7-18)

38 Kennedy, H.G., 'Therapeutic Uses of Security: Mapping Forensic Mental Health Services by Stratifying Risk' *Advances in Psychiatric Treatment* (2002; 8: 433-443)

Introduction

1   Kelly, B.D., 'Criminal Insanity in Nineteenth-Century Ireland, Europe and the United States: Cases, Contexts and Controversies', *International Journal of Law and Psychiatry* (2009; 32: 362–8)

2   Kelly, B.D., 'Intellectual Disability, Mental Illness and Offending Behaviour: Forensic Cases from Early Twentieth-Century Ireland', *Irish Journal of Medical Science* (2010; 179: 409–16)

3   Walsh, O., 'Gender and Insanity in Nineteenth-Century Ireland', *Clio Medica* (2004; 73: 69–93)

4   See also: Prior, P.M., *Madness and Gender: Gender, Crime and Mental Disorder in Nineteenth-Century Ireland* (Dublin and Portland, Oregon: Irish Academic Press, 2008)

5   Stone, J., K. O'Shea, S. Roberts, J. O'Grady and A. Taylor (eds), *Faulk's Basic Forensic Psychiatry* (3rd edition) (Oxford: Blackwell Sciences, 2000). Part of this chapter is from: Kelly, B.D. 'Poverty, Crime and Mental Illness: Female Forensic Psychiatric Committal in Ireland, 1910–1948', *Social History of Medicine* (2008; 21: 311–28)

6   Croudace, T.J., R. Kayne, P.B. Jones and G.L. Harrison, 'Non-Linear Relationship Between an Index of Social Deprivation, Psychiatric Admission, Prevalence and the Incidence of Psychosis', *Psychological Medicine* (2000; 30: 177–85)

7   Taylor, P.J. and J. Gunn, 'Violence and Psychosis, I: Risk of Violence Among Psychotic Men', *British Medical Journal (Clinical Research Edition)* (1984; 288: 1945–49); Teplin, L.A., 'Criminalizing Mental Disorder: The Comparative Arrest Rate of the Mentally Ill', *American Psychologist* (1984; 39: 794–803)

8   Fazel, S. and J. Danesh, 'Serious Mental Disorder in 23,000 Prisoners: A Systematic Review of 62 Surveys', *The Lancet* (2002; 359: 545–50); Duffy, D., S. Linehan and H.G. Kennedy, 'Psychiatric Morbidity in the Male Sentenced Irish Prisons Population', *Irish Journal of Psychological Medicine* (2006; 23: 54–62)

9   O'Neill, C., H. Sinclair, A. Kelly and H. Kennedy, 'Interaction of Forensic and General Psychiatric Services in Ireland: Learning the Lessons or Repeating the Mistakes?', *Irish Journal of Psychological Medicine* (2002; 19: 48–54)

10 Scull, A., *The Most Solitary of Afflictions: Madness and Society in Britain, 1700–1900* (New Haven and London: Yale University Press, 1993); Shorter,

E., *A History of Psychiatry: From the Era of the Asylum to the Age of Prozac* (New York: John Wiley & Sons, 1997); Kelly, B.D., 'Structural Violence and Schizophrenia', *Social Science and Medicine* (2005; 61: 721–30); Kelly, B.D., 'The Power Gap: Freedom, Power and Mental Illness', *Social Science and Medicine* (2006; 63: 2118–28)

11 Condrau, F., 'The Patient's View Meets the Clinical Gaze', *Social History of Medicine* (2007; 20: 525–40; p. 525)

12 Inspectors of Lunatics, *The Forty-Second Report (With Appendices) of the Inspector of Lunatics (Ireland)* (Dublin: Thom & Co. for Her Majesty's Stationary Office, 1893)

13 Kelly, B.D., 'Mental Health Law in Ireland, 1945 to 2000: Reformation and Renewal?', *Medical-Legal Journal* (2008; 76: 65–72)

1. Mental Health Care in Nineteenth-Century Ireland

1 Torrey, E.F. and J. Miller, *The Invisible Plague: The Rise of Mental Illness from 1750 to the Present* (New Brunswick, New Jersey: Rutgers University Press, 2001); Psychiatrist, 'Insanity in Ireland', *The Bell* (1944; 7: 303–10)

2 Kelly, B.D., 'Dr William Saunders Hallaran and Psychiatric Practice in Nineteenth-Century Ireland', *Irish Journal of Medical Science* (2008; 177: 79–84)

3 Kelly, B.D., 'Mental Illness in Nineteenth Century Ireland: A Qualitative Study of Workhouse Records', *Irish Journal of Medical Science* (2004; 173: 53–5)

4 Robins, J., *Fools and Mad: A History of the Insane in Ireland* (Dublin: Institute of Public Administration, 1986)

5 Quoted in Shorter, E., *A History of Psychiatry: From the Era of the Asylum to the Age of Prozac* (New York: John Wiley & Sons, 1997); pp. 1–2

6 Porter, R., *Madness: A Brief History* (Oxford: Oxford University Press, 2002)

7 Stone, M.H., *Healing the Mind: A History of Psychiatry from Antiquity to the Present* (London: Pimlico, 1998)

8 Robins, J., *Fools and Mad: A History of the Insane in Ireland* (Dublin: Institute of Public Administration, 1986); Williamson, A.P., 'Psychiatry, Moral Management and the Origins of Social Policy for Mentally Ill People in Ireland', *Irish Journal of Medical Science* (1992; 161: 556–8); Shorter, E., *A History of Psychiatry: From the Era of the Asylum to the Age of Prozac* (New York: John Wiley & Sons, 1997)

9 Reynolds, J., *Grangegorman: Psychiatric Care in Dublin since 1815* (Dublin: Institute of Public Administration in association with Eastern Health Board, 1992)

10 Esquirol, J-É., *Des Passions* (Paris: Didot Jeune, 1805)

11 Carlson, E.T. and N. Dain, 'The Psychotherapy that was Moral Treatment', *American Journal of Psychiatry* (1960; 117: 519–24)

12 Kelly, B.D., 'Dr William Saunders Hallaran and Psychiatric Practice
    in Nineteenth-Century Ireland', *Irish Journal of Medical Science*
    (2008; 177: 79–84)

13 Kelly, B.D., 'Dr William Saunders Hallaran and Psychiatric Practice
    in Nineteenth-Century Ireland', *Irish Journal of Medical Science*
    (2008; 177: 79–84)

14 Hallaran, W.S., *An Enquiry into the Causes Producing the Extraordinary
    Addition to the Number of Insane together with Extended Observations on the
    Cure of Insanity with Hints as to the Better Management of Public Asylums
    for Insane Persons* (Cork: Edwards and Savage, 1810)

15 Hunter, R. and I. Macalpine, *Three Hundred Years of Psychiatry, 1535–1860:
    A History Presented in Selected English Texts* (London: Oxford University
    Press, 1963) pp. 648–55; Laffey, P., 'Two Registers of Madness in
    Enlightenment Britain. Part 2', *History of Psychiatry* (2003; 14: 63–81)

16 Stone, M.H., *Healing the Mind: A History of Psychiatry from Antiquity to
    the Present* (London: Pimlico, 1998)

17 Prestwich, P.E., 'Family Strategies and Medical Power: "Voluntary"
    Committal in a Parisian Asylum, 1876–1914' in R. Porter and D. Wright
    (eds), *The Confinement of the Insane: International Perspectives, 1800–1965*
    (Cambridge: Cambridge University Press, 2003) pp. 79–99

18 Dörries, A. and T. Beddies, 'The Wittenauer Heilstätten in Berlin:
    A Case Record Study of Psychiatric Patients in Germany, 1919–1960'
    in R. Porter and D. Wright (eds), *The Confinement of the Insane:
    International Perspectives, 1800–1965* (Cambridge: Cambridge University
    Press, 2003) pp. 149–172

19 Hallaran, W.S., *Practical Observations on the Causes and Cures of Insanity*
    (2nd edition) (Cork: Edwards and Savage, 1818); Fleetwood, J.F.,
    The History of Medicine in Ireland (2nd edition) (Dublin: Skellig Press, 1983)

20 Torrey, E.F. and J. Miller, *The Invisible Plague: The Rise of Mental Illness
    from 1750 to the Present* (New Brunswick, New Jersey: Rutgers University
    Press, 2001)

21 Malcolm, E., *Swift's Hospital: A History of St Patrick's Hospital, Dublin,
    1746–1989* (Dublin: Gill and Macmillan, 1989)

22 Finnane, M., *Insanity and the Insane in Post-Famine Ireland* (London:
    Croon Helm, 1981); Robins, J., *Fools and Mad: A History of the Insane
    in Ireland* (Dublin: Institute of Public Administration, 1986)

23 Tuke, D.H., 'Increase of Insanity in Ireland', *Journal of Mental Science*
    (1894; 40: 549–58)

24 Kelly, B.D., 'Mental Illness in Nineteenth Century Ireland:
    A Qualitative Study of Workhouse Records', *Irish Journal of Medical
    Science* (2004; 173: 53–5)

25 Inspector of Lunatics (Ireland), *The Forty-Second Report (With
    Appendices) of the Inspector of Lunatics (Ireland)* (Dublin: Thom & Co./
    Her Majesty's Stationery Office, 1893); Prior, P., 'Dangerous Lunacy:

The Misuse of Mental Health Law in Nineteenth-Century Ireland',
Journal of Forensic Psychiatry and Psychology (2003; 14: 525–541)

26 Smith, C., 'The Central Mental Hospital, Dundrum, Dublin' in
R. Bluglass and P. Bowden (eds), *Principles and Practice of Forensic
Psychiatry* (Edinburgh: Churchill Livingstone, 1990) pp. 1351–3

27 Torrey, E.F. and J. Miller, *The Invisible Plague: The Rise of Mental Illness
from 1750 to the Present* (New Brunswick, New Jersey: Rutgers University
Press, 2001)

28 Reynolds, J., *Grangegorman: Psychiatric Care in Dublin since 1815*
(Dublin: Institute of Public Administration in association with Eastern
Health Board, 1992)

29 Williamson, A.P., 'Psychiatry, Moral Management and the Origins
of Social Policy for Mentally Ill People in Ireland', *Irish Journal of
Medical Science* (1992; 161: 556–8); Reuber, M., 'The Architecture of
Psychological Management: The Irish Asylums (1801–1922)', *Psychological
Medicine* (1996; 26: 1179–89); Walsh, D., 'Mental Illness in Ireland and its
Management' in D. McCluskey (ed.), *Health Policy and Practice in Ireland*
(Dublin: University College Dublin Press, 2006) pp. 29–43

30 World Health Organization, *The ICD-Classification of Mental and
Behavioural Disorders* (Geneva: World Health Organization, 1992)

31 Appleby, L., 'Suicide and Self-Harm' in R. Murray, P. Hill and P.
McGuffin (eds), *The Essentials of Postgraduate Psychiatry* (3rd edition)
(Cambridge: Cambridge University Press, 1997) pp. 551–62

32 Kerridge, I.H. and M. Lowe, 'Bloodletting: The Story of a Therapeutic
Technique', *Medical Journal of Australia* (1995; 163: 631–33)

33 Millon, T., *Masters of the Mind: Exploring the Story of Mental Illness from
Ancient Times to the New Millennium* (Hoboken, New Jersey: John Wiley
& Sons, 2004)

34 Stone, M.H., *Healing the Mind: A History of Psychiatry from Antiquity to
the Present* (London: Pimlico, 1998)

35 Farmar, T., *Patients, Potions and Physicians: A Social History of Medicine in
Ireland* (Dublin: A & A Farmar in association with the Royal College of
Physicians of Ireland, 2004)

36 Tuomy, M., *Treatise on the Principal Diseases of Dublin* (Dublin: William
Folds, 1810)

37 Stone, M.H., *Healing the Mind: A History of Psychiatry from Antiquity to
the Present* (London: Pimlico, 1998)

38 Farmar, T., *Patients, Potions and Physicians: A Social History of Medicine in
Ireland* (Dublin: A & A Farmar in association with the Royal College of
Physicians of Ireland, 2004)

39 Stone, M.H., *Healing the Mind: A History of Psychiatry from Antiquity to
the Present* (London: Pimlico, 1998)

40 Millon, T., *Masters of the Mind: Exploring the Story of Mental Illness from
Ancient Times to the New Millennium* (Hoboken, New Jersey: John Wiley

& Sons, 2004); Stone, M.H., *Healing the Mind: A History of Psychiatry from Antiquity to the Present* (London: Pimlico, 1998)

41 Tuomy, M., *Treatise on the Principal Diseases of Dublin* (Dublin: William Folds, 1810); Farmar, T., *Patients, Potions and Physicians: A Social History of Medicine in Ireland* (Dublin: A & A Farmar in association with the Royal College of Physicians of Ireland, 2004)

42 Stone, M.H., *Healing the Mind: A History of Psychiatry from Antiquity to the Present* (London: Pimlico, 1998); Porter, R., *Madmen: A Social History of Madhouses, Mad-Doctors and Lunatics* (Gloucestershire, UK: Tempus Publishing, 2004)

43 Cox, J.M., *Practical Observations on Insanity* (London: Baldwin and Murray, 1804)

44 Wade, N.J., U. Norrsell and A. Presly, 'Cox's Chair: A Moral and a Medical Mean in the Treatment of Maniacs', *History of Psychiatry* (2005; 16: 73–88)

45 Wade, N.J., 'The Original Spin Doctors – The Meeting of Perception and Insanity', *Perception* (2005; 34: 253–60)

46 Torrey, E.F. and J. Miller, *The Invisible Plague: The Rise of Mental Illness from 1750 to the Present* (New Brunswick, New Jersey: Rutgers University Press, 2001); Wade, N.J., U. Norrsell and A. Presly, 'Cox's Chair: A Moral and a Medical Mean in the Treatment of Maniacs', *History of Psychiatry* (2005; 16: 73–88)

47 United Nations, *Principles for the Protection of Persons with Mental Illness and the Improvement of Mental Health Care* (New York: United Nations, Secretariat Centre For Human Rights, 1991)

48 Scull, A., *The Most Solitary of Afflictions: Madness and Society in Britain, 1700–1900* (New Haven and London: Yale University Press, 1993); Shorter, E., *A History of Psychiatry: From the Era of the Asylum to the Age of Prozac* (New York: John Wiley & Sons, 1997); Porter, R., *Madness: A Brief History* (Oxford: Oxford University Press, 2002)

49 Cox, J.M., *Practical Observations on Insanity* (London: Baldwin and Murray, 1804)

50 Kelly, B.D., 'Mental Health and Human Rights: Challenges for a New Millennium', *Irish Journal of Psychological Medicine* (2001; 18: 114–5)

51 Farmar, T., *Patients, Potions and Physicians: A Social History of Medicine in Ireland* (Dublin: A & A Farmar in association with the Royal College of Physicians of Ireland, 2004)

52 Leonard, E.C. Jr, 'Did some 18th and 19th Century Treatments for Mental Disorders Act on the Brain?', *Medical Hypotheses* (2004; 62: 219–21)

53 Breckenridge, A., 'William Withering's Legacy – For the Good of the Patient', *Clinical Medicine* (2006; 6: 393–97)

54 Farmar, T., *Patients, Potions and Physicians: A Social History of Medicine in Ireland* (Dublin: A & A Farmar in association with the Royal College of Physicians of Ireland, 2004)

55 Weber, M.M. and H.M. Emrich, 'Current and Historical Concepts of Opiate Treatment in Psychiatric Disorders', *International Journal of Clinical Psychopharmacology* (1988; 3: 255–66)

56 Sneader, W., 'The Prehistory of Psychotherapeutic Agents', *Journal of Psychopharmacology* (1990; 4: 115–9)

57 Shorter, E., *A History of Psychiatry: From the Era of the Asylum to the Age of Prozac* (New York: John Wiley & Sons, 1997)

58 Guthrie, D., *A History of Medicine* (London: Nelson, 1945); Fleetwood, J.F., *The History of Medicine in Ireland* (2nd edition) (Dublin: Skellig Press, 1983); Farmar, T., *Patients, Potions and Physicians: A Social History of Medicine in Ireland* (Dublin: A & A Farmar in association with the Royal College of Physicians of Ireland, 2004)

59 Merrit, H.H., R. Adams and H.C. Solomon, *Neurosyphilis* (Oxford: Oxford University Press, 1946); Brown, E.M., 'Why Wagner-Jauregg Won the Nobel Prize for Discovering Malaria Therapy for General Paralysis of the Insane', *History of Psychiatry* (2000; 11: 371–82)

60 Waugh, M.A., 'Alfred Fournier, 1832–1914: His Influence on Venereology', *British Journal of Venereal Disease* (1974; 50: 232–6)

61 Shorter, E., *A History of Psychiatry: From the Era of the Asylum to the Age of Prozac* (New York: John Wiley & Sons, 1997)

62 Williamson, A.P., 'Psychiatry, Moral Management and the Origins of Social Policy for Mentally Ill People in Ireland', *Irish Journal of Medical Science* (1992; 161: 556–58); McCarthy, A., 'Hearths, Bodies and Minds: Gender Ideology and Women's Committal to Enniscorthy Lunatic Asylum, 1916–1925' in A. Hayes and D. Urguhart (eds), *Irish Women's History* (Dublin and Portland: Irish Academic Press, 2004) pp. 115–36; Prior, P., 'Prisoner or Lunatic? The Official Debate on the Criminal Lunatic in Nineteenth-Century Ireland', *History of Psychiatry* (2004; 15: 177–92)

63 Reuber, M., 'The Architecture of Psychological Management: The Irish Asylums (1801–1922)', *Psychological Medicine* (1996; 26: 1179–89); Reuber, M., 'Moral Management and the "Unseen Eye": Public Lunatic Asylums in Ireland, 1800–1845' in E. Malcolm and G. Jones (eds), *Medicine, Disease and the State in Ireland, 1650–1940* (Cork: Cork University Press, 1999) pp. 208–33

64 Gabbard, G.O. and J. Kay, 'The Fate of Integrated Treatment: Whatever Happened to the Biopsychosocial Psychiatrist?', *American Journal of Psychiatry* (2001; 158: 1956–63); Kelly, B.D., 'Mental Health Law in Ireland, 1945 to 2001: Reformation and Renewal?' *Medico-Legal Journal* (2008; 76: 65–72)

65 Kelly, B.D., 'Mental Illness in Nineteenth Century Ireland: A Qualitative Study of Workhouse Records', *Irish Journal of Medical Science* (2004; 173: 53–55)

66 Kennedy, L., P.S. Ell, E.M. Crawford and L.A. Clarkson, *Mapping the Great Irish Famine* (Dublin: Four Courts Press Ltd, 1999)

67 Mokyr, J., *Why Ireland Starved: A Quantitative and Analytical History of the Irish Economy, 1800–1850* (London: Unwin Hyman, 1985)

68 Reuber, M., 'The Architecture of Psychological Management: The Irish Asylums (1801–1922)', *Psychological Medicine* (1996; 26: 1179–89)

69 Robins, J., *Fools and Mad: A History of the Insane in Ireland* (Dublin: Institute of Public Administration, 1986)

70 Kelly, B.D., 'Mental Illness in Nineteenth Century Ireland: A Qualitative Study of Workhouse Records', *Irish Journal of Medical Science* (2004; 173: 53–5). In this paper, original workhouse records and minutes uncovered from the Ballinrobe Poor Law Union, County Mayo, Ireland were examined so as to extract all information relevant to the provision of health care and accommodation to the mentally ill in Ireland between 1845 and 1900.

71 Stone, M., *Healing the Mind: A History of Psychiatry from Antiquity to the Present* (London: Pimico, 1998)

72 Robins, J., *Fools and Mad: A History of the Insane in Ireland* (Dublin: Institute of Public Administration, 1986)

73 Clare, A.W., 'St Patrick's Hospital', *American Journal of Psychiatry* (1998; 155: 1599); Clare, A.W., 'Swift, Mental Illness and St Patrick's Hospital', *Irish Journal of Psychological Medicine* (1998; 15: 100–4)

74 Williamson, A.P., 'Psychiatry, Moral Management and the Origins of Social Policy for Mentally Ill People in Ireland', *Irish Journal of Medical Science* (1992; 161: 556–8)

75 Reuber, M., 'The Architecture of Psychological Management: The Irish Asylums (1801–1922)', *Psychological Medicine* (1996; 26: 1179–89)

76 Kennedy, L., P.S. Ell, E.M. Crawford and L.A. Clarkson, *Mapping the Great Irish Famine* (Dublin: Four Courts Press Ltd, 1999)

77 Finnane, M., *Insanity and the Insane in Post-Famine Ireland* (London: Croon Helm, 1981); Torrey, E.F. and J. Miller, *The Invisible Plague: The Rise of Mental Illness from 1750 to the Present* (New Brunswick, New Jersey: Rutgers University Press, 2001); Walsh, D., 'The Ennis District Lunatic Asylum and the Clare Workhouse Lunatic Asylums in 1901', *Irish Journal of Psychological Medicine* (2010; 26: 206–11)

78 George, S.L., N.J. Shanks and L. Westlake, 'Census of Single Homeless People in Sheffield', *British Medical Journal* (1991; 302: 1387–9); Holohan, T.W., 'Health and Homelessness in Dublin', (Irish Medical Journal 2000; 93: 41–3)

79 World Health Organisation, *The World Health Report 2001: Mental Health: New Understanding, New Hope* (Geneva: World Health Organisation, 2001)

2. Creating the Asylums and the Insanity Defence

1 Kelly, B.D., 'Mental Health Law in Ireland, 1945 to 2001: Reformation and Renewal?' *Medico-Legal Journal* (2008; 76: 65–72)

2 Psychiatrist, 'Insanity in Ireland', *The Bell* (1944; 7: 303–10)

3 Shorter, E., .*A History of Psychiatry: From the Era of the Asylum to the Age of Prozac* (New York: John Wiley & Sons, 1997)

4 Malcolm, E., *Swift's Hospital: A History of St Patrick's Hospital, Dublin, 1746–1989* (Dublin: Gill and Macmillan, 1989)

5 Finnane, M., *Insanity and the Insane in Post-Famine Ireland* (London: Croon Helm, 1981)

6 Williamson, A., 'The Beginnings of State Care for the Mentally Ill in Ireland', *Economic and Social Review* (1970; 10: 281–90)

7 Williamson, A., 'The Beginnings of State Care for the Mentally Ill in Ireland', *Economic and Social Review* (1970; 10: 281–90)

8 Tuke, D.H., 'Increase of Insanity in Ireland', *Journal of Mental Science* (1894; 40: 549–58); Smith, C., 'The Central Mental Hospital, Dundrum, Dublin' in R. Bluglass and P. Bowden (eds), *Principles and Practice of Forensic Psychiatry* (Edinburgh: Churchill Livingstone, 1990) pp. 1351–3; Torrey, E.F. and J. Miller, *The Invisible Plague: The Rise of Mental Illness from 1750 to the Present* (New Brunswick, New Jersey: Rutgers University Press, 2001); Prior, P., 'Dangerous Lunacy: The Misuse of Mental Health Law in Nineteenth-Century Ireland', *Journal of Forensic Psychiatry and Psychology* (2003; 14: 525–41); Kelly, B.D., 'Mental Illness in Nineteenth Century Ireland: A Qualitative Study of Workhouse Records', *Irish Journal of Medical Science* (2004; 173: 53–5)

9 O'Neill, A-M., *Irish Mental Health Law* (Dublin: First Law, 2005)

10 Jones, K., *Lunacy, Law and Conscience* (London: Routledge and Kegan Paul, 1955)

11 Reynolds, J., *Grangegorman: Psychiatric Care in Dublin since 1815* (Dublin: Institute of Public Administration in association with Eastern Health Board, 1992)

12 Kelly, B.D., 'One Hundred Years Ago: The Richmond Asylum, Dublin in 1907', *Irish Journal of Psychological Medicine* (2007; 24: 108–14)

13 O'Neill, A-M., *Irish Mental Health Law* (Dublin: First Law, 2005)

14 Esquirol, J-É., *Des Passions* (Paris: DidotJeune, 1805)

15 Hallaran, W.S., *An Enquiry into the Causes Producing the Extraordinary Addition to the Number of Insane together with Extended Observations on the Cure of Insanity with Hints as to the Better Management of Public Asylums for Insane Persons* (Cork: Edwards and Savage, 1810); Kelly, B.D., 'Dr William Saunders Hallaran and Psychiatric Practice in Nineteenth-Century Ireland', *Irish Journal of Medical Science* (2008; 177: 79–84)

16 Reuber, M., 'The Architecture of Psychological Management: The Irish Asylums (1801–1922)', *Psychological Medicine* (1996; 26: 1179–89); Reuber, M., 'Moral Management and the "Unseen Eye": Public Lunatic Asylums in Ireland, 1800–1845' in E. Malcolm and G. Jones (eds), *Medicine, Disease and the State in Ireland, 1650–1940* (Cork: Cork University Press, 1999) pp. 208–33; Reynolds, J., *Grangegorman: Psychiatric Care in Dublin since 1815*

(Dublin: Institute of Public Administration in association with Eastern
Health Board, 1992); Williamson, A.P., 'Psychiatry, Moral Management
and the Origins of Social Policy for Mentally Ill People in Ireland', *Irish
Journal of Medical Science* (1992; 161: 556–8)

17 Williamson, A., 'The Beginnings of State Care for the Mentally Ill in
Ireland', *Economic and Social Review* (1970; 10: 281–90)

18 Robins, J., *Fools and Mad: A History of the Insane in Ireland*
(Dublin: Institute of Public Administration, 1986)

19 Williamson, A., 'The Beginnings of State Care for the Mentally Ill in
Ireland', *Economic and Social Review* (1970; 10: 281–90)

20 Williamson, A.P., 'Psychiatry, Moral Management and the Origins of
Social Policy for Mentally Ill People in Ireland', *Irish Journal of Medical
Science* (1992; 161: 556–8)

21 Reuber, M., 'The Architecture of Psychological Management: The Irish
Asylums (1801–1922)', *Psychological Medicine* (1996; 26: 1179–89)

22 Inspector of Lunatics (Ireland), *The Forty-Second Report (With
Appendices) of the Inspector of Lunatics (Ireland)* (Dublin: Thom & Co./Her
Majesty's Stationery Office, 1893)

23 O'Neill, A-M., *Irish Mental Health Law* (Dublin: First Law, 2005)

24 Smith, C., 'The Central Mental Hospital, Dundrum, Dublin' in
R. Bluglass and P. Bowden (eds), *Principles and Practice of Forensic
Psychiatry* (Edinburgh: Churchill Livingstone, 1990) pp. 1351–3

25 Gibbons, P., N. Mulryan and A. O'Connor, 'Guilty but Insane:
The Insanity Defence in Ireland, 1850–1995', *British Journal of Psychiatry*
(1997; 170: 467–72); Mulryan, N., P. Gibbons and A. O'Connor,
'Infanticide and Child Murder – Admissions to the Central Mental
Hospital, 1850–2000', *Irish Journal of Psychological Medicine* (2002; 19: 8–12)

26 Kelly, B.D., 'One Hundred Years Ago: The Richmond Asylum, Dublin
in 1907', *Irish Journal of Psychological Medicine* (2007; 24: 108–14); Kelly,
B.D., 'Tuberculosis in the Nineteenth-Century Asylum: Clinical Cases
from the Central Criminal Lunatic Asylum, Dundrum, Dublin' in
P. Prior (ed.), *Asylums, Mental Health Care and the Irish, 1800–2010*
(Dublin and Portland, Oregon: Irish Academic Press, 2012) pp. 205–20

27 Robins, J., *Fools and Mad: A History of the Insane in Ireland*
(Dublin: Institute of Public Administration, 1986)

28 Wright, D., J.E. Moran and S. Gouglas, 'The Confinement of the Insane
in Victorian Canada: The Hamilton and Toronto Asylums, *c.* 1861–1891'
in R. Porter and D. Wright (eds), *The Confinement of the Insane:
International Perspectives, 1800–1965* (Cambridge: Cambridge University
Press, 2003) pp. 100–28

29 Coleborne, C., 'Passage to the Asylum: The Role of the Police in
Committals of the Insane in Victoria, Australia, 1848–1900' in R. Porter
and D. Wright (eds), *The Confinement of the Insane: International
Perspectives, 1800–1965* (Cambridge: Cambridge University Press, 2003)

pp. 129–48

30 Gasser, J. and G. Heller, 'The Confinement of the Insane in Switzerland,
     1900–1970: Cery (Vaud) and Bel-Air (Geneva) Asylums' in R. Porter
     and D. Wright (eds), *The Confinement of the Insane: International
     Perspectives, 1800–1965* (Cambridge: Cambridge University Press, 2003)
     pp. 54–78

31 Prestwich, P.E., 'Family Strategies and Medical Power: "Voluntary"
     Committal in a Parisian Asylum, 1876–1914' in R. Porter and D. Wright
     (eds), *The Confinement of the Insane: International Perspectives, 1800–1965*
     (Cambridge: Cambridge University Press, 2003) pp. 79–99

32 Prior, P., 'Dangerous Lunacy: The Misuse of Mental Health Law in
     Nineteenth-Century Ireland', *Journal of Forensic Psychiatry and Psychology*
     (2003; 14: 525–41)

33 Dillon, W., 'Law Adviser's Report on the Liability of the Joint
     Committee of Management of the Richmond District Asylum
     to Maintain Lunatics Sent from Workhouses and as to their
     Powers to Erect and Maintain Auxiliary Asylums for Harmless
     and Chronic Lunatics' in *Richmond Asylum Joint Committee Minutes*
     (Dublin: Richmond Asylum, 1907)

34 Kelly, B.D., 'One Hundred Years Ago: The Richmond Asylum, Dublin in
     1907', *Irish Journal of Psychological Medicine* (2007; 24: 108–14)

35 Norman, C., 'Report of Dr Norman' in *Richmond Asylum Joint
     Committee Minutes* (Dublin: Richmond Asylum, 1907)

36 Robins, J., *Fools and Mad: A History of the Insane in Ireland*
     (Dublin: Institute of Public Administration, 1986)

37 Inspector of Lunatics (Ireland). *The Forty-Second Report (With
     Appendices) of the Inspector of Lunatics (Ireland)* (Dublin: Thom and Co./
     Her Majesty's Stationery Office, 1893)

38 O'Neill, A-M., *Irish Mental Health Law* (Dublin: First Law, 2005)

39 Williamson, A.P., 'Psychiatry, Moral Management and the Origins of
     Social Policy for Mentally Ill People in Ireland', *Irish Journal of Medical
     Science* (1992; 161: 556–8)

40 Hallaran, W.S., *An Enquiry into the Causes Producing the Extraordinary
     Addition to the Number of Insane together with Extended Observations on the
     Cure of Insanity with Hints as to the Better Management of Public Asylums
     for Insane Persons* (Cork: Edwards and Savage, 1810); Kelly, B.D., 'Dr
     William Saunders Hallaran and Psychiatric Practice in Nineteenth-
     Century Ireland', *Irish Journal of Medical Science* (2008; 177: 79–84)

41 Shorter, E., *A History of Psychiatry: From the Era of the Asylum to the Age
     of Prozac* (New York: John Wiley & Sons, 1997)

42 Thorne, M.L., 'Colonizing the New World of NHS Management:
     The Shifting Power of Professionals. Health Services Management
     Research' (2002; 15, 14–26); Connolly, M. and N. Jones, 'Constructing
     Management Practice in the New Public Management: The Case

of Mental Health Managers', *Health Services Management Research*
(2003; 16: 203–10); Tempest, M., *The Future of the NHS* (Hertfordshire:
XPL Publishing, 2006)

43 Anonymous, 'Increase in insanity', *American Journal of Insanity* (1861; 18: 95);
Tuke, D.H., 'Increase of Insanity in Ireland', *Journal of Mental Science*
(1894; 40: 549–58); Smith, C., 'The Central Mental Hospital, Dundrum,
Dublin' in R. Bluglass and P. Bowden (eds), *Principles and Practice of Forensic
Psychiatry* (Edinburgh: Churchill Livingstone, 1990) pp. 1351–3; Torrey,
E.F. and J. Miller, *The Invisible Plague: The Rise of Mental Illness from 1750 to
the Present* (New Brunswick, New Jersey: Rutgers University Press, 2001)

44 Healy, D., 'Irish Psychiatry in the Twentieth Century' in H. Freeman
and G.E. Berrios (eds), *150 Years of British Psychiatry. Volume II:
The Aftermath* (London: Athlone Press, 1996) pp. 268–91

45 Hallaran, W.S., *An Enquiry into the Causes Producing the Extraordinary
Addition to the Number of Insane together with Extended Observations on the
Cure of Insanity with Hints as to the Better Management of Public Asylums
for Insane Persons* (Cork: Edwards and Savage, 1810) p. 10

46 Inspector of Lunatics (Ireland), *The Forty-Second Report (With
Appendices) of the Inspector of Lunatics (Ireland)* (Dublin: Thom and Co./
Her Majesty's Stationery Office, 1893)

47 Tuke, D.H., 'Increase of Insanity in Ireland', *Journal of Mental Science*
(1894; 40: 549–58)

48 Anonymous, 'Increase in Insanity', *American Journal of Insanity* (1861; 18:
95); Torrey, E.F. and J. Miller, *The Invisible Plague: The Rise of Mental Illness
from 1750 to the Present* (New Brunswick, New Jersey: Rutgers University
Press, 2001)

49 Walsh, D., 'The Ups and Downs of Schizophrenia in Ireland', *Irish
Journal of Psychiatry* (1992; 13: 12–6)

50 Shorter, E., *A History of Psychiatry: From the Era of the Asylum to the Age
of Prozac* (New York: John Wiley & Sons, 1997)

51 Jones, K., *Lunacy, Law and Conscience* (London: Routledge and Kegan
Paul, 1955); Torrey, E.F. and J. Miller, *The Invisible Plague: The Rise of
Mental Illness from 1750 to the Present* (New Brunswick, New Jersey:
Rutgers University Press, 2001)

52 O'Neill, A-M., *Irish Mental Health Law* (Dublin: First Law, 2005)

53 Reynolds, J., *Grangegorman: Psychiatric Care in Dublin since 1815*
(Dublin: Institute of Public Administration in association with Eastern
Health Board, 1992)

54 Hallaran, W.S., *An Enquiry into the Causes Producing the Extraordinary
Addition to the Number of Insane together with Extended Observations on the
Cure of Insanity with Hints as to the Better Management of Public Asylums
for Insane Persons* (Cork: Edwards and Savage, 1810)

55 Walsh, D., 'The Ups and Downs of Schizophrenia in Ireland', *Irish
Journal of Psychiatry* (1992; 13: 12–6)

56 Tuke, D.H., 'Increase of Insanity in Ireland', *Journal of Mental Science*
    (1894; 40: 549–58)

57 Williamson, A., 'The Beginnings of State Care for the Mentally Ill in
    Ireland', *Economic and Social Review* (1970; 10: 281–90)

58 Walsh, D., 'The Ups and Downs of Schizophrenia in Ireland', *Irish
    Journal of Psychiatry* (1992; 13: 12–6)

59 Inspector of Lunatics (Ireland), *The Forty-Second Report (With
    Appendices) of the Inspector of Lunatics (Ireland)* (Dublin: Thom and Co./
    Her Majesty's Stationery Office, 1893)

60 Prior, P., 'Dangerous Lunacy: The Misuse of Mental Health Law in
    Nineteenth-Century Ireland', *Journal of Forensic Psychiatry and Psychology*
    (2003; 14: 525–41)

61 Walsh, D., 'The Ups and Downs of Schizophrenia in Ireland',
    Irish Journal of Psychiatry (1992; 13: 12–6)

62 Walsh, O., 'Gender and Insanity in Nineteenth-Century Ireland',
    Clio Medica (2004; 73: 69–93)

63 Jones, G., 'The Campaign Against Tuberculosis in Ireland, 1899–1914' in
    E. Malcolm and G. Jones (eds), *Medicine, Disease and the State in Ireland,
    1650–1940* (Cork: Cork University Press, 1999) pp. 158–76

64 McCandless, P., 'Curative Asylum, Custodial Hospital: The South
    Carolina Lunatic Asylum and State Hospital, 1828–1920' in R. Porter
    and D. Wright (eds), *The Confinement of the Insane: International Perspectives,
    1800–1965* (Cambridge: Cambridge University Press, 2003) pp. 173–92

65 Walsh, D., 'The Ups and Downs of Schizophrenia in Ireland', *Irish
    Journal of Psychiatry* (1992; 13: 12–6)

66 Mulryan, N., P. Gibbons and A. O'Connor, 'Infanticide and Child
    Murder – Admissions to the Central Mental Hospital, 1850–2000', *Irish
    Journal of Psychological Medicine* (2002; 19: 8–12)

67 Walsh, D., 'The Ups and Downs of Schizophrenia in Ireland', *Irish
    Journal of Psychiatry* (1992; 13: 12–6)

68 Inspector of Lunatics (Ireland), *The Forty-Second Report (With Appendices)
    of the Inspector of Lunatics (Ireland)* (Dublin: Thom and Co./Her Majesty's
    Stationery Office, 1893)

69 Powell, R., 'Observations upon the Comparative Prevalence of Insanity
    at Different Periods', *Medical Transactions* (1813; 4: 131–59)

70 Walsh, D., 'The Ups and Downs of Schizophrenia in Ireland', *Irish
    Journal of Psychiatry* (1992; 13: 12–6)

71 Torrey, E.F. and J. Miller, *The Invisible Plague: The Rise of Mental Illness
    from 1750 to the Present* (New Brunswick, New Jersey: Rutgers University
    Press, 2001)

72 Torrey, E.F. and J. Miller, *The Invisible Plague: The Rise of Mental
    Illness from 1750 to the Present* (New Brunswick, New Jersey: Rutgers
    University Press, 2001)

73 Healy, D., 'Irish Psychiatry in the Twentieth Century' in H. Freeman

and G.E. Berrios (eds), *150 Years of British Psychiatry. Volume II: The Aftermath* (London: Athlone Press, 1996) pp. 268–91

74   Hallaran, W.S., *An Enquiry into the Causes Producing the Extraordinary Addition to the Number of Insane together with Extended Observations on the Cure of Insanity with Hints as to the Better Management of Public Asylums for Insane Persons* (Cork: Edwards and Savage, 1810)

75   Norman, C., 'Report of Dr Norman' in *Richmond Asylum Joint Committee Minutes* (Dublin: Richmond Asylum, 1907)

76   Walsh, D. and A. Daly, *Mental Illness in Ireland 1750–2002: Reflections on the Rise and Fall of Institutional Care* (Dublin: Health Research Board, 2004)

77   O'Neill, A-M., *Irish Mental Health Law* (Dublin: First Law, 2005)

78   Boyd, Barrett, E., 'Modern Psycho-Therapy and our Asylums', *Studies* (1924; 8: 29–43)

79   O'Neill, A-M., *Irish Mental Health Law* (Dublin: First Law, 2005)

80   Gasser, J. and G. Heller, 'The Confinement of the Insane in Switzerland, 1900–1970: Cery (Vaud) and Bel-Air (Geneva) Asylums' in R. Porter and D. Wright (eds), *The Confinement of the Insane: International Perspectives, 1800–1965* (Cambridge: Cambridge University Press, 2003) pp. 54–78

81   Prestwich, P.E., 'Family Strategies and Medical Power: "Voluntary" Committal in a Parisian Asylum, 1876–1914' in R. Porter and D. Wright (eds), *The Confinement of the Insane: International Perspectives, 1800–1965* (Cambridge: Cambridge University Press, 2003) pp. 79–99

82   Reynolds, J., *Grangegorman: Psychiatric Care in Dublin since 1815* (Dublin: Institute of Public Administration in association with Eastern Health Board, 1992)

83   Williamson, A.P., 'Psychiatry, Moral Management and the Origins of Social Policy for Mentally Ill People in Ireland', *Irish Journal of Medical Science* (1992; 161: 556–8); Reuber, M., 'The Architecture of Psychological Management: The Irish Asylums (1801–1922)', *Psychological Medicine* (1996; 26: 1179–89); Walsh, D., 'Mental Illness in Ireland and its Management' in D. McCluskey (ed.) *Health Policy and Practice in Ireland* (Dublin: University College Dublin Press, 2006) pp. 29–43

84   Reynolds, J., *Grangegorman: Psychiatric Care in Dublin since 1815* (Dublin: Institute of Public Administration in association with Eastern Health Board, 1992)

85   Inspector of Lunatic Asylums in Ireland, *Report of the District, Local, and Private Lunatic Asylums in Ireland, 1846 (With Appendices)* (Dublin: Alexander Thom for Her Majesty's Stationery Office, 1847)

86   Robins, J., *Fools and Mad: A History of the Insane in Ireland* (Dublin: Institute of Public Administration, 1986); Kelly, B.D., 'Mental Health Law in Ireland, 1821–1902: Building the Asylums', *Medico-Legal Journal* (2008; 76: 19–25); Kelly, B.D., 'Mental Health Law in Ireland,

1821–1902: Dealing with the "Increase of Insanity in Ireland", *Medico-Legal Journal* (2008; 76: 26–33)

87 Inspector of Lunatics (Ireland), *The Forty-Second Report (With Appendices) of the Inspector of Lunatics (Ireland)* (Dublin: Thom and Co./ Her Majesty's Stationery Office, 1893)

88 *Ibid*, p. 9

89 The 1907 volume of 'Richmond Asylum Joint Committee Minutes' contains minutes from the Richmond District Asylum 'Joint Committee' (referring to both Richmond and Portrane), the 'Richmond Visiting Committee' (referring to Richmond) and the 'Portrane Visiting Committee' (referring to Portrane). Despite their differing titles, these committees tended to be concerned with similar issues. The topics covered at the meeting of the Portrane Visiting Committee on 4 September 1907, for example, included reports from the medical superintendent, storekeeper, agricultural manager and engineer, as well as updates on water supply works, wages of engine drivers, recent correspondence and other general issues (pp. 411–418). Quotations from meeting minutes for all three committees are used throughout this chapter to illustrate relevant points.

90 Reynolds, J., *Grangegorman: Psychiatric Care in Dublin since 1815* (Dublin: Institute of Public Administration in association with Eastern Health Board, 1992)

91 Walsh, D. and A. Daly, *Mental Illness in Ireland 1750–2002: Reflections on the Rise and Fall of Institutional Care* (Dublin: Health Research Board, 2004)

92 Anonymous, 'Increase in insanity', *American Journal of Insanity* (1861; 18: 95); MacCabe, F., 'On the Alleged Increase in Lunacy', *Journal of Mental Science* (1869; 15: 363–6); Drapes, T., 'On the Alleged Increase in Insanity in Ireland', *Journal of Mental Science* (1894; 40: 519–43); Torrey, E.F. and J. Miller, *The Invisible Plague: The Rise of Mental Illness from 1750 to the Present* (New Brunswick, New Jersey: Rutgers University Press, 2001)

93 Hallaran, W.S., *An Enquiry into the Causes Producing the Extraordinary Addition to the Number of Insane together with Extended Observations on the Cure of Insanity with Hints as to the Better Management of Public Asylums for Insane Persons* (Cork: Edwards and Savage, 1810)

94 Tuke, D.H., 'Increase of Insanity in Ireland', *Journal of Mental Science* (1894; 40: 549–58)

95 Smith, C., 'The Central Mental Hospital, Dundrum, Dublin' in R. Bluglass and P. Bowden (eds), *Principles and Practice of Forensic Psychiatry* (Edinburgh: Churchill Livingstone, 1990) pp. 1351–3; Torrey, E.F. and J. Miller, *The Invisible Plague: The Rise of Mental Illness from 1750 to the Present* (New Brunswick, New Jersey: Rutgers University Press, 2001); Prior, P., 'Dangerous Lunacy: The Misuse of Mental Health Law in Nineteenth-Century Ireland', *Journal of Forensic Psychiatry and Psychology* (2003; 14: 525–41)

96 Inspectors of Lunatics (Ireland), 1893; p. 9.

97 Walsh, D. and A. Daly, *Mental Illness in Ireland 1750–2002: Reflections on the Rise and Fall of Institutional Care* (Dublin: Health Research Board, 2004); Kelly, B.D., 'Mental Illness in Nineteenth Century Ireland: A Qualitative Study of Workhouse Records', *Irish Journal of Medical Science* (2004; 173: 53–5)

98 Reynolds, J., *Grangegorman: Psychiatric Care in Dublin since 1815* (Dublin: Institute of Public Administration in association with Eastern Health Board, 1992)

99 St Brendan's Hospital (Richmond Asylum), Rathdown Road, Phibsborough, Dublin 7, Ireland, *Richmond Asylum Joint Committee Minutes, 1907*, pp. 206–7

100 Jones, G., 'The Campaign Against Tuberculosis in Ireland, 1899–1914' in E. Malcolm and G. Jones (eds), *Medicine, Disease and the State in Ireland, 1650–1940* (Cork: Cork University Press, 1999) pp. 158–76

101 Finnane, M., *Insanity and the Insane in Post-Famine Ireland* (London: Croon Helm, 1981).

102 McCandless, P., 'Curative Asylum, Custodial Hospital: The South Carolina Lunatic Asylum and State Hospital, 1828–1920' in R. Porter and D. Wright (eds), *The Confinement of the Insane: International Perspectives, 1800–1965* (Cambridge: Cambridge University Press, 2003) pp. 173–92

103 Cherry, S. and R. Munting, '"Exercise is the Thing"? Sport and the Asylum c.1850–1950', *International Journal of the History of Sport* (2005; 22: 42–58)

104 Walsh, D., 'The Ennis District Lunatic Asylum and the Clare Workhouse Lunatic Asylums in 1901', *Irish Journal of Psychological Medicine* (2010; 26: 206–11)

105 Tuke, D.H., 'Increase of Insanity in Ireland', *Journal of Mental Science* (1894; 40: 549–58)

106 Walsh, D. and A. Daly, *Mental Illness in Ireland 1750–2002: Reflections on the Rise and Fall of Institutional Care* (Dublin: Health Research Board, 2004)

107 Kelly, B.D., 'Mental Illness in Nineteenth Century Ireland: A Qualitative Study of Workhouse Records', *Irish Journal of Medical Science* (2004; 173: 53–5)

108 Walsh, D. and A. Daly, *Mental Illness in Ireland 1750–2002: Reflections on the Rise and Fall of Institutional Care* (Dublin: Health Research Board, 2004)

109 McCauley, M., S. Rooney, C. Clarke, T. Carey and J. Owens, 'Home-Based Treatment in Monaghan: The First Two Years', *Irish Journal of Psychological Medicine* (2003; 20: 11–4)

110 Holohan, T.W., 'Health and Homelessness in Dublin', *Irish Medical Journal* (2000; 93: 41–3); Teesson, M., T. Hodder and N. Buhrich, 'Psychiatric Disorders in Homeless Men and Women in Inner Sydney', *Australian and New Zealand Journal of Psychiatry* (2004; 38: 162–8)

111 Ritson, E.B., J.D. Chick and I. Strang, 'Dependence on Alcohol and Other Drugs' in R.E. Kendell and A.K. Zealley (eds), *Companion to Psychiatric Studies* (5th edition) (Edinburgh: Churchill Livingstone, 1996) pp. 359–96

112 Inspector of Mental Health Services, *Report of the Inspector of Mental Health Services 2004* (Dublin: Mental Health Commission, 2005); Kelly, B.D., 'Mental Health Need among the Intellectually Disabled', *Irish Journal of Medical Science* (2013; 182: 359)

113 Kelly, B.D., 'Criminal Insanity in Nineteenth-Century Ireland, Europe and the United States: Cases, Contexts and Controversies', *International Journal of Law and Psychiatry* (2009; 32: 362–8); Robinson, D., *Wild Beasts and Idle Humors: The Insanity Defence from Antiquity to the Present* (Cambridge, Massachusetts: Harvard University Press, 1998).

114 Ray, I., *A Treatise on the Medical Jurisprudence of Insanity* [1838] [Reprint, W. Overholser (ed.)]. (Cambridge, Massachusetts: Harvard University Press, 1962); Quen, J.M., 'Isaac Ray: Have we Learned his Lessons?', *Bulletin of the American Academy of Psychiatry and the Law* (1974; 2: 137–47); Payne, H. and R. Luthe, 'Isaac Ray and Forensic Psychiatry in the United States', *Forensic Science International* (1980; 15: 115–27); Quen, J.M., 'Isaac Ray and the Development of American Psychiatry and the Law', *Psychiatric Clinics of North America* (1983; 6: 527–37); Hughes, J.S., 'Isaac Ray's "Project of a Law" and the 19th-Century Debate over Involuntary Commitment', *International Journal of Law and* Psychiatry (1986; 9: 191–200); Quen, J.M., 'Law and Psychiatry in America over the Past 150 years', *Hospital and Community Psychiatry* (1994; 45: 1005–10)

115 Ray, I., *A Treatise on the Medical Jurisprudence of Insanity* (3rd edition, with additions) (Cambridge, Massachusetts: Little, Brown and Company, 1853) pp. iiv–iv

116 Ray, I., *A Treatise on the Medical Jurisprudence of Insanity* (3rd edition, with additions) (Cambridge, Massachusetts: Little, Brown and Company, 1853) p. 2

117 Finnane, M., *Insanity and the Insane in Post-Famine Ireland* (London: Croon Helm, 1981); Prior, P., 'Dangerous Lunacy: The Misuse of Mental Health Law in Nineteenth-Century Ireland', *Journal of Forensic Psychiatry and Psychology* (2003; 14: 525–41); Prior, P., 'Prisoner or Lunatic? The Official Debate on the Criminal Lunatic in Nineteenth-Century Ireland', *History of Psychiatry* (2004; 15: 177–92)

118 Hallaran, W.S., *An Enquiry into the Causes Producing the Extraordinary Addition to the Number of Insane together with Extended Observations on the Cure of Insanity with Hints as to the Better Management of Public Asylums for Insane Persons* (Cork: Edwards and Savage, 1810) p. 10

119 Williamson, A., 'The Beginnings of State Care for the Mentally Ill in Ireland', *Economic and Social Review* (1970; 10: 281–90)

120 Ray, I., *A Treatise on the Medical Jurisprudence of Insanity* [1838] [Reprint,

W. Overholser (ed.),]. (Cambridge, Massachusetts: Harvard University Press, 1962)

121 O'Neill, A-M., *Irish Mental Health Law* (Dublin: First Law, 2005)

122 Prior, P., 'Dangerous Lunacy: The Misuse of Mental Health Law in Nineteenth-Century Ireland', *Journal of Forensic Psychiatry and Psychology* (2003; 14: 525–41)

123 Gasser, J. and G. Heller, 'The Confinement of the Insane in Switzerland, 1900–1970: Cery (Vaud) and Bel-Air (Geneva) Asylums' in R. Porter and D. Wright (eds), *The Confinement of the Insane: International Perspectives, 1800–1965* (Cambridge: Cambridge University Press, 2003) pp. 54–78

124 Prestwich, P.E., 'Family Strategies and Medical Power: "Voluntary" Committal in a Parisian Asylum, 1876–1914' in R. Porter and D. Wright (eds), *The Confinement of the Insane: International Perspectives, 1800–1965* (Cambridge: Cambridge University Press, 2003) pp. 79–99

125 Ray, I., 'Confinement of the Insane', *American Law Review* (1869; 3: 193–221)

126 Quen, J.M., 'Law and Psychiatry in America over the Past 150 years', *Hospital and Community Psychiatry* (1994; 45: 1005–10)

127 Carlson, E.T. and N. Dain, 'The Psychotherapy that was Moral Treatment', *American Journal of Psychiatry* (1960; 117: 519–24); Esquirol, J-É., *Des Passions* (Paris: DidotJeune, 1805); McCandless, P., 'Curative Asylum, Custodial Hospital: The South Carolina Lunatic Asylum and State Hospital, 1828–1920' in R. Porter and D. Wright (eds), *The Confinement of the Insane: International Perspectives, 1800–1965* (Cambridge: Cambridge University Press, 2003) pp. 173–92

128 Wright, D., J.E. Moran and S. Gouglas, 'The Confinement of the Insane in Victorian Canada: The Hamilton and Toronto Asylums, *c.*1861–1891' in R. Porter and D. Wright (eds), *The Confinement of the Insane: International Perspectives, 1800–1965* (Cambridge: Cambridge University Press, 2003) pp. 100–28

129 Torrey, E.F. and J. Miller, *The Invisible Plague: The Rise of Mental Illness from 1750 to the Present* (New Brunswick, New Jersey: Rutgers University Press, 2001)

130 Smith, C., 'The Central Mental Hospital, Dundrum, Dublin' in R. Bluglass and P. Bowden (eds), *Principles and Practice of Forensic Psychiatry* (Edinburgh: Churchill Livingstone, 1990) pp. 1351–3

131 Robinson, D., *Wild Beasts and Idle Humors: The Insanity Defence from Antiquity to the Present* (Cambridge, Massachusetts: Harvard University Press, 1998).

132 Moran, R., *Knowing Right from Wrong: The Insanity Defence of Daniel McNaughtan* (New York: Free Press, 1981)

133 Slovenko, R., *Psychiatry in Law / Law in Psychiatry* (New York: Routledge, 2002) p. 219

134 Ray, I., *A Treatise on the Medical Jurisprudence of Insanity* [1838] [Reprint, W. Overholser (ed.)] (Cambridge, Massachusetts: Harvard University

Press, 1962)

135 Quen, J.M., 'Law and Psychiatry in America over the Past 150 years',
    Hospital and Community Psychiatry (1994; 45: 1005–10)

136 McAuley, F., *Insanity, Psychiatry and Criminal Responsibility*
    (Dublin: Round Hall Press, 1993); Moran, R., *Knowing Right from Wrong:
    The Insanity Defence of Daniel McNaughtan* (New York: Free Press, 1981)

137 Spiegel, A.D., 'Abraham Lincoln and the Insanity Plea', *Journal of
    Community Health* (1994; 19: 201–20); Spiegel, A.D. and F. Kavaler,
    'A. Lincoln, Esquire Defends the Murderer of a Physician', *Journal of
    Community Health* (2005; 30: 309–24)

138 Watson, A.S., 'The Evolution of Legal Methods for Dealing with
    Mind-States in Crimes', *Bulletin of the American Academy of Psychiatry
    and the Law* (1992; 20: 211–20); White, R., 'The Trial of Abner
    Baker, Jr., MD: Monomania and McNaughtan Rules in Antebellum
    America', *Bulletin of the American Academy of Psychiatry and the Law*
    (1990; 18: 223–34); Spiegel, A.D. and M.B. Spiegel, 'The Insanity Plea
    in Early Nineteenth-Century America', *Journal of Community Health*
    (1998; 23: 227–47)

139 Spiegel, A.D. and F. Kavaler, 'The Differing Views on Insanity of Two
    Nineteenth-Century Forensic Psychiatrists', *Journal of Community
    Health* (2006; 31: 430–51)

140 Allan, C., 'Blame Game Players are Thoughtless and Ill-Informed',
    Guardian (2008, 6 February); Perr, I.N., 'The Insanity Defence: A Tale of
    Two Cities', *American Journal of Psychiatry* (1983; 140: 873–4)

141 More detailed considerations of the evolution of court practices and
    verdicts in this context are provided by: McAuley, F., *Insanity, Psychiatry
    and Criminal Responsibility* (Dublin: Round Hall Press, 1993); Gibbons, P.,
    N. Mulryan and A. O'Connor, 'Guilty but Insane: The Insanity Defence
    in Ireland, 1850–1995', *British Journal of Psychiatry* (1997; 170: 467–72)

142 Walsh, O., 'Gender and Insanity in Nineteenth-Century Ireland',
    Clio Medica (2004; 73: 69–93)

143 Gibbons, P., N. Mulryan and A. O'Connor, 'Guilty but Insane:
    The Insanity Defence in Ireland, 1850–1995', *British Journal of Psychiatry*
    (1997; 170: 467–72)

144 Mulryan, N., P. Gibbons and A. O'Connor, 'Infanticide and Child
    Murder – Admissions to the Central Mental Hospital, 1850–2000', *Irish
    Journal of Psychological Medicine* (2002; 19: 8–12)

145 Wright, D., J.E. Moran and S. Gouglas, 'The Confinement of the Insane
    in Victorian Canada: The Hamilton and Toronto Asylums, c.1861–1891'
    in R. Porter and D. Wright (eds), *The Confinement of the Insane:
    International Perspectives, 1800–1965* (Cambridge: Cambridge University
    Press, 2003) pp. 100–28

146 Gibbons, P., N. Mulryan and A. O'Connor, 'Guilty but Insane:
    The Insanity Defence in Ireland, 1850–1995', *British Journal of Psychiatry*

(1997; 170: 467–72)

147 Walsh, O., 'Gender and Insanity in Nineteenth-Century Ireland',
     Clio Medica (2004; 73: 69–93)

148 Deacon, H., 'Insanity, Institutions and Society: The Case of the
     Robben Island Lunatic Asylum, 1846–1910' in R. Porter and D. Wright
     (eds), *The Confinement of the Insane: International Perspectives, 1800–1965*
     (Cambridge: Cambridge University Press, 2003) pp. 20–53

149 Torrey, E.F. and J. Miller, *The Invisible Plague: The Rise of Mental Illness
     from 1750 to the Present* (New Brunswick, New Jersey: Rutgers University
     Press, 2001)

150 Hallaran, W.S. *An Enquiry into the Causes Producing the Extraordinary
     Addition to the Number of Insane together with Extended Observations on
     the Cure of Insanity with Hints as to the Better Management of Public
     Asylums for Insane Persons* (Cork: Edwards and Savage, 1810); Hallaran,
     W.S. *Practical Observations on the Causes and Cures of Insanity* (2nd
     edition) (Cork: Edwards and Savage, 1818)

151 Inspector of Lunatics (Ireland), *The Forty-Second Report (With
     Appendices) of the Inspector of Lunatics (Ireland)* (Dublin: Thom & Co./Her
     Majesty's Stationery Office, 1893)

152 Tuke, D.H., 'Increase of Insanity in Ireland', *Journal of Mental Science*
     (1894; 40, 549–58) p. 555

153 Healy, D., 'Irish Psychiatry in the Twentieth Century' in H. Freeman and
     G.E. Berrios (eds), *150 Years of British Psychiatry. Volume II: The Aftermath*
     (London: Athlone Press, 1996) pp. 268–91; Smith, C., 'The Central Mental
     Hospital, Dundrum, Dublin' in R. Bluglass and P. Bowden (eds), *Principles
     and Practice of Forensic Psychiatry* (Edinburgh: Churchill Livingstone, 1990)
     pp. 1351–3; Torrey, E.F. and J. Miller, *The Invisible Plague: The Rise of Mental
     Illness from 1750 to the Present* (New Brunswick, New Jersey: Rutgers
     University Press, 2001); Walsh, D., 'The Ups and Downs of Schizophrenia
     in Ireland', *Irish Journal of Psychiatry* (1992; 13: 12–6)

154 Gibbons, P., N. Mulryan and A. O'Connor, 'Guilty but Insane:
     The Insanity Defence in Ireland, 1850–1995', *British Journal of Psychiatry*
     (1997; 170: 467–72)

155 Kelly, B.D., 'One Hundred Years Ago: The Richmond Asylum, Dublin in
     1907', *Irish Journal of Psychological Medicine* (2007; 24: 108–14); McCandless,
     P., 'Curative Asylum, Custodial Hospital: The South Carolina Lunatic
     Asylum and State Hospital, 1828–1920' in R. Porter and D. Wright
     (eds), *The Confinement of the Insane: International Perspectives, 1800–1965*
     (Cambridge: Cambridge University Press, 2003) pp. 173–192

156 Inspector of Lunatics (Ireland), *The Forty-Second Report (With
     Appendices) of the Inspector of Lunatics (Ireland)* (Dublin: Thom & Co./Her
     Majesty's Stationery Office, 1893)

157 Deacon, H., 'Insanity, Institutions and Society: The Case of the
     Robben Island Lunatic Asylum, 1846–1910' in R. Porter and D. Wright

(eds), *The Confinement of the Insane: International Perspectives, 1800–1965* (Cambridge: Cambridge University Press, 2003) pp. 20–53; Gibbons, P., N. Mulryan and A. O'Connor, 'Guilty but Insane: The Insanity Defence in Ireland, 1850–1995', *British Journal of Psychiatry* (1997; 170: 467–72); Mulryan, N., P. Gibbons and A. O'Connor, 'Infanticide and Child Murder – Admissions to the Central Mental Hospital, 1850–2000', *Irish Journal of Psychological Medicine* (2002; 19: 8–12); Walsh, O., 'Gender and Insanity in Nineteenth-Century Ireland', *Clio Medica* (2004; 73: 69–93); Wright, D., J.E. Moran and S. Gouglas, 'The Confinement of the Insane in Victorian Canada: The Hamilton and Toronto Asylums, c.1861–1891' in R. Porter and D. Wright (eds), *The Confinement of the Insane: International Perspectives, 1800–1965* (Cambridge: Cambridge University Press, 2003) pp. 100–28

158 Jones, G., 'The Campaign Against Tuberculosis in Ireland, 1899–1914' in E. Malcolm and G. Jones (eds), *Medicine, Disease and the State in Ireland, 1650–1940* (Cork: Cork University Press, 1999) pp. 158–76

159 Finnane, M., *Insanity and the Insane in Post-Famine Ireland* (London: Croon Helm, 1981); Kelly, B.D., 'One Hundred Years Ago: The Richmond Asylum, Dublin in 1907', *Irish Journal of Psychological Medicine* (2007; 24: 108–14)

160 McCandless, P., 'Curative Asylum, Custodial Hospital: The South Carolina Lunatic Asylum and State Hospital, 1828–1920' in R. Porter and D. Wright (eds), *The Confinement of the Insane: International Perspectives, 1800–1965* (Cambridge: Cambridge University Press, 2003) pp. 173–92

161 Jones, G., 'The Campaign Against Tuberculosis in Ireland, 1899–1914' in E. Malcolm and G. Jones (eds), *Medicine, Disease and the State in Ireland, 1650–1940* (Cork: Cork University Press, 1999) pp. 158–76

162 Lyons, F.S.L., *Ireland Since the Famine* (London: Fontana, 1985)

163 Breathnach, C.S. and J.B. Moynihan, 'An Irish Statistician's Analysis of the National Tuberculosis Problem – Robert Charles Geary (1896–1983)', *Irish Journal of Medical Science* (2003; 172: 149–53)

164 Inspector of Lunatics (Ireland), *The Forty-Second Report (With Appendices) of the Inspector of Lunatics (Ireland)* (Dublin: Thom & Co./Her Majesty's Stationery Office, 1893)

165 Inspector of Lunatics (Ireland), *The Forty-Second Report (With Appendices) of the Inspector of Lunatics (Ireland)* (Dublin: Thom & Co./Her Majesty's Stationery Office, 1893) p. 6

166 Inspector of Lunatics (Ireland), *The Forty-Second Report (With Appendices) of the Inspector of Lunatics (Ireland)* (Dublin: Thom & Co./Her Majesty's Stationery Office, 1893); Kelly, B.D., 'One Hundred Years Ago: The Richmond Asylum, Dublin in 1907', *Irish Journal of Psychological Medicine* (2007; 24: 108–114)

167 McCandless, P., 'Curative Asylum, Custodial Hospital: The South Carolina Lunatic Asylum and State Hospital, 1828–1920' in R. Porter

and D. Wright (eds), *The Confinement of the Insane: International Perspectives,*
1800–1965 (Cambridge: Cambridge University Press, 2003) pp. 173–192

168   Wright, D., J.E. Moran and S. Gouglas, 'The Confinement of the Insane
in Victorian Canada: The Hamilton and Toronto Asylums, *c.* 1861–1891'
in R. Porter and D. Wright (eds), *The Confinement of the Insane:*
International Perspectives, 1800–1965 (Cambridge: Cambridge University
Press, 2003) pp. 100–28

169   Gibbons, P., N. Mulryan and A. O'Connor, 'Guilty but Insane:
The Insanity Defence in Ireland, 1850–1995', *British Journal of Psychiatry*
(1997; 170: 467–72)

170   Mulryan, N., P. Gibbons and A. O'Connor, 'Infanticide and Child
Murder – Admissions to the Central Mental Hospital, 1850–2000', *Irish*
Journal of Psychological Medicine (2002; 19: 8–12)

171   McCarthy, A., 'Hearths, Bodies and Minds: Gender Ideology and Women's
Committal to Enniscorthy Lunatic Asylum, 1916–1925' in A. Hayes
and D. Urguhart (eds), *Irish Women's History* (Dublin and Portland:
Irish Academic Press, 2004) pp. 115–36; Prior, P., 'Murder and Madness:
Gender and the Insanity Defence in Nineteenth-Century Ireland',
New Hibernia Review (2005; 9: 19–36); Prior, P., 'Roasting a Man
Alive: The Case of Mary Reilly, Criminal Lunatic', *Éire-Ireland* (2006;
41: 169–91); Walsh, O., '"A Lightness of Mind": Gender and Insanity
in Nineteenth-Century Ireland' in M. Kelleher and J.H. Murphy
(eds), *Gender Perspectives in 19th Century Ireland: Public and Private*
Spheres (Dublin: Irish Academic Press, 1997) pp. 159–67; Walsh, O.,
'"The Designs of Providence": Race, Religion and Irish Insanity'
in J. Melling and B. Forsythe (eds), *Insanity Institutions and Society,*
1800–1914: A Social History of Madness in Comparative Perspective (London
and New York: Routledge, 1999) pp. 223–42; Walsh, O., 'Gender and
Insanity in Nineteenth-Century Ireland', *Clio Medica* (2004; 73: 69–93)

172   Gibbons, P., N. Mulryan and A. O'Connor, 'Guilty but Insane:
The Insanity Defence in Ireland, 1850–1995', *British Journal of Psychiatry*
(1997; 170: 467–72); Kelly, B.D., 'Clinical and Social Characteristics of
Women Committed to Inpatient Forensic Psychiatric Care in Ireland,
1868–1908', *Journal of Forensic Psychiatry and Psychology* (2008; 19: 261–73);
Mulryan, N., P. Gibbons and A. O'Connor, 'Infanticide and Child
Murder – Admissions to the Central Mental Hospital, 1850–2000', *Irish*
Journal of Psychological Medicine (2002; 19: 8–12)

173   Kelly, B.D., 'Clinical and Social Characteristics of Women Committed
to Inpatient Forensic Psychiatric Care in Ireland, 1868–1908', *Journal of*
Forensic Psychiatry and Psychology (2008; 19: 261–73)

174   More detailed considerations of infanticide in its societal, medical and
judicial contexts are provided in: Guilbride, A., 'Infanticide: The Crime
of Motherhood' in P. Kennedy (ed.), *Motherhood in Ireland* (Cork: Mercier
Press, 2004) pp. 170–80; Kelly, B.D., 'Murder, Mercury and Mental Illness:

Infanticide in Nineteenth-Century Ireland', *Irish Journal of Medical Science*
(2007; 176: 149–52); Kelly, B.D., 'Clinical and Social Characteristics of
Women Committed to Inpatient Forensic Psychiatric Care in Ireland,
1868–1908', *Journal of Forensic Psychiatry and Psychology* (2008; 19: 261–73);
Marland, H., *Dangerous Motherhood: Insanity and Childbirth in Victorian
Britain* (Basingstoke: Palgrave MacMillan, 2004)

175   Churchill, F., 'On the Mental Disorders of Pregnancy and Childbed',
Dublin Quarterly Journal of Medical Science (1850; 17: 39)

176   Maudsley, H., 'Homicidal Insanity', *Journal of Mental Science* (1863; 47:
327–43)

177   Meehan, E. and K. MacRae, 'Legal Implications of Premenstrual
Syndrome: A Canadian Perspective', *Canadian Medical Association Journal*
(1986; 135: 601–8); Spiegel, A.D., 'Temporary Insanity and Premenstrual
Syndrome: Medical Testimony in an 1865 Murder Trial', *New York State
Journal of Medicine* (1988; 88: 482–92)

178   Spiegel, A.D. and M.B. Spiegel, 'Was it Murder or Insanity? Reactions
to a Successful Paroxysmal Insanity Plea in 1865', *Women and Health*
(1992; 18: 69–86)

179   Ray, I., *A Treatise on the Medical Jurisprudence of Insanity* (3rd edition,
with additions) (Cambridge, Massachusetts: Little, Brown and Company,
1853) p. 198

180   Marland, H., *Dangerous Motherhood: Insanity and Childbirth in Victorian
Britain* (Basingstoke: Palgrave MacMillan, 2004)

181   Friedman, S.H., S.M. Horowitz and P.J. Resnick, 'Child Murder by
Mothers: A Critical Analysis of the Current State of Knowledge and
a Research Agenda', *American Journal of Psychiatry* (2005;162: 1578–87);
Putkonen, H., J. Collander, M.L. Honkaslo and J. Lonnqvist, 'Finnish
Female Homicide Offenders, 1982–1992', *Journal of Forensic Psychiatry*
(1998; 9: 672–84); Schwartz L.L., N.K. Isser, *Endangered Children:
Neonaticide, Infanticide and Filicide* (Pacific Institute Series on Forensic
Psychology) (Boca Raton, FL: CRC Press Inc., 2000)

182   Allan, C., 'Blame Game Players are Thoughtless and Ill-Informed',
Guardian (6 February 2008)

183   Perr, I.N., 'The Insanity Defence: A Tale of Two Cities' *American Journal
of Psychiatry* 1983; 140: 873–4

184   Quen, J.M., 'Law and Psychiatry in America over the Past 150 years',
Hospital and Community Psychiatry (1994; 45: 1005–10)

185   Mulryan, N., P. Gibbons and A. O'Connor, 'Infanticide and Child
Murder – Admissions to the Central Mental Hospital, 1850–2000', *Irish
Journal of Psychological Medicine* (2002; 19: 8–12)

186   Amnesty International, *Amnesty International Report 2006: The State of the
World's Human Rights* (London: Amnesty International UK, 2006)

187   Edemariam, A., 'I'm Ready', Guardian (20 September, 2006)

188   Cunningham, M.D. & M.P. Vigen, 'Death Row Inmate Characteristics,

Adjustment, and Confinement: A Critical Review of the Literature',
Behavioural Sciences and the Law (2002; 20: 191-210); Lewis D.O., J.H.
Pincus, M. Feldman, L. Jackson & B. Bard, 'Psychiatric, Neurological,
and Psychoeducational Characteristics of 15 Death Row Inmates in the
United States' *American Journal of Psychiatry* (1986; 143: 838-45)

189   Foley S.R., B.D. Kelly, 'Psychological Concomitants of Capital
Punishment: Thematic Analysis of Last Statements from Death Row',
American Journal of Forensic Psychiatry (2007; 28: 7-13); Kelly, B.D. & S.R.
Foley, 'The Price of Life', *British Medical Journal* (2007; 335: 938); Kelly,
B.D. & S.R. Foley, 'Love, Spirituality and Regret: Thematic Analysis
of Last Statements from Death Row, Texas (2006–2011)' *International
Journal of Psychiatry and Law* (2013; 41: 540–50).

190   Friedman, S.H., S.M. Horowitz and P.J. Resnick, 'Child Murder by
Mothers: A Critical Analysis of the Current State of Knowledge
and a Research Agenda', *American Journal of Psychiatry* (2005;162:
1578–87); Putkonen, H., J. Collander, M.L. Honkaslo and
J. Lonnqvist, 'Finnish Female Homicide Offenders, 1982–1992',
Journal of Forensic Psychiatry (1998; 9: 672–84); Schwartz, L.L. and
N.K. Isser, *Endangered Children: Neonaticide, Infanticide and Filicide
(Pacific Institute Series on Forensic Psychology)* (Boca Raton, FL:
CRC Press Inc., 2000)

191   Benedek, E.P., 'Premenstrual Syndrome: A View from the Bench',
Journal of Clinical Psychiatry (1988; 49: 498–502)

192   Downs, L.L., 'PMS, Psychosis and Culpability: Sound or Misguided
Defence?', *Journal of Forensic Sciences* (2002; 47: 1083–9)

193   Meehan, E. and K. MacRae, 'Legal Implications of Premenstrual
Syndrome: A Canadian Perspective', *Canadian Medical Association Journal*
(1986; 135: 601–8)

194   Meehan, E. and K. MacRae, 'Legal Implications of Premenstrual
Syndrome: A Canadian Perspective', *Canadian Medical Association Journal*
(1986; 135: 601–8)

3. Women in the Central Criminal Lunatic Asylum, Dublin, 1868-1948

1   Chapter 3 uses material from: Kelly, B.D., 'Murder, Mercury and
Mental Illness: Infanticide in Nineteenth-Century Ireland', *Irish Journal
of Medical Science* (2007; 176: 149–52); Kelly, B.D., 'Clinical and Social
Characteristics of Women Committed to Inpatient Forensic Psychiatric
Care in Ireland, 1868–1908', *Journal of Forensic Psychiatry and Psychology*
(2008; 19: 261–73); Kelly, B.D., 'Poverty, Crime and Mental Illness:
Female Forensic Psychiatric Committal in Ireland, 1910–1948', *Social
History of Medicine* (2008; 21: 311–28)

2   Pearsall, J. and B. Trumble, *The Oxford English Reference Dictionary* (2nd
Edition) (Oxford and New York: Oxford University Press, 1996)

3 Jackson, M. (ed.). *Infanticide: Historical Perspectives on Child Murder and Concealment, 1550–2000* (Hampshire, England: Ashgate, 2002)

4 Schwartz, L.L. and N.K. Isser, *Endangered Children: Neonaticide, Infanticide and Filicide (Pacific Institute Series on Forensic Psychology)* (Boca Raton, FL: CRC Press Inc., 2000)

5 This case is drawn from: Kelly, B.D., 'Murder, Mercury and Mental Illness: Infanticide in Nineteenth-Century Ireland', *Irish Journal of Medical Science* (2007; 176: 149–52). The case is based on original archival material from the Central Criminal Lunatic Asylum (Central Mental Hospital), Dublin. In order to maintain patient confidentiality, the woman whose case is described is referred to as 'Dora' (not her real name).

6 Resnick, P., 'Murder of the Newborn: A Psychiatric Review of Neonaticide', *American Journal of Psychiatry* (1970; 126: 1414–20); Finkelhor, D., 'The Homicides of Children and Youth: A Developmental Perspective' in G.K. Kantor and J.L. Jasinski (eds), *Out of the Darkness: Contemporary Perspectives on Family Violence* (Thousand Oaks, CA: Sage Publications, 1997) pp. 17–34; Hesketh, T. and W.X. Zhu, 'The One Child Family Policy: The Good, the Bad, and the Ugly', *British Medical Journal* (1997; 314: 1685–7); Wu, Z., K. Viisainen, Y. Wang and E. Hemminki, 'Perinatal Mortality in Rural China: A Retrospective Cohort Study', *British Medical Journal* (2003; 327: 1319); Hesketh, T., L. Lu and Z.W. Xing, 'The Effect of China's One-Child Family Policy after 25 Years', *New England Journal of Medicine* (2005; 353: 1171–6)

7 Mulryan, N., P. Gibbons and A. O'Connor, 'Infanticide and Child Murder – Admissions to the Central Mental Hospital, 1850–2000', *Irish Journal of Psychological Medicine* (2002; 19: 8–12)

8 Finkelhor, D., 'The Homicides of Children and Youth: A Developmental Perspective' in G.K. Kantor and J.L. Jasinski (eds), *Out of the Darkness: Contemporary Perspectives on Family Violence* (Thousand Oaks, CA: Sage Publications, 1997) pp. 17–34

9 Guilbride, A., 'Infanticide: The Crime of Motherhood' in P. Kennedy (ed.), *Motherhood in Ireland* (Cork: Mercier Press, 2004) pp. 170–80

10 Friedman, S.H., S.M. Horowitz and P.J. Resnick, 'Child Murder by Mothers: A Critical Analysis of the Current State of Knowledge and a Research Agenda', *American Journal of Psychiatry* (2005; 162: 1578–87)

11 Smith, C., 'The Central Mental Hospital, Dundrum, Dublin' in R. Bluglass and P. Bowden (eds), *Principles and Practice of Forensic Psychiatry* (Edinburgh: Churchill Livingstone, 1990) pp. 1351–3

12 Mulryan, N., P. Gibbons and A. O'Connor, 'Infanticide and Child Murder – Admissions to the Central Mental Hospital, 1850–2000', *Irish Journal of Psychological Medicine* (2002; 19: 8–12)

13 Mulryan, N., P. Gibbons and A. O'Connor, 'Infanticide and Child Murder – Admissions to the Central Mental Hospital, 1850–2000', *Irish*

Journal of Psychological Medicine (2002; 19: 8–12)

14 Williamson, A.P., 'Psychiatry, Moral Management and the Origins of Social Policy for Mentally Ill People in Ireland', *Irish Journal of Medical Science* (1992; 161: 556–8); Reuber, M., 'The Architecture of Psychological Management: The Irish Asylums (1801–1922)', *Psychological Medicine* (1996; 26: 1179–89); Reuber, M., 'Moral Management and the "Unseen Eye": Public Lunatic Asylums in Ireland, 1800–1845' in E. Malcolm and G. Jones (eds), *Medicine, Disease and the State in Ireland, 1650–1940* (Cork: Cork University Press, 1999) pp. 208–33; McCarthy, A., 'Hearths, Bodies and Minds: Gender Ideology and Women's Committal to Enniscorthy Lunatic Asylum, 1916–1925' in A. Hayes and D. Urguhart (eds), *Irish Women's History* (Dublin and Portland: Irish Academic Press, 2004) pp. 115–36; Prior, P., 'Prisoner or Lunatic? The Official Debate on the Criminal Lunatic in Nineteenth-Century Ireland', *History of Psychiatry* (2004; 15: 177–92)

15 Merrit, H.H., R. Adams and H.C. Solomon, *Neurosyphilis* (Oxford: Oxford University Press, 1946); Brown, E.M., 'Why Wagner-Jauregg Won the Nobel Prize for Discovering Malaria Therapy for General Paralysis of the Insane', *History of Psychiatry* (2000; 11: 371–82)

16 Guthrie, D., *A History of Medicine* (London: Nelson, 1945)

17 Prestwich, P.E., 'Family Strategies and Medical Power: "Voluntary" Committal in a Parisian Asylum, 1876–1914' in R. Porter and D. Wright (eds), *The Confinement of the Insane: International Perspectives, 1800–1965* (Cambridge: Cambridge University Press, 2003) pp. 79–99

18 Hallaran, W.S., *Practical Observations on the Causes and Cures of Insanity* (2nd edition) (Cork: Edwards and Savage, 1818); Fleetwood, J.F., *The History of Medicine in Ireland* (2nd edition) (Dublin: Skellig Press, 1983)

19 Mulryan, N., P. Gibbons and A. O'Connor, 'Infanticide and Child Murder – Admissions to the Central Mental Hospital, 1850–2000', *Irish Journal of Psychological Medicine* (2002; 19: 8–12)

20 Gibbons, P., N. Mulryan and A. O'Connor, 'Guilty but Insane: The Insanity Defence in Ireland, 1850–1995', *British Journal of Psychiatry* (1997; 170: 467–72)

21 Walsh, O., 'Gender and Insanity in Nineteenth-Century Ireland', *Clio Medica* (2004; 73: 69–93)

22 Finnane, M., *Insanity and the Insane in Post-Famine Ireland* (London: Croon Helm, 1981); Scull, A., *The Most Solitary of Afflictions: Madness and Society in Britain, 1700–1900* (New Haven and London: Yale University Press, 1993); Porter, R., *A Social History of Madness: Stories of the Insane* (London: Phoenix, 1996); Torrey, E.F. and J. Miller, *The Invisible Plague: The Rise of Mental Illness from 1750 to the Present* (New Brunswick, New Jersey: Rutgers University Press, 2001)

23 Bynum, W.F., 'Rationales for Therapy in British Psychiatry: 1780–1835', *Medical History* (1964; 18: 317–34); Porter, R., *A Social History of Madness:*

Stories of the Insane (London: Phoenix, 1996)

24 Gibbons, P., N. Mulryan and A. O'Connor, 'Guilty but Insane:
    The Insanity Defence in Ireland, 1850–1995', *British Journal of Psychiatry*
    (1997; 170: 467–72); Prior, P., 'Dangerous Lunacy: The Misuse of
    Mental Health Law in Nineteenth-Century Ireland', *Journal of Forensic
    Psychiatry and Psychology* (2003; 14: 525–41); Andrews, J. and A. Digby,
    'Introduction: Gender and Class in the Historiography of British and
    Irish Psychiatry', *Clio Medica* (2004; 73: 7–44); Walsh, O., 'Gender and
    Insanity in Nineteenth-Century Ireland', *Clio Medica* (2004; 73: 69–93)

25 This section of the book is largely drawn from: Kelly, B.D., 'Clinical
    and Social Characteristics of Women Committed to Inpatient Forensic
    Psychiatric Care in Ireland, 1868–1908', *Journal of Forensic Psychiatry and
    Psychology* (2008; 19: 261–73). For this paper, a single researcher (BDK)
    studied all medical case-records of women admitted to the Central
    Criminal Lunatic Asylum (Central Mental Hospital), Dublin between
    1868 and 1908 (n=70). This period was chosen because complete medical
    records were available for all women admitted during this time, medical
    records prior to 1868 and for 1909 being unavailable. Medical records
    for each woman included personal details (e.g. age, marital status), details
    of offence (e.g. date of conviction, crime, sentence), clinical notes on
    admission (e.g. mental health, physical status) and follow-up notes
    (e.g. significant medical events, progress in the asylum). The Statistical
    Package for the Social Sciences was used for the description and analysis
    of quantitative data. A narrative approach was used for the study of
    medical follow-up notes; three anonymised case histories are presented.
    This paper formed part of a broader programme of historical and
    archival research based at the Department of Adult Psychiatry, Mater
    Misericordiae University Hospital, Dublin; the National Forensic
    Psychiatry Service, Central Mental Hospital, Dundrum, Dublin; and
    University College Dublin, Ireland. This programme of research was
    approved by the Health Service Executive (Dublin, Mid-Leinster)
    Research Ethics Committee. In order to maintain patient confidentiality,
    names were changed so as to render specific individuals unidentifiable.

26 Kelly, B.D. 'Poverty, Crime and Mental Illness: Female Forensic
    Psychiatric Committal in Ireland, 1910–1948', *Social History of Medicine*
    (2008; 21: 311–28)

27 Prior, P., 'Dangerous Lunacy: The Misuse of Mental Health Law in
    Nineteenth-Century Ireland', *Journal of Forensic Psychiatry and Psychology*
    (2003; 14: 525–41)

28 Langan-Egan, M., *Galway Women in the Nineteenth Century*
    (Dublin: Open Air (Four Courts Press), 1999)

29 D'Orban, P.T., 'Women Who Kill their Children', *British Journal
    of Psychiatry* (1979; 134: 560–71); Putkonen, H., J. Collander,
    M.L. Honkaslo and J. Lonnqvist, 'Finnish Female Homicide Offenders,

1982–1992', *Journal of Forensic Psychiatry* (1998; 9: 672–84); Schwartz, L.L. and N.K. Isser, *Endangered Children: Neonaticide, Infanticide and Filicide (Pacific Institute Series on Forensic Psychology)* (Boca Raton, FL: CRC Press Inc., 2000)

30   Friedman, S.H., S.M. Horowitz and P.J. Resnick, 'Child Murder by Mothers: A Critical Analysis of the Current State of Knowledge and a Research Agenda', *American Journal of Psychiatry* (2005; 162: 1578–87)

31   Mulryan, N., P. Gibbons and A. O'Connor, 'Infanticide and Child Murder – Admissions to the Central Mental Hospital, 1850–2000', *Irish Journal of Psychological Medicine* (2002; 19: 8–12)

32   Kelly, B.D., 'Murder, Mercury and Mental Illness: Infanticide in Nineteenth-Century Ireland', *Irish Journal of Medical Science* (2007; 176: 149–52)

33   Rehman, A.U., D. St Clair and C. Platz, 'Puerperal Insanity in the 19th and 20th Centuries', *British Journal of Psychiatry* (1990; 156: 861–5)

34   Tschinkel, S., M. Harris, J. Le Noury and D. Healy, 'Postpartum Psychosis: Two Cohorts Compared, 1875–1924 and 1994–2005', *Psychological Medicine* (2007; 37: 529–36)

35   Marland, H., *Dangerous Motherhood: Insanity and Childbirth in Victorian Britain* (Basingstoke: Palgrave MacMillan, 2004)

36   Tschinkel, S., M. Harris, J. Le Noury and D. Healy, 'Postpartum Psychosis: Two Cohorts Compared, 1875–1924 and 1994–2005', *Psychological Medicine* (2007; 37: 529–36)

37   Mulryan, N., P. Gibbons and A. O'Connor, 'Infanticide and Child Murder – Admissions to the Central Mental Hospital, 1850–2000', *Irish Journal of Psychological Medicine* (2002; 19: 8–12)

38   Gibbons, P., N. Mulryan and A. O'Connor, 'Guilty but Insane: The Insanity Defence in Ireland, 1850–1995', *British Journal of Psychiatry* (1997; 170: 467–72)

39   Mulryan, N., P. Gibbons and A. O'Connor, 'Infanticide and Child Murder – Admissions to the Central Mental Hospital, 1850–2000', *Irish Journal of Psychological Medicine* (2002; 19: 8–12)

40   Inspector of Lunatics (Ireland), *The Forty-Second Report (With Appendices) of the Inspector of Lunatics (Ireland)* (Dublin: Thom and Co./Her Majesty's Stationery Office, 1893); Torrey, E.F. and J. Miller, *The Invisible Plague: The Rise of Mental Illness from 1750 to the Present* (New Brunswick, New Jersey: Rutgers University Press, 2001); Prior, P., 'Dangerous Lunacy: The Misuse of Mental Health Law in Nineteenth-Century Ireland', *Journal of Forensic Psychiatry and Psychology* (2003; 14: 525–41)

41   Smith, C., 'The Central Mental Hospital, Dundrum, Dublin' in R. Bluglass and P. Bowden (eds), *Principles and Practice of Forensic Psychiatry* (Edinburgh: Churchill Livingstone, 1990) pp. 1351–3

42   Smith, R., 'Scientific Thought and the Boundary of Insanity and Criminal Responsibility', *Psychological Medicine* (1980; 10: 15–23); Smith,

R., 'The Victorian Controversy about the Insanity Defence', *Journal of the Royal Society of Medicine* (1988; 81: 70–3); Eigen, J.P., 'Delusion in the Courtroom: the Role of Partial Insanity in Early Forensic Testimony', *Medical History* (1991; 35: 25–49); Clark, M. and C. Crawford (eds), *Legal Medicine in History (Cambridge Studies in the History of Medicine)* (Cambridge: Cambridge University Press, 1994); Eigen, J.P., *Witnessing Insanity: Madness and Mad-Doctors in the English Court* (New Haven, CT: Yale University Press, 1995); Eigen, J.P. 'Criminal Lunacy in Early Modern England: Did Gender Make a Difference? *International Journal of Law and Psychiatry* (1998; 21: 409-19); Eigen, J.P., *Unconscious Crime: Mental Absence and Criminal Responsibility in Victorian London* (Baltimore, MD: Johns Hopkins University Press, 2003); Eigen, J.P., 'Delusion's Odyssey: Charting the Course of Victorian Forensic Psychiatry', *International Journal of Law and Psychiatry* (2004; 27: 395–412); Skalevag, S.A., 'The Matter of Forensic Psychiatry: A Historical Enquiry', *Medical History* (2006; 50: 49–68)

43 Smith, R., 'The Victorian Controversy about the Insanity Defence', *Journal of the Royal Society of Medicine* (1988; 81: 70–3)

44 Skalevag, S.A., 'The Matter of Forensic Psychiatry: A Historical Enquiry', *Medical History* (2006; 50: 49–68)

45 Eigen, J.P., *Witnessing Insanity: Madness and Mad-Doctors in the English Court* (New Haven, CT: Yale University Press, 1995)

46 Harris, R., *Murders and Madness: Medicine, Law and Society in the 'Fin de Siècle'* (Oxford: Oxford University Press, 1989)

47 Kelly, B.D., 'Criminal Insanity in Nineteenth-Century Ireland, Europe and the United States: Cases, Contexts and Controversies', *International Journal of Law and Psychiatry* (2009; 32: 362–8)

48 Gibbons, P., N. Mulryan and A. O'Connor, 'Guilty but Insane: The Insanity Defence in Ireland, 1850–1995', *British Journal of Psychiatry* (1997; 170: 467–72)

49 Walsh, D. and A. Daly, *Mental Illness in Ireland 1750–2002: Reflections on the Rise and Fall of Institutional Care* (Dublin: Health Research Board, 2004)

50 O'Neill, A-M., *Irish Mental Health Law* (Dublin: First Law, 2005)

51 Psychiatrist, 'Insanity in Ireland', *The Bell* (1944; 7: 303–10)

52 Kelly, B.D., 'The Mental Treatment Act 1945 in Ireland: An Historical Enquiry', *History of Psychiatry* (2008; 19: 47–67)

53 This section of this chapter is drawn from: Kelly, B.D., 'Poverty, Crime and Mental Illness: Female Forensic Psychiatric Committal in Ireland, 1910–1948', *Social History of Medicine* (2008; 21: 311–28). For this study, a single researcher (BDK) studied medical case-records of all women admitted to the Central Criminal Lunatic Asylum, Dublin between 1910 and 1948 (n=42). Medical records for 1909 were missing and the methods of record keeping changed following 1948,

reducing comparability. Up until 1948, medical admission records for each woman included personal details (marital status), details of offence (offence, sentence), clinical notes on admission (mental and physical status) and follow-up notes (progress in the asylum).

This paper formed part of a programme of archival and historical research at the Department of Adult Psychiatry, Mater Misericordiae University Hospital, Dublin; the National Forensic Psychiatry Service, Central Mental Hospital, Dundrum, Dublin; and University College Dublin, Ireland.

54 Walsh, D., 'The Ups and Downs of Schizophrenia in Ireland', *Irish Journal of Psychiatry* (1992; 13: 12–6)

55 Finnane, M., *Insanity and the Insane in Post-Famine Ireland* (London: Croon Helm, 1981)

56 Scull, A., *The Most Solitary of Afflictions: Madness and Society in Britain, 1700–1900* (New Haven and London: Yale University Press, 1993)

57 Walsh, D., 'The Ups and Downs of Schizophrenia in Ireland', *Irish Journal of Psychiatry* (1992; 13: 12–6)

58 Kelly, B.D., 'Mental Illness in Nineteenth Century Ireland: A Qualitative Study of Workhouse Records', *Irish Journal of Medical Science* (2004; 173: 53–5)

59 Reynolds, J., *Grangegorman: Psychiatric Care in Dublin since 1815* (Dublin: Institute of Public Administration in association with Eastern Health Board, 1992)

60 Boyd, Barrett, E., 'Modern Psycho-Therapy and our Asylums', *Studies* (1924; 8: 29–43)

61 Psychiatrist, 'Insanity in Ireland', *The Bell* (1944; 7: 303–10)

62 Ferriter, D., *The Transformation of Ireland 1900–2000* (London: Profile Books, 2004)

63 Bardon, J., *A History of Ulster* (Belfast: Blackstaff Press, 1993)

64 McClelland, R.J., 'The Madhouses and Mad Doctors of Ulster', *Ulster Medical Journal* (1988; 57: 101–20)

65 Mulholland, M., *To Comfort Always: A History of Holywell Hospital, 1898–1998* (Ballymena: Homefirst Community Trust, 1998)

66 Barrington, R., *Health, Medicine and Politics in Ireland 1900–1970* (Dublin: Institute of Public Administration, 1987)

67 Healy, D., 'Irish Psychiatry in the Twentieth Century' in H. Freeman and G.E. Berrios (eds), *150 Years of British Psychiatry. Volume II: The Aftermath* (London: Athlone Press, 1996) pp. 268–91; O'Neill, A-M., *Irish Mental Health Law* (Dublin: First Law, 2005); Kelly, B.D., 'The Mental Treatment Act 1945 in Ireland: An Historical Enquiry', *History of Psychiatry* (2008; 19: 47–67)

68 Mulryan, N., P. Gibbons and A. O'Connor, 'Infanticide and Child Murder – Admissions to the Central Mental Hospital, 1850–2000', *Irish Journal of Psychological Medicine* (2002; 19: 8–12)

69 Kelly, B.D., 'Clinical and Social Characteristics of Women Committed to Inpatient Forensic Psychiatric Care in Ireland, 1868–1908', *Journal of Forensic Psychiatry and Psychology* (2008; 19: 261–73); Kelly, B.D. 'Poverty, Crime and Mental Illness: Female Forensic Psychiatric Committal in Ireland, 1910–1948', *Social History of Medicine* (2008; 21: 311–28). See also: Andrews, J., 'The Boundaries of her Majesty's Pleasure: Discharging Child-Murderers from Broadmoor and Perth Criminal Lunatic Department, *c.*1860–1920' in M. Jackson (ed.), *Infanticide: Historical Perspectives on Child Murder and Concealment* (Aldershot: Ashgate, 2002) pp. 216–48

70 Ryan, L. 'The Press and Prosecution: Perspectives on Infancide in the 1920s' in A. Hayes and D. Urquhart (eds.), *Irish Women's History* (Dublin and Portland, OR: Irish Academic Press, 2004) pp. 137–51

71 Wright, D., ;'"Childlike in his Innocence": Lay Attitudes to "Idiots" and "Imbeciles" in Victorian England' in D. Wright and A. Digby (eds), *From Idiocy to Mental Deficiency: Historical Perspectives on People with Learning Disabilities* (London and New York: Routledge, 1996) pp. 118–33

72 Marland, H., *Dangerous Motherhood: Insanity and Childbirth in Victorian Britain* (Basingstoke: Palgrave MacMillan, 2004)

73 Marland, H., '"Destined to a Perfect Recovery": The Confinement of Puerperal Insanity in the Nineteenth Century' in J. Melling and B. Forsythe (eds), *Insanity Institutions and Society, 1800–1914: A Social History of Madness in Comparative Perspective* (London and New York: Routledge, 1999) pp. 137–56

74 Jackson, M., (ed.), *Infanticide: Historical Perspectives on Child Murder and Concealment, 1550–2000* (Hampshire, England: Ashgate, 2002)

75 Wright, D., J.E. Moran and S. Gouglas, 'The Confinement of the Insane in Victorian Canada: The Hamilton and Toronto Asylums, *c.*1861–1891' in R. Porter and D. Wright (eds), *The Confinement of the Insane: International Perspectives, 1800–1965* (Cambridge: Cambridge University Press, 2003) pp. 100–28

76 Coleborne, C., 'Passage to the Asylum: The Role of the Police in Committals of the Insane in Victoria, Australia, 1848–1900' in R. Porter and D. Wright (eds), *The Confinement of the Insane: International Perspectives, 1800–1965* (Cambridge: Cambridge University Press, 2003) pp. 129–48

77 Walsh, O., '"The Designs of Providence": Race, Religion and Irish Insanity' in J. Melling and B. Forsythe (eds), *Insanity Institutions and Society, 1800–1914: A Social History of Madness in Comparative Perspective* (London and New York: Routledge, 1999) pp. 223–42; Andrews, J. and A. Digby (eds), *Sex and Seclusion, Class and Custody: Perspectives on Gender and Class in the History of British and Irish Psychiatry* (Amsterdam: Rodopi, 2004); Michael, P., 'Class, Gender and Insanity in Nineteenth-Century Wales', *Clio Medica* (2004; 73: 95–122); Walsh, O., 'Gender and Insanity in Nineteenth-Century Ireland', *Clio Medica* (2004; 73: 69–93); Prior, P., 'Murder and Madness: Gender and the Insanity Defence in Nineteenth-Century Ireland', *New Hibernia Review*

(2005; 9: 19–36); Prior, P., 'Roasting a Man Alive: The Case of Mary Reilly, Criminal Lunatic', *Éire-Ireland* (2006; 41: 169–91)

78 Walsh, O., 'Gender and Insanity in Nineteenth-Century Ireland', *Clio Medica* (2004; 73: 69–93)

79 Walsh, O., '"A Lightness of Mind": Gender and Insanity in Nineteenth-Century Ireland' in M. Kelleher and J.H. Murphy (eds), *Gender Perspectives in 19th Century Ireland: Public and Private Spheres* (Dublin: Irish Academic Press, 1997) pp. 159–67

80 McCarthy, A., 'Hearths, Bodies and Minds: Gender Ideology and Women's Committal to Enniscorthy Lunatic Asylum, 1916–1925' in A. Hayes and D. Urquhart (eds), *Irish Women's History* (Dublin and Portland: Irish Academic Press, 2004) pp. 115–36

81 Harris, R., '"Risk", Law and Hygiene in Late Nineteenth-Century France', *Society for the Social History of Medicine Bulletin* (1987; 40: 86–9)

82 Torrey, E.F. and J. Miller, *The Invisible Plague: The Rise of Mental Illness from 1750 to the Present* (New Brunswick, New Jersey: Rutgers University Press, 2001); Malcolm, E., '"Ireland's Crowded Madhouses": The Institutional Confinement of the Insane in Nineteenth- and Twentieth-Century Ireland' in R. Porter and D. Wright (eds), *The Confinement of the Insane: International Perspectives, 1800–1965* (Cambridge: Cambridge University Press, 2003) pp. 315–33

83 Churchill, F., 'On the Mental Disorders of Pregnancy and Childbed', *Dublin Quarterly Journal of Medical Science* (1850; 17: 39); Maudsley, H., 'Homicidal Insanity', *Journal of Mental Science* (1863; 47: 327–43); Oppenheim, J., *Shattered Nerves: Doctors, Patients and Depression in Victorian England* (New York and Oxford: Oxford University Press, 1991)

84 Andrews, J. and A. Scull, *Customers and Patrons of the Mad-Trade: The Management of Lunacy in Eighteenth-Century London, with the Complete Text of John Munro's 1766 Case Book* (Berkeley CA: University of California Press, 2002)

85 Michael, P. and D. Hirst, 'Establishing the "Rule of Kindness": The Foundation of the North Wales Lunatic Asylum, Denbigh' in J. Melling and B. Forsythe (eds), *Insanity, Institutions and Society, 1800–1914: A Social History of Madness in Comparative Perspective (Studies in the Social History of Medicine)* (London & New York: Routledge/Taylor & Francis Group, 1999) pp. 159–79; Michael, P., *Care and Treatment of the Mentally Ill in North Wales, 1800–2000* (Cardiff: University of Wales Press, 2003)

86 Walsh, O., '"The Designs of Providence": Race, Religion and Irish Insanity' in J. Melling and B. Forsythe (eds), *Insanity Institutions and Society, 1800–1914: A Social History of Madness in Comparative Perspective* (London and New York: Routledge, 1999) pp. 223–42

87 Marland, H., *Dangerous Motherhood: Insanity and Childbirth in Victorian Britain* (Basingstoke: Palgrave MacMillan, 2004)

4. Clinical Aspects of Criminal Insanity in Nineteenth- and Twentieth-Century Ireland

1 Kelly, B.D., 'Folie à Plusieurs: Forensic Cases from Nineteenth-Century Ireland', *History of Psychiatry* (2009; 20: 47–60)

2 Enoch, D. and H. Ball, *Uncommon Psychiatric Syndromes* (4th edition) (London: Hodder Arnold, 2001); Ireland, W.W., 'Folie à Deux – A Mad Family' in Ireland W.W., *The Blot upon the Brain* (1st edition) (Edinburgh: Bell & Bradfute, 1885) pp. 201–8; Lasègue, C. and J. Falret, 'La Folie à Deux ou Folie Communiquée', *Annales Medico-Psychologiques* (1877; 18: 321–55); Mickaud, R., 'Translation of Lasègue and Farlet's paper of 1877: Le folie à ou folie communiquée', *American Journal of Psychiatry* (1964; 121 (suppl. 4))

3 World Health Organization, *The ICD-Classification of Mental and Behavioural Disorders* (Geneva: World Health Organization, 1992)

4 Berrios, G.E., *The History of Mental Symptoms. Descriptive Psychopathology since the 19th Century* (Cambridge: Cambridge University Press, 1996); Berrios, G.E., 'Introduction. Classic Text No. 35: Folie à deux – A Mad Family', *History of Psychiatry* (1998; 9: 383–95)

5 Berrios, G.E., 'Introduction. Classic Text No. 35: Folie à Deux – A Mad Family', *History of Psychiatry* (1998; 9: 383–95); Dewhurst, K. and J. Todd, 'The Psychosis of Association – Folie à Deux', *Journal of Nervous and Mental Disease* (1987; 74: 451–9); Enoch, D. and H. Ball, *Uncommon Psychiatric Syndromes* (4th Edition) (London: Hodder Arnold, 2001); Franzini, L.R. and J.M. Grossberg, *Eccentric and Bizarre Behaviours* (New York: John Wiley, 1995); Gralnick, A., 'Folie à deux', *Psychiatric Quarterly* (1942; 16: 230–63); Halberstadt, G., *La Folie par Contagion Mentale* (Paris: Baillière, 1906)

6 Enoch, D. and H. Ball, *Uncommon Psychiatric Syndromes* (4th edition) (London: Hodder Arnold, 2001)

7 Mentjox, R., C.A. van Houten and C.G. Kooiman, 'Induced Psychotic Disorder: Clinical Aspects, Theoretical Considerations, and some Guidelines for Treatment', *Comprehensive Psychiatry* (1993; 34: 120–6)

8 Enoch, D. and H. Ball, *Uncommon Psychiatric Syndromes* (4th edition) (London: Hodder Arnold, 2001); Munro, A., *Delusional Disorder: Paranoia and Related Illnesses* (Cambridge: Cambridge University Press, 1999)

9 Kraya, N.A.F. and C. Patrick, 'Folie à deux in Forensic Setting', *Australian and New Zealand Journal of Psychiatry* (1997; 31: 883–8); Mela, M., 'Folie à Trios in a Multilevel Security Forensic Treatment Center: Forensic and Ethics-Related implications', *Journal of the American Academy of Psychiatry and the Law* (2005; 33: 310–6)

10 Enoch, D. and H. Ball, *Uncommon Psychiatric Syndromes* (4th edition) (London: Hodder Arnold, 2001)

11 Bourgeois, M.L, P. Duhamel and H. Verdoux, 'Delusional Parasitosis:

folie à deux and Attempted Murder of a Family Doctor', *British Journal of Psychiatry* (1992; 161: 709–11)

12 Ireland, W.W., 'Folie à Deux – A Mad Family', in W.W. Ireland, *The Blot upon the Brain* (1st edition) (Edinburgh: Bell & Bradfute, 1885) pp. 201–8

13 Woods, O.T., 'Notes of a Case of Folie à Deux in Five Members of One Family', *Journal of Mental Science* (1889; 34: 535–9)

14 Woods, O.T., 'Notes of a Case of Folie à Deux in Five Members of One Family', *Journal of Mental Science* (1889; 34: 535–9)

15 Gibbons, P., N. Mulryan and A. O'Connor, 'Guilty but Insane: The Insanity Defence in Ireland, 1850–1995', *British Journal of Psychiatry* (1997; 170: 467–72)

16 McCarthy, A., 'Hearths, Bodies and Minds: Gender Ideology and Women's Committal to Enniscorthy Lunatic Asylum, 1916–1925' in A. Hayes and D. Urquhart (eds), *Irish Women's History* (Dublin and Portland: Irish Academic Press, 2004) pp. 115–136; Williamson, A.P., 'Psychiatry, Moral Management and the Origins of Social Policy for Mentally Ill People in Ireland', *Irish Journal of Medical Science* (1992; 161: 556–8)

17 Reuber, M., 'The Architecture of Psychological Management: The Irish Asylums (1801–1922)', *Psychological Medicine* (1996; 26: 1179–89); Reuber, M., 'Moral Management and the 'Unseen Eye': Public Lunatic Asylums in Ireland, 1800–1845' in E. Malcolm and G. Jones (eds), *Medicine, Disease and the State in Ireland, 1650–1940* (Cork: Cork University Press, 1999) pp. 208–233

18 Prior, P., 'Prisoner or Lunatic? The Official Debate on the Criminal Lunatic in Nineteenth-Century Ireland', *History of Psychiatry* (2004; 15: 177–92)

19 Jones, G., 'The Campaign Against Tuberculosis in Ireland, 1899–1914' in E. Malcolm and G. Jones (eds), *Medicine, Disease and the State in Ireland, 1650–1940* (Cork: Cork University Press, 1999) pp. 158–76; McCandless, P., 'Curative Asylum, Custodial Hospital: The South Carolina Lunatic Asylum and State Hospital, 1828–1920' in R. Porter and D. Wright (eds), *The Confinement of the Insane: International Perspectives, 1800–1965* (Cambridge: Cambridge University Press, 2003) pp. 173–92

20 Jones, G., 'The Campaign Against Tuberculosis in Ireland, 1899–1914' in E. Malcolm and G. Jones (eds), *Medicine, Disease and the State in Ireland, 1650–1940* (Cork: Cork University Press, 1999) pp. 158–76

21 Lyons, F.S.L., *Ireland Since the Famine* (London: Fontana, 1985)

22 Breathnach, C.S. and J.B. Moynihan, 'An Irish Statistician's Analysis of the National Tuberculosis Problem – Robert Charles Geary (1896–1983)', *Irish Journal of Medical Science* (2003; 172: 149–53)

23 Inspector of Lunatics (Ireland), *The Forty-Second Report (With Appendices) of the Inspector of Lunatics (Ireland)*, Dublin: Thom & Co./ Her Majesty's Stationery Office, 1893); Torrey, E.F. and J. Miller, *The Invisible Plague: The Rise of Mental Illness from 1750 to the Present* (New Brunswick, New Jersey: Rutgers University Press, 2001);

Prior, P., 'Dangerous Lunacy: The Misuse of Mental Health Law in Nineteenth-Century Ireland', *Journal of Forensic Psychiatry and Psychology* (2003; 14: 525–41)

24 Kelly, B.D., 'Tuberculosis in the Nineteenth-Century Asylum: Clinical Cases from the Central Criminal Lunatic Asylum, Dundrum, Dublin' in P. Prior (ed.) *Asylums, Mental Health Care and the Irish, 1800–2010* (Dublin and Portland, Oregon: Irish Academic Press, 2012) pp. 205–20.

25 Woods, O.T., 'Notes of a Case of Folie à Deux in Five Members of One Family', *Journal of Mental Science* (1889; 34: 535–9)

26 Eberly, S.S., 'Fairies and the Folklore of Disability: Changelings, Hybrids and the Solitary Fairy', *Folklore* (1988; 99: 58–77); M'Manus, L., 'Folk-Tales from Western Ireland', *Folklore* (1914; 25: 324–41)

27 Bourke, A., *The Burning of Bridget Cleary: A True Story* (London: Pimlico, 1999); Hoff, J. and M. Yeates, *The Cooper's Wife is Missing: The Ritual Murder of Bridget Cleary* (New York: Basic Books, 2000)

28 Wilde, F.S., *Ancient Legends, Mystic Charms, and Superstitions of Ireland* (London: Ward and Downey, 1887)

29 Yeats, W.B., *Irish Fairy Tales* (New York: Scott, 1907)

30 Goodey, C.F. and T. Stainton, 'Intellectual Disability and the Myth of the Changeling', *Journal of the History of the Behavioural Sciences* (2001; 37: 223–40)

31 Leask, J., A. Leask and N. Silove, 'Evidence for Autism in Folklore?', *Archives of Disease in Childhood* (2005; 90: 271)

32 Muir, R., 'The Changeling Myth and the Pre-Psychology of Parenting', *British Journal of Medical Psychology* (1982; 55: 97–104)

33 Cawte, J. and M. Tarrant, 'Capgras' Syndrome: Outmoded term for Changeling Delusions?' *Australian and New Zealand Journal of Psychiatry* (1984; 18: 388–90)

34 Bourke, A., *The Burning of Bridget Cleary: A True Story* (London: Pimlico, 1999)

35 Woods, O.T., 'Notes of a Case of Folie à Deux in Five Members of One Family', *Journal of Mental Science* (1889; 34: 535–9)

36 Ireland, W.W., 'Folic à Deux   A Mad Family' in W.W. Ireland, *The Blot upon the Brain* (1st edition) (Edinburgh: Bell & Bradfute, 1885) pp. 201–8

37 Anonymous, 'Obituary: Daniel Hack Tuke', *The Lancet* (1895; 145: 718–9)

38 Tuke, D.H. 'Folie à Deux', *Brain* (1888; 10: 408–421)

39 Ireland, W.W., 'Folie à Deux – A Mad Family' in W.W. Ireland, *The Blot upon the Brain* (1st edition) (Edinburgh: Bell & Bradfute, 1885) pp. 201–208

40 Woods, O.T., 'Notes of a Case of Folie à Deux in Five Members of One Family', *Journal of Mental Science* (1889; 34: 535–9)

41 Enoch, D. and H. Ball, *Uncommon Psychiatric Syndromes* (4th edition) (London: Hodder Arnold, 2001); Munro, A., *Delusional Disorder: Paranoia and Related Illnesses* (Cambridge: Cambridge University Press, 1999)

42 Bourgeois, M.L., P. Duhamel and H. Verdoux, 'Delusional Parasitosis: Folie à Deux and Attempted Murder of a Family Doctor', *British*

Journal of Psychiatry (1992; 161: 709–11); Kraya, N.A.F. and C. Patrick, 'Folie à Deux in Forensic Setting', *Australian and New Zealand Journal of Psychiatry* (1997; 31: 883–8)

43 Mela, M., 'Folie à Trios in a Multilevel Security Forensic Treatment Center: Forensic and Ethics-Related implications', *Journal of the American Academy of Psychiatry and the Law* (2005; 33: 310–6).

44 Kraya, N.A.F. and C. Patrick, 'Folie à Deux in Forensic Setting', *Australian and New Zealand Journal of Psychiatry* (1997; 31: 883–8); Mela, M., 'Folie à Trios in a Multilevel Security Forensic Treatment Center: Forensic and Ethics-Related implications', *Journal of the American Academy of Psychiatry and the Law* (2005; 33: 310–6)

45 Enoch, D. and H. Ball, *Uncommon Psychiatric Syndromes* (4th edition) (London: Hodder Arnold, 2001); Munro, A., *Delusional Disorder: Paranoia and Related Illnesses* (Cambridge: Cambridge University Press, 1999)

46 Irish College of Psychiatrists, *People With a Learning Disability Who Offend: Forgiven But Forgotten? (Occasional Paper OP63)* (Dublin: Irish College of Psychiatrists, 2008)

47 Myers, F., *On the Borderline? People with Learning Disabilities and/or Autism Spectrum Disorders in Secure Forensic and Other Specialist Settings* (Edinburgh: The Stationery Office/Scottish Development Centre for Mental Health, 2004)

48 Digby, A., 'Contexts and Perspectives' in D. Wright and A. Digby (eds), *From Idiocy to Mental Deficiency: Historical Perspectives on People with Learning Disabilities (Studies in the Social History of Medicine)* (London & New York: Routledge, 1996) pp 1–21

49 Smith, C., 'The Central Mental Hospital, Dundrum, Dublin' in R. Bluglass and P. Bowden (eds), *Principles and Practice of Forensic Psychiatry* (Edinburgh: Churchill Livingstone, 1990) pp. 1351–3

50 Kelly, B.D., 'Learning Disability and Forensic Mental Healthcare in Nineteenth-Century Ireland', *Irish Journal of Psychological Medicine* (2008; 25: 116–8)

51 Atkinson, D., M. Jackson and J. Walmsley, 'Introduction: Methods and Themes' in D. Atkinson, M. Jackson and J. Walmsley (eds), *Forgotten Lives: Exploring the History of Learning Disability* (Worcestershire: British Institute of Learning Disabilities (BILD), 1997) pp. 1–20; Dale, P. and J. Melling, 'The Politics of Mental Welfare: Fresh Perspectives on the History of Institutional Care for the Mentally Ill and Disabled' in P. Dale and J. Melling (eds), *Mental Illness and Learning Disability: Finding a Place for Mental Disorder in the United Kingdom* (Routledge Studies in the *Social History of Medicine*) (London & New York: Routledge/Taylor & Francis Group, 2006) pp. 1–23; Digby, A., 'Contexts and Perspectives' in D. Wright and A. Digby (eds), *From Idiocy to Mental Deficiency: Historical Perspectives on People with Learning Disabilities (Studies in the Social History of Medicine)* (London & New York: Routledge, 1996) pp. 1–21

52 Crompton, F., 'Needs and Desires in the Care of Pauper Lunatics: Admissions to Worcester Asylum, 1852–72' in P. Dale and J. Melling (eds), *Mental Illness and Learning Disability: Finding a Place for Mental Disorder in the United Kingdom* (Routledge Studies in the *Social History of Medicine*) (London & New York: Routledge/Taylor & Francis Group, 2006) pp. 46–64; Inspector of Lunatics (Ireland), *The Forty-Second Report (With Appendices) of the Inspector of Lunatics (Ireland)* (Dublin: Thom & Co./Her Majesty's Stationery Office, 1893); Michael, P. and D. Hirst, 'Establishing the "Rule of Kindness": The Foundation of the North Wales Lunatic Asylum, Denbeigh' in Melling, J. and B. Forsythe (eds), *Insanity, Institutions and Society, 1800–1914: A Social History of Madness in Comparative Perspective (Studies in the Social History of Medicine)* (London & New York: Routledge/Taylor & Francis Group, 1999) pp. 159–79

53 Deb, S., M. Thomas and C. Bright, 'Mental Disorder in Adults with Intellectual Disability. I: Prevalence of Functional Psychiatric Illness among a Community-Based Population Aged between 16 and 64 Years', *Journal of Intellectual Disability Research* (2001; 45: 495–505); White, P., D. Chant, N. Edwards, C. Townsend and G. Waghorn, 'Prevalence of Intellectual Disability and Comorbid Mental Illness in an Australian Community Sample', *Australian and New Zealand Journal of Psychiatry* (2005; 39: 395–400)

54 Glaser, W. and D. Flood, 'Beyond Specialist Programmes: A Study of the Needs of Offenders with Intellectual Disability Requiring Psychiatric Attention', *Journal of Intellectual Disability Research* (2004; 48: 591–602); Holland, T., I.C. Claire and T. Mukhopadhyay, Prevalence of Criminal Offending by Men and Women with Intellectual Disability and the Characteristics of Offenders: Implications for Research and Service Development', *Journal of Intellectual Disability Research* (2002; 46 (Suppl. 1): 6–20); Johnston, S.J., 'Risk Assessment in Offenders with Intellectual Disability: The Evidence Base', *Journal of Intellectual Disability Research* (2002; 46 (Suppl. 1): 47–56); Lindsay, W.R., A.H. Smith, K. Quinn, A. Anderson, A. Smith, R. Allan and J. Law, 'Women with Intellectual Disability who have Offended: Characteristics and Outcome', *Journal of Intellectual Disability Research* (2004; 48: 580–90); Riches, V.C., T.R. Parmenter, M. Wiese and R.J. Stancliffe, 'Intellectual Disability and Mental Illness in the NSW Criminal Justice System', *International Journal of Law and Psychiatry* (2006; 29: 386–96)

55 Kelly, B.D., 'Murder, Mercury, Mental Illness: Infanticide in Nineteenth-Century Ireland', *Irish Journal of Medical Science* (2007; 176: 149–52); Mulryan, N., P. Gibbons and A. O'Connor, 'Infanticide and Child Murder – Admission to the Central Mental Hospital 1850–2000', *Irish Journal of Psychological Medicine* (2002; 19: 8–12)

56 Andrews, J. and A. Digby, 'Introduction: Gender and Class in the Historiography of British and Irish Psychiatry', *Clio Medica* (2004; 73:

7–44); Prior, P., 'Dangerous Lunacy: The Misuse of Mental Health Law in Nineteenth-Century Ireland', *Journal of Forensic Psychiatry and Psychology* (2003; 14: 525–41); Walsh, O., 'Gender and Insanity in Nineteenth-Century Ireland', *Clio Medica* (2004; 73: 69–93)

57   Reuber, M., 'The Architecture of Psychological Management: The Irish Asylums', *Psychological Medicine* (1996; 26: 1179–89); Williamson, A., 'Psychiatry, Moral Management and the Origins of Social Policy for Mentally Ill People in Ireland', *Irish Journal of Medical Science* (1992; 161: 556–8)

58   Kelly, B.D., 'One Hundred Years Ago: The Richmond Asylum, Dublin in 1907', *Irish Journal of Psychological Medicine* (2007; 24: 108–114)

59   Inspector of Lunatics (Ireland), *The Forty-Second Report (With Appendices) of the Inspector of Lunatics (Ireland)* (Dublin: Thom & Co./Her Majesty's Stationery Office, 1893); Torrey, E.F. and J. Miller, *The Invisible Plague: The Rise of Mental Illness from 1750 to the Present* (New Brunswick, New Jersey: Rutgers University Press, 2001); Walsh, D., 'The Ups and Downs of Schizophrenia in Ireland,' *Irish Journal of Psychiatry* (1992; 13: 12–16)

60   Smith, C., 'The Central Mental Hospital, Dundrum, Dublin' in R. Bluglass and P. Bowden (eds), *Principles and Practice of Forensic Psychiatry* (Edinburgh: Churchill Livingstone, 1990) pp. 1351–3

61   Finnane, M., *Insanity and the Insane in Post-Famine Ireland* (London: Croon Helm, 1981)

62   Buckingham, J., *Bitter Nemesis: The Intimate History of Strychnine* (Boca Raton, Florida: CRC Press (Taylor and Francis Group), 2008)

63   Aronson, J.K., *An Account of the Foxglove and Its Medical Uses, 1785–1985: Incorporating a Facsimile of William Withering's 'An Account of the Foxglove and Some of Its Uses' (1785)* (Oxford: Oxford University Press, 1985)

64   Hodgson, B., *In the Arms of Morpheus: The Tragic History of Morphine, Laudanum and Patent Medicines* (Buffalo, New York: Firefly Books (US) Inc., 2001); McGarry, R.C. and P. McGarry, 'Please Pass the Strychnine: The Art of Victorian Pharmacy', *Canadian Medical Association Journal* (1999; 161: 1556–8)

65   Simmons, H.G., 'Explaining Social Policy: The English Mental Deficiency Act of 1913', *Journal of Social History* (1978; 11: 387–403)

66   Kelly, B.D., 'Murder, Mercury, Mental Illness: Infanticide in Nineteenth-Century Ireland', *Irish Journal of Medical Science* (2007; 176: 149–52)

67   Conley, C.A., 'No Pedestals: Women and Violence in Late Nineteenth Century Ireland', *Journal of Social History* (1995; 28: 801–8); Kennedy, L., *Bastardy and the Great Famine: Ireland, 1845–1850* (Continuity and Change 1999; 14: 429–52)

68   Conley, C.A., 'No Pedestals: Women and Violence in Late Nineteenth Century Ireland', *Journal of Social History* (1995; 28: 801–8)

69   Jones, G., 'The Campaign Against Tuberculosis in Ireland, 1899–1914' in

E. Malcolm and G. Jones (eds), *Medicine, Disease and the State in Ireland, 1650–1940* (Cork: Cork University Press, 1999) pp. 158–76

70 McCandless, P., 'Curative Asylum, Custodial Hospital: The South Carolina Lunatic Asylum and State Hospital, 1828–1920' in R. Porter and D. Wright (eds), *The Confinement of the Insane: International Perspectives, 1800–1965* (Cambridge: Cambridge University Press, 2003) pp. 173–92

71 Dale, P. and J. Melling, 'The Politics of Mental Welfare: Fresh Perspectives on the History of Institutional Care for the Mentally Ill and Disabled' in Dale P and J. Melling (eds), *Mental Illness and Learning Disability: Finding a Place for Mental Disorder in the United Kingdom (Routledge Studies in the Social History of Medicine)* (London & New York: Routledge/Taylor & Francis Group, 2006) pp. 1–23; Scull, A.T., *Museums of Madness: The Social Organization of Insanity in Nineteenth-Century England* (London: Allen Lane, 1979); Walsh, D. and A. Daly, *Mental Illness in Ireland 1750–2002: Reflections on the Rise and Fall of Institutional Care* (Dublin: Health Research Board, 2004)

72 Anonymous, 'Increase in Insanity', *American Journal of Insanity* (1861; 18: 95); Inspector of Lunatics (Ireland), *The Forty-Second Report (With Appendices) of the Inspector of Lunatics (Ireland)* (Dublin: Thom & Co./ Her Majesty's Stationery Office, 1893); Tuke, D.H., 'Increase of Insanity in Ireland', *Journal of Mental Science* (1894; 40: 549–58); Walsh, O., 'Gender and Insanity in Nineteenth-Century Ireland', *Clio Medica* (2004; 73: 69–93)

73 Crompton, F., 'Needs and Desires in the Care of Pauper Lunatics: Admissions to Worcester Asylum, 1852–72' in P. Dale and J. Melling (eds), *Mental Illness and Learning Disability: Finding a Place for Mental Disorder in the United Kingdom (Routledge Studies in the Social History of Medicine)* (London & New York: Routledge/Taylor & Francis Group, 2006) pp. 46–64; Inspector of Lunatics (Ireland), *The Forty-Second Report (With Appendices) of the Inspector of Lunatics (Ireland)* (Dublin: Thom & Co./Her Majesty's Stationery Office, 1893)

74 Ireland, W.W., *The Blot upon the Brain* (1st edition) (Edinburgh: Bell & Bradfute, 1885); Michael, P. and D. Hirst, 'Establishing the "Rule of Kindness": The Foundation of the North Wales Lunatic Asylum, Denbeigh' in J. Melling and B. Forsythe (eds), *Insanity, Institutions and Society, 1800–1914: A Social History of Madness in Comparative Perspective (Studies in the Social History of Medicine)* (London & New York: Routledge/Taylor & Francis Group, 1999) pp. 159–79

75 Simmons, H.G., 'Explaining Social Policy: The English Mental Deficiency Act of 1913', *Journal of Social History* (1978; 11: 387–403)

76 Inspectors of Lunatics, *Special Report from the Inspectors of Lunatics to the Chief Secretary: Alleged Increasing Prevalence of Insanity in Ireland* (Dublin: Her Majesty's Stationery Office, 1894); Walsh, D. and A. Daly, *Mental Illness in Ireland 1750–2002: Reflections on the Rise and Fall of Institutional Care* (Dublin: Health Research Board, 2004)

77 Egan, M., 'The "Manufacture" of Mental Defectives: Why the Number
    of Mental Defectives increased in Scotland, 1857–1939' in P. Dale and
    J. Melling (eds), *Mental Illness and Learning Disability: Finding a Place
    for Mental Disorder in the United Kingdom (Routledge Studies in the Social
    History of Medicine)* (London & New York: Routledge/Taylor & Francis
    Group, 2006) pp. 131–53; Gladstone, D., 'The Changing Dynamic of
    Institutional Care: The Western Counties Idiot Asylum, 1864–1914' in
    D. Wright and A. Digby (eds), *From Idiocy to Mental Deficiency: Historical
    Perspectives on People with Learning Disabilities (Studies in the Social History
    of Medicine)* (London & New York: Routledge, 1996) pp. 134–60; Jackson,
    M., 'Institutional Provision for the Feeble-Minded in Edwardian
    England: Sandlebridge and the Scientific Morality of Permanent Care' in
    D. Wright and A. Digby (eds), *From Idiocy to Mental Deficiency: Historical
    Perspectives on People with Learning Disabilities (Studies in the Social History of
    Medicine)* (London & New York: Routledge, 1996) pp. 161–83

78 Inspectors of Lunatics, *Special Report from the Inspectors of Lunatics to
    the Chief Secretary: Alleged Increasing Prevalence of Insanity in Ireland*
    (Dublin: Her Majesty's Stationery Office, 1894); Walsh, D., and A. Daly,
    *Mental Illness in Ireland 1750–2002: Reflections on the Rise and Fall of
    Institutional Care* (Dublin: Health Research Board, 2004)

79 Finnane, M., *Insanity and the Insane in Post-Famine Ireland*
    (London: Croon Helm, 1981)

80 Andrews, J. and A. Digby, 'Introduction: Gender and Class in the
    Historiography of British and Irish Psychiatry', *Clio Medica* (2004; 73:
    7–44); Gibbons, P., N. Mulryan and A. O'Connor, 'Guilty but Insane:
    The Insanity Defence in Ireland, 1850–1995', *British Journal of Psychiatry*
    (1997; 170: 467–72)

81 Mulryan, N., P. Gibbons and A. O'Connor, 'Infanticide and Child
    Murder – Admissions to the Central Mental Hospital, 1850–2000', *Irish
    Journal of Psychological Medicine* (2002; 19: 8–12)

82 Gibbons, P., N. Mulryan and A. O'Connor, 'Guilty but Insane:
    The Insanity Defence in Ireland, 1850–1995', *British Journal of Psychiatry*
    (1997; 170: 467–72); Mulryan, N., P. Gibbons and A. O'Connor,
    'Infanticide and Child Murder – Admissions to the Central Mental
    Hospital, 1850–2000', *Irish Journal of Psychological Medicine* (2002; 19:
    8–12)

83 Glaser, W. and D. Flood, 'Beyond Specialist Programmes: A Study of the
    Needs of Offenders with Intellectual Disability Requiring Psychiatric
    Attention', *Journal of Intellectual Disability Research* (2004; 48: 591–602);
    Holland, T., I.C. Claire and T. Mukhopadhyay, 'Prevalence of Criminal
    Offending by Men and Women with Intellectual Disability and the
    Characteristics of Offenders: Implications for Research and Service
    Development', *Journal of Intellectual Disability Research* (2002; 46 (Suppl.
    1): 6–20); Lindsay, W.R., A.H. Smith, K. Quinn, A. Anderson, A. Smith,

R. Allan and J. Law, 'Women with Intellectual Disability who have Offended: Characteristics and Outcome', *Journal of Intellectual Disability Research* (2004; 48: 580–90)

84 Johnston, S.J., 'Risk Assessment in Offenders with Intellectual Disability: The Evidence Base', *Journal of Intellectual Disability Research* (2002; 46 (Suppl. 1): 47–56)

85 Fraser, W.I., 'Forensic Learning Disabilities: The Evidence Base: Executive summary', *Journal of Intellectual Disability Research* (2002; 46 (Suppl. 1): 1–5); Riches, V.C., T.R. Parmenter, M. Wiese and R.J. Stancliffe, 'Intellectual Disability and Mental Illness in the NSW Criminal Justice System', *International Journal of Law and Psychiatry* (2006; 29: 386–96)

86 Richmond Asylum Joint Committee, *Richmond Asylum Joint Committee Minutes* (Dublin: Richmond Asylum, 1907); Kelly, B.D., 'One Hundred Years Ago: The Richmond Asylum, Dublin in 1907', *Irish Journal of Psychological Medicine* (2007; 24: 108–114)

87 Walsh, O., 'Gender and Insanity in Nineteenth-Century Ireland', *Clio Medica* (2004; 73: 69–93)

88 Digby, A., 'Contexts and Perspectives' in D. Wright and A. Digby (eds), *From Idiocy to Mental Deficiency: Historical Perspectives on People with Learning Disabilities (Studies in the Social History of Medicine)* (London & New York: Routledge, 1996) pp. 1–21; Atkinson, D., M. Jackson and J. Walmsley, 'Introduction: Methods and Themes' in D. Atkinson, M. Jackson and J. Walmsley (eds), *Forgotten Lives: Exploring the History of Learning Disability* (Worcestershire, UK: British Institute of Learning Disabilities (BILD), 1997) pp. 1–20; Dale, P. and J. Melling, 'The Politics of Mental Welfare: Fresh Perspectives on the History of Institutional Care for the Mentally Ill and Disabled' in P. Dale and J. Melling (eds), *Mental Illness and Learning Disability: Finding a Place for Mental Disorder in the United Kingdom (Routledge Studies in the Social History of Medicine)* (London and New York: Routledge/Taylor & Francis Group, 2006) pp. 1–23

89 Simmons, H.G., 'Explaining Social Policy: The English Mental Deficiency Act of 1913', *Journal of Social History* (1978; 11: 387–403); Gladstone, D., 'The Changing Dynamic of Institutional Care: The Western Counties Idiot Asylum, 1864–1914' in D. Wright and A. Digby (eds), *From Idiocy to Mental Deficiency: Historical Perspectives on People with Learning Disabilities (Studies in the Social History of Medicine)* (London & New York: Routledge, 1996) pp. 134–160

90 Jackson, M., 'Institutional Provision for the Feeble-Minded in Edwardian England: Sandlebridge and the Scientific Morality of Permanent Care' in D. Wright and A. Digby (eds), *From Idiocy to Mental Deficiency: Historical Perspectives on People with Learning Disabilities (Studies in the Social History of Medicine)* (London & New York: Routledge, 1996)

pp. 161–183

91 Digby, A., 'Contexts and Perspectives' in D. Wright and A. Digby (eds), *From Idiocy to Mental Deficiency: Historical Perspectives on People with Learning Disabilities (Studies in the Social History of Medicine)* (London & New York: Routledge, 1996) pp 1–21

92 Irish College of Psychiatrists, *People With a Learning Disability who Offend: Forgiven but Forgotten? (Occasional Paper OP63)* (Dublin: Irish College of Psychiatrists, 2008)

93 Expert Group on Mental Health Policy, *A Vision for Change* (Dublin: The Stationery Office, 2006)

94 Dayan, L. and C. Ooi, 'Syphilis Treatment: Old and New', *Expert Opinion in Pharmacotherapy* (2005; 6: 2271–80); Fleetwood, J.F., *The History of Medicine in Ireland* (2nd edition) (Dublin: Skellig Press, 1983); Hutto, B., 'Syphilis in Clinical Psychiatry: A Review. Psychosomatics', (2001; 42: 453–60); Quetel, C., *The History of Syphilis* (Oxford: Polity Press, 1990); Rothschild, B.M., 'History of Syphilis', *Clinical Infectious Diseases* (2005; 40: 1454–63); Shorter, E., *A History of Psychiatry: From the Era of the Asylum to the Age of Prozac* (New York: John Wiley & Sons, 1997)

95 Prestwich, P.E., 'Family Strategies and Medical Power: "Voluntary" Committal in a Parisian Asylum, 1876–1914' in R. Porter and D. Wright (eds), *The Confinement of the Insane: International Perspectives, 1800–1965* (Cambridge: Cambridge University Press, 2003) pp. 79–99

96 Dörries, A. and T. Beddies, 'The Wittenauer Heilstätten in Berlin: A Case Record Study of Psychiatric Patients in Germany, 1919–1960' in R. Porter and D. Wright (eds), *The Confinement of the Insane: International Perspectives, 1800–1965* (Cambridge University Press, Cambridge, 2003) pp. 149–172

97 Fleetwood, J.F., *The History of Medicine in Ireland* (2nd edition) (Dublin: Skellig Press, 1983)

98 Kelly, B.D., 'Dr William Saunders Hallaran and Psychiatric Practice in Nineteenth-Century Ireland', *Irish Journal of Medical Science* (2008; 177: 79–84)

99 Hallaran, W.S., *Practical Observations on the Causes and Cures of Insanity* (2nd edition) (Cork: Edwards and Savage, 1818)

100 Finnane, M., *Insanity and the Insane in Post-Famine Ireland* (London: Croon Helm, 1981)

101 Dörries, A. and T. Beddies, 'The Wittenauer Heilstätten in Berlin: A Case Record Study of Psychiatric Patients in Germany, 1919–1960' in R. Porter and D. Wright (eds), *The Confinement of the Insane: International Perspectives, 1800–1965* (Cambridge: Cambridge University Press, 2003) pp. 149–72; Prestwich, P.E., 'Family Strategies and Medical Power: "Voluntary" Committal in a Parisian Asylum, 1876–1914' in R. Porter and D. Wright (eds), *The Confinement of the Insane: International Perspectives,*

1800–1965 (Cambridge: Cambridge University Press, 2003) pp. 79–99;
Torrey, E.F. and J. Miller, *The Invisible Plague: The Rise of Mental Illness
from 1750 to the Present* (New Brunswick, New Jersey: Rutgers University
Press, 2001)

102 Kelly, B.D., 'Syphilis, Psychiatry and Offending Behaviour: Clinical
Cases from Nineteenth-Century Ireland', *Irish Journal of Medical Science*
(2009; 178: 73–7)

103 Gibbons, P., N. Mulryan and A. O'Connor, 'Guilty but Insane:
The Insanity Defence in Ireland, 1850–1995', *British Journal of Psychiatry*
(1997; 170: 467–72); Mulryan, N., P. Gibbons and A. O'Connor,
'Infanticide and Child Murder – Admissions to the Central Mental
Hospital, 1850–2000', *Irish Journal of Psychological Medicine* (2002; 19:
8-12); Smith, C., 'The Central Mental Hospital, Dundrum, Dublin' in
R. Bluglass and P. Bowden (eds), *Principles and Practice of Forensic Psychiatry*
(Edinburgh: Churchill Livingstone, Edinburgh, 1990) pp. 1351–1353

104 Farthing, M.J.G., D.J. Jeffries and J.M. Parkin, 'Infectious Diseases,
Tropical Medicine and Sexually Transmitted Diseases' in P. Kumar
and M. Clark (eds), *Clinical Medicine* (3rd edition) (London: Baillière
Tindall, 1994) pp. 1–105

105 Ances, B.M., R. Shelhaus, M.J. Brown, O.V. Rios, S.T. Herman and
J.A. French, 'Neurosyphilis and Status Epilepticus: Case Report and
Literature Review', *Epilepsy Research* (2004; 59: 67–70); Clarke, C.R.A.,
'Neurological Diseases and Diseases of Voluntary Muscle' in P. Kumar
and M. Clark (eds), *Clinical Medicine* (3rd edition) (London: Baillière
Tindall, 1994) pp. 871–955; Gürses, C., M. Kürtüncü, J. Jirsch,
N. Yeşilot, H. Hanağasi, N. Bebek, B. Baykan, M. Emre, A. Gökyiğit
and F. Andermann, 'Neurosyphilis Presenting with Status Epilepticus',
Epileptic Disorders (2007; 9: 51–6)

106 Kaplan, H.I. and B.J. Saddock, *Concise Textbook of Clinical Psychiatry*
(Baltimore: Williams and Wilkins, 1996)

107 Farthing, M.J.G., D.J. Jeffries and J.M. Parkin, 'Infectious Diseases,
Tropical Medicine and Sexually Transmitted Diseases' in P. Kumar
and M. Clark (eds), *Clinical Medicine* (3rd edition) (London: Baillière
Tindall, 1994) pp. 1–105

108 Clarke, C.R.A., 'Neurological Diseases and Diseases of Voluntary
Muscle' in P. Kumar and M. Clark (eds), *Clinical Medicine* (3rd edition)
(London: Baillière Tindall, 1994) pp. 871–955

109 Walsh, O., 'Gender and Insanity in Nineteenth-Century Ireland',
Clio Med (2004; 73: 69–93)

110 Walsh, D., 'The Ups and Downs of Schizophrenia in Ireland',
Irish Journal of Psychiatry (1992; 13: 12–6)

111 Jones, G., 'The Campaign Against Tuberculosis in Ireland, 1899–1914' in
E. Malcolm and G. Jones (eds), *Medicine, Disease and the State in Ireland,
1650–1940* (Cork: Cork University Press, 1999) pp. 158–76

112   Finnane, M., *Insanity and the Insane in Post-Famine Ireland* (London: Croon Helm, 1981); Kelly, B.D., 'One Hundred Years Ago: The Richmond Asylum, Dublin in 1907', *Irish Journal of Psychological Medicine* (2007; 24: 108–14)

113   Brown, E.M., 'Why Wagner-Jauregg Won the Nobel Prize for Discovering Malaria Therapy for General Paralysis of the Insane', *History of Psychiatry* (2000; 11: 371–82); Fleetwood, J.F., *The History of Medicine in Ireland* (2nd edition) (Dublin: Skellig Press, 1983); Guthrie, D., *A History of Medicine* (London: Nelson, 1945); Merrit, H.H., R. Adams and H.C. Solomon, *Neurosyphilis* (Oxford: Oxford University Press, 1946)

114   Fleetwood, J.F., *The History of Medicine in Ireland* (2nd edition) (Dublin: Skellig Press, 1983)

115   Kelly, B.D., 'Murder, Mercury and Mental Illness: Infanticide in Nineteenth-Century Ireland', *Irish Journal of Medical Science* (2007; 176: 149–52)

116   Malcolm, E., *Swift's Hospital: A History of St Patrick's Hospital, Dublin, 1746–1989* (Dublin: Gill and Macmillan, 1989)

117   Gordon, A.G., 'Swift's Pocky Queen', *Journal of the Royal Society of Medicine* (1998; 92: 102)

118   Bewley, T.H., 'The Health of Jonathan Swift', *Journal of the Royal Society of Medicine* (1998; 91: 602–5); Bewley, T.H., 'Swift's Pocky Queen', *Journal of the Royal Society of Medicine* (1998; 92: 216)

119   Ferris, K., *James Joyce and the Burden of Disease* (Lexington: University Press of Kentucky, 1996)

120   Waisbren, B.A. and F.L. Walzl, 'Paresis and the Priest. James Joyce's Symbolic use of Syphilis in "The Sisters"', *Annals of Internal Medicine* (1974; 80: 758–62)

121   Prestwich, P.E., 'Family Strategies and Medical Power: "Voluntary" Committal in a Parisian Asylum, 1876–1914' in R. Porter and D. Wright (eds), *The Confinement of the Insane: International Perspectives, 1800–1965* (Cambridge: Cambridge University Press, 2003) pp. 79–99

122   Hutto, B., 'Syphilis in Clinical Psychiatry: A Review', *Psychosomatics* (2001; 42: 453–60)

123   Dayan, L. and C. Ooi, 'Syphilis Treatment: Old and New', *Expert Opinion in Pharmacotherapy* (2005; 6: 2271–80)

124   Hook, E.W. and R.W. Peeling, 'Syphilis Control – A Continuing Challenge', *New England Journal of Medicine* (2004; 351: 122–4)

135   Doherty, L., K.A. Fenton, J. Jones, T.C. Paine, S.P. Higgins, D. Williams and A. Palfreeman, 'Syphilis: Old Problem, New Strategy', *British Medical Journal* (2002; 325: 153–6)

126   Cronin, M., L. Domegan, L. Thornton, M. Fitzgerald, P. O'Lorcain, E. Creamer and D. O'Flanagan, 'The Epidemiology of Infectious

Syphilis in the Republic of Ireland', *Euro surveillance: Bulletin Européen sur les Maladies Transmissibles (European Communicable Disease Bulletin)* (2004; 9: 14–7); Hopkins, S., F. Lyons, F. Mulcahy and C. Bergin, 'The Great Pretender Returns to Dublin, Ireland', *Sexually Transmitted Infections* (2001; 77: 316–8); Hopkins, S., F. Lyons, C. Coleman, G. Courtney, C. Bergin and F. Mulcahy, 'Resurgence in Infectious Syphilis in Ireland: An Epidemiological Study', *Sexually Transmitted Diseases* (2004; 31: 317–21)

127 Gerbase, A.C., J.T. Rowley, T.E. Mertens, 'Global Epidemiology of Sexually Transmitted Diseases', *The Lancet* (1998; 351(suppl. 3): 2–4)

128 Ashton, M., W. Sopwith, P. Clark, D. McKelvey, L. Lighton and D. Mandal, 'An Outbreak No Longer: Factors Contributing to the Return of Syphilis in Greater Manchester', *Sexually Transmitted Infections* (2003; 79: 291–3)

129 Singh, A.E., K. Sutherland, B. Lee, J.L. Robinson and T. Wong, 'Resurgence of Congenital Syphilis in Alberta', *Canadian Medical Association Journal* (2007; 177: 33–6)

130 Tikhonova, L., E. Salakhov, K. Southwick, A. Shakarishvili, C. Ryan and S. Hillis, for the Congenital Syphilis Investigation Team, 'Congenital Syphilis in the Russian Federation: Magnitude, Determinants, and Consequences', *Sexually Transmitted Infections* (2003; 79: 106–10)

5. Reformation and Renewal: Into the Twentieth Century

1 Chapter 5 uses material from: Kelly, B.D., 'Physical Sciences and Psychological Medicine: The Legacy of Prof John Dunne', *Irish Journal of Psychological Medicine* (2005; 22: 67–72); Kelly, B.D., 'Mental Health Law in Ireland, 1945 to 2001: Reformation and Renewal?' *Medico-Legal Journal* (2008; 76: 65–72); Kelly, B.D., 'The Mental Treatment Act 1945 in Ireland: An Historical Enquiry', *History of Psychiatry* (2008; 19: 47–67); Kelly, B.D., 'Poverty, Crime and Mental Illness: Female Forensic Psychiatric Committal in Ireland, 1910–1948', *Social History of Medicine* (2008; 21: 311–28)

2 Kelly, B.D., 'The Mental Treatment Act 1945 in Ireland: An Historical Enquiry', *History of Psychiatry* (2008; 19: 47–67)

3 Ferriter, D., *The Transformation of Ireland 1900–2000* (London: Profile Books, 2004)

4 Finnane, M., *Insanity and the Insane in Post-Famine Ireland* (London: Croon Helm, 1981)

5 Barrington, R., *Health, Medicine and Politics in Ireland 1900–1970* (Dublin: Institute of Public Administration, 1987)

6 Healy, D., 'Irish Psychiatry in the Twentieth Century' in H. Freeman and G.E. Berrios (eds), *150 Years of British Psychiatry. Volume II: The Aftermath* (London: Athlone Press, 1996) pp. 268–91

7 Jones, G., 'The Campaign Against Tuberculosis in Ireland, 1899–1914' in

E. Malcolm and G. Jones (eds), *Medicine, Disease and the State in Ireland, 1650–1940* (Cork: Cork University Press, 1999) pp. 158–76

8   Barrington, R., *Health, Medicine and Politics in Ireland 1900–1970* (Dublin: Institute of Public Administration, 1987)

9   Barrington, R., *Health, Medicine and Politics in Ireland 1900–1970* (Dublin: Institute of Public Administration, 1987)

10 Psychiatrist, 'Insanity in Ireland', *The Bell* (1944; 7: 303–10)

11 O'Neill, A-M., *Irish Mental Health Law* (Dublin: First Law, 2005)

12 Prior, P., 'Dangerous Lunacy: The Misuse of Mental Health Law in Nineteenth-Century Ireland', *Journal of Forensic Psychiatry and Psychology* (2003; 14: 525–41)

13 Quotations from the Official Report of Dáil Éireann are Copyright Houses of Oireachtas

14 O'Neill, A-M., *Irish Mental Health Law* (Dublin: First Law, 2005)

15 Inspector of Lunatics (Ireland), *The Forty-Second Report (With Appendices) of the Inspector of Lunatics (Ireland)* (Dublin: Thom and Co./ Her Majesty's Stationery Office, 1893)

16 Kelly, B.D., 'Mental Illness in Nineteenth Century Ireland: A Qualitative Study of Workhouse Records', *Irish Journal of Medical Science* (2004; 173: 53–5)

17 Bartlett, P., *The Poor Law of Lunacy* (London and Washington, DC: Leicester University Press, 1999)

18 Inspector of Lunatics (Ireland), *The Forty-Second Report (With Appendices) of the Inspector of Lunatics (Ireland)* (Dublin: Thom and Co./ Her Majesty's Stationery Office, 1893)

19 Tuke, D.H., 'Increase of Insanity in Ireland', *Journal of Mental Science* (1894; 40: 549–58)

20 Anonymous, 'Increase in insanity', *American Journal of Insanity* (1861; 18: 95)

21 Torrey, E.F. and J. Miller, *The Invisible Plague: The Rise of Mental Illness from 1750 to the Present* (New Brunswick, New Jersey: Rutgers University Press, 2001)

22 Boyd, Barrett, E., 'Modern Psycho-Therapy and our Asylums', *Studies* (1924; 8: 29–43); Quotations from 'Modern Psycho-Therapy and Out Asylums' by E. Boyd Barrett (Studies 1924: 8: 29–43) are reproduced by kind permission of the editor of *Studies: An Irish Quarterly Review*

23 Psychiatrist, 'Insanity in Ireland', *The Bell* (1944; 7: 303–10)

24 O'Neill, A-M., *Irish Mental Health Law* (Dublin: First Law, 2005)

25 Healy, D., 'Irish Psychiatry in the Twentieth Century' in H. Freeman and G.E. Berrios (eds), *150 Years of British Psychiatry. Volume II: The Aftermath* (London: Athlone Press, 1996) pp. 268–91

26 Reynolds, J., *Grangegorman: Psychiatric Care in Dublin since 1815* (Dublin: Institute of Public Administration in association with Eastern Health Board, 1992)

27 Reynolds, J., *Grangegorman: Psychiatric Care in Dublin since 1815* (Dublin: Institute of Public Administration in association with Eastern Health Board, 1992)

28 Williamson, A.P., 'Psychiatry, Moral Management and the Origins of Social Policy for Mentally Ill People in Ireland', *Irish Journal of Medical Science* (1992; 161: 556–8); Reuber, M., 'The Architecture of Psychological Management: The Irish Asylums (1801–1922)', *Psychological Medicine* (1996; 26: 1179–89)

29 Walsh, D., 'Mental Illness in Ireland and its Management' in D. McCluskey (ed.) *Health Policy and Practice in Ireland* (Dublin: University College Dublin Press, 2006) pp. 29–43

30 Walsh, D. and A. Daly, *Mental Illness in Ireland 1750–2002: Reflections on the Rise and Fall of Institutional Care* (Dublin: Health Research Board, 2004)

31 See also: Kelly, B.D., 'Poverty, Crime and Mental Illness: Female Forensic Psychiatric Committal in Ireland, 1910–1948', *Social History of Medicine* (2008; 21: 311–28)

32 Shorter, E., *A History of Psychiatry: From the Era of the Asylum to the Age of Prozac* (New York: John Wiley & Sons, 1997).

33 United States, 'Bureau of the Census. Historical Statistics of the United States: Colonial Times to 1970', *Bicentennial Edition, Part 2* (Washington, DC: GPO, 1975)

34 See also: Scull, A., *The Most Solitary of Afflictions: Madness and Society in Britain, 1700–1900* (New Haven and London: Yale University Press, 1993); Shorter, E., *A History of Psychiatry: From the Era of the Asylum to the Age of Prozac* (New York: John Wiley & Sons, 1997); Stone, M.H., *Healing the Mind: A History of Psychiatry from Antiquity to the Present.* (London: Pimlico, 1998); Torrey, E.F. and J. Miller, *The Invisible Plague: The Rise of Mental Illness from 1750 to the Present* (New Brunswick, New Jersey: Rutgers University Press, 2001); Porter, R., *Madmen: A Social History of Madhouses, Mad-Doctors and Lunatics* (Gloucestershire, UK: Tempus Publishing, 2004)

35 Walsh, D., 'Mental Illness in Ireland and its Management' in D. McCluskey (ed.), *Health Policy and Practice in Ireland* (Dublin: University College Dublin Press, 2006) pp. 29–43

36 Kelly, B.D., 'Poverty, Crime and Mental Illness: Female Forensic Psychiatric Committal in Ireland, 1910–1948', *Social History of Medicine* (2008; 21: 311–28)

37 Lyons, F.S.L., *Ireland Since the Famine* (London: Fontana, 1985); Healy, D., 'Irish Psychiatry in the Twentieth Century' in H. Freeman and G.E. Berrios (eds), *150 Years of British Psychiatry. Volume II: The Aftermath* (London: Athlone Press, 1996) pp. 268–91

38 Viney, M., 'Mental illness: An Enquiry', *The Irish Times* (1968; October 23–30)

39 Dunne, J., 'Survey of Modern Physical Methods of Treatment for
    Mental Illness carried out in Grangegorman Mental Hospital', *Journal
    of the Medical Association of Eire* (1950; 27: 4–9)

40 O'Neill, A-M., *Irish Mental Health Law* (Dublin: First Law, 2005)

41 Gasser, J. and G. Heller, 'The Confinement of the Insane in Switzerland,
    1900–1970: Cery (Vaud) and Bel-Air (Geneva) Asylums' in R. Porter
    and D. Wright (eds), *The Confinement of the Insane: International
    Perspectives, 1800–1965* (Cambridge: Cambridge University Press, 2003)
    pp. 54–78

42 Suzuki, A., 'The State, Family, and the Insane in Japan, 1900–1945'
    in R. Porter and D. Wright (eds), *The Confinement of the Insane:
    International Perspectives, 1800–1965* (Cambridge: Cambridge University
    Press, 2003) pp. 193–225

43 Jain, S., 'Psychiatry and Confinement in India' in R. Porter
    and D. Wright (eds), *The Confinement of the Insane: International
    Perspectives, 1800–1965* (Cambridge: Cambridge University
    Press, 2003) pp. 273–98

44 Brand, J.L., 'The National Mental Health Act of 1946: A Retrospect',
    Bulletin of the History of Medicine (1965; 39: 231–45)

45 Bush, V., *Science: The Endless Frontier. A Report to the President*
    (Washington, DC: US Government Printing Office, 1945)

46 Beers, C.W., *A Mind That Found Itself: An Autobiography* (reprint)
    (Pittsburgh: Pittsburgh: University of Pittsburgh Press, 1981) (originally
    published in 1908)

47 Brand, J.L., 'The National Mental Health Act of 1946: A Retrospect',
    Bulletin of the History of Medicine (1965; 39: 231–45)

48 Menninger, W.C., 'Lessons from Military Psychiatry for Civilian
    Psychiatry', *Mental Hygiene* (1946; 30: 577–82)

49 Brand, J.L., 'The National Mental Health Act of 1946: A Retrospect',
    Bulletin of the History of Medicine (1965; 39: 231–45)

50 Clare, A., R.J. Daly, T.G. Dinan, D. King, B.E. Leonard, C. O'Boyle,
    J. O'Connor, J. Waddington, N. Walsh and M. Webb, 'Advancement of
    Psychiatric Research in Ireland: Proposal for a National Body', *Irish
    Journal of Psychological Medicine* (1990; 7: 93); Daly, R.J., 'Community
    Psychiatry and the National Institute of Mental Health', *Irish Journal of
    Psychological Medicine* (1990; 7: 5)

51 Ishay, M.R., *The History of Human Rights* (Berkeley and Los Angeles:
    University of California Press, 2004)

52 United Nations, *Principles for the Protection of Persons with Mental Illness
    and the Improvement of Mental Health Care* (New York: United Nations,
    Secretariat Centre For Human Rights, 1991)

53 Cooney, T. and O. O'Neill, *Psychiatric Detention: Civil Commitment in
    Ireland (Kritik 1)* (Wicklow, Ireland: Baikonur, 1996)

54 Kelly, B.D., 'Ireland's Mental Health Act 2001', *Psychiatric Bulletin* (2007; 31:

21–4); Ní Mhaoláin, Á. and B.D. Kelly, 'Ireland's Mental Health Act 2001: Where Are We Now?', *Psychiatric Bulletin* (2009; 33: 161–4)

55 Blehein, V., *The Minister for Health and Children and Others* [2008] (IESC 40); Madden, E., 'Section of Mental Health Act was Unconstitutional', *Irish Medical Times* (2009; 30: 15)

56 This section uses material from: Kelly, B.D., 'Physical Sciences and Psychological Medicine: The Legacy of Prof John Dunne', *Irish Journal of Psychological Medicine* (2005; 22: 67–72). Professor John Dunne's Presidential Address was delivered to annual meeting of the Royal Medico-Psychological Association (RMPA), the forerunner of the Royal College of Psychiatrists, on the 13 July 1955 and was reprinted in the *Journal of Mental Science* in the following year (Dunne, J., 'The Contribution of the Physical Sciences to Psychological Medicine', *Journal of Mental Science* (1956; 102: 209–20). Quotations from this paper are reprinted with the kind permission of the Royal College of Psychiatrists, and with the consent of Dr David Dunne. The author is grateful for the co-operation of the Royal College of Psychiatrists and Dr David Dunne.

57 Bewley, T., *Madness to Mental Illness: A History of the Royal College of Psychiatrists* (London: Royal College of Psychiatrists, 2008)

58 Bewley, T., *Madness to Mental Illness: A History of the Royal College of Psychiatrists* (London: Royal College of Psychiatrists, 2008); Collins, A., 'Eleonora Fleury Captured', *British Journal of Psychiatry* (2013; 203: 5)

59 Dunne, J., 'The Contribution of the Physical Sciences to Psychological Medicine', *Journal of Mental Science* (1956; 102: 209–20)

60 Reynolds, J., *Grangegorman: Psychiatric Care in Dublin since 1815* (Dublin: Institute of Public Administration in Association with Eastern Health Board, 1992)

61 Stone, M.H., *Healing the Mind: A History of Psychiatry from Antiquity to the Present* (London: Pimlico, 1998)

62 Dunne, J., 'Survey of Modern Physical Methods of Treatment for Mental Illness carried out in Grangegorman Mental Hospital', *Journal of the Medical Association of Eire* (1950; 27: 4–9)

63 Reynolds, J., *Grangegorman: Psychiatric Care in Dublin since 1815* (Dublin: Institute of Public Administration in association with Eastern Health Board, 1992)

64 Shorter, E., *A History of Psychiatry: From the Era of the Asylum to the Age of Prozac* (New York: John Wiley & Sons, 1997)

65 Reynolds, J., *Grangegorman: Psychiatric Care in Dublin since 1815* (Dublin: Institute of Public Administration in association with Eastern Health Board, 1992)

66 Dunne, J,. 'Survey of Modern Physical Methods of Treatment for Mental Illness carried out in Grangegorman Mental Hospital', *Journal of the Medical Association of Eire* (1950; 27: 4–9)

67   Reynolds, J., *Grangegorman: Psychiatric Care in Dublin since 1815* (Dublin: Institute of Public Administration in association with Eastern Health Board, 1992)

68   Dunne, J., 'The Contribution of the Physical Sciences to Psychological Medicine', *Journal of Mental Science* (1956; 102: 209–20)

69   Claes, S.J., 'Corticotropin-Releasing Hormone (CRH) in Psychiatry: From Stress to Psychopathology', *Annals of Medicine* (2004; 36: 50–61). Current evidence suggests that CRH is not only critical for the regulation of the hypothalamic pituitary adrenal (HPA) axis, but also acts as a neurotransmitter in several brain regions. In addition to mediating reactions to stress, however, CRH can also produce psycho-pathological effects in the context of chronic stress. Given these strong emerging relationships between CRH and HPA axis abnormalities in major depression and other mental illnesses, it is suggested that this field of enquiry may radically change our understanding of much human psycho-pathology in the years to come.

70   Fleshner, M. and M.L. Laudenslager, 'Psychoneuroimmunology: Then and Now', *Behavioral and Cognitive Neuroscience Reviews* (2004; 3: 114–30)

71   Germine, M., 'Information and Psychopathology', *Journal of Nervous and Mental Disease* (1993; 181: 382–7)

72   Stone, M.H., *Healing the Mind: A History of Psychiatry from Antiquity to the Present* (London: Pimlico, 1998)

73   Jeffery, K.J. and I.C. Reid, 'Modifiable Neuronal Connections: An Overview for Psychiatrists', *American Journal of Psychiatry* (1997; 154: 156–64)

74   Horwitz, B. and A.R. Braun, 'Brain Network Interactions in Auditory, Visual and Linguistic Processing. Brain and Language' (2004; 89: 377–84)

75   Grossberg, S. and J.W. Merrill, 'A Neural Network Model of Adaptively Timed Reinforcement Learning and Hippocampal Dynamics', *Brain Research. Cognitive Brain Research* (1992; 1: 3–38)

76   Gustafsson, L. and A.P. Paplinski, 'Self-Organization of an Artificial Neural Network Subjected to Attention Shift Impairments and Familiarity Preference, Characteristics Studied in Autism', *Journal of Autism and Developmental Disorders* (2004; 34: 189–98)

77   Ward, N.S., 'Functional Reorganization of the Cerebral Motor System after Stroke', *Current Opinion in Neurology* (2004; 17: 725–30)

78   Friedel, R.O., 'Dopamine Dysfunction in Borderline Personality Disorder: A Hypothesis', *Neuropsychopharmacology* (2004; 29: 1029–39)

79   Dennett, D., *Consciousness Explained* (Boston: Little, Brown, 1991); Damasio, A., *The Feeling of What Happens: Body, Emotion and the Making of Consciousness* (London: Vintage, 2000)

80   Shorter, E., *A History of Psychiatry: From the Era of the Asylum to the Age of Prozac* (New York: John Wiley & Sons, 1997).

81   Millon, T., *Masters of the Mind: Exploring the Story of Mental Illness from*

Ancient Times to the New Millennium (Hoboken, New Jersey: John Wiley & Sons, 2004)

82 Edelman, G., *The Remembered Present* (New York: Basic Books, 1989); Dennett, D., *Consciousness Explained* (Boston: Little, Brown, 1991); Damasio, A., *The Feeling of What Happens: Body, Emotion and the Making of Consciousness* (London: Vintage, 2000)

83 Gabbard, G.O. and J. Kay, 'The Fate of Integrated Treatment: Whatever Happened to the Biopsychosocial Psychiatrist?', *American Journal of Psychiatry* (2001; 158:1956–63)

84 Reynolds, J., *Grangegorman: Psychiatric Care in Dublin since 1815* (Dublin: Institute of Public Administration in association with Eastern Health Board, 1992)

85 Wiglesworth, J., 'The Presidential Address, Delivered at the Sixty-first Annual Meeting of the Medico-Psychological Association, Held at Liverpool on July 24th, 1902', *Journal of Mental Science* (1902; XLVIII: 611–45); Smith, R.P., 'The Presidential Address, on Paranoia, Delivered at the Sixty-Third Annual Meeting of the Medico-Psychological Association, Held in London on July 21 and 22, 1904', *Journal of Mental Science* (1904; L: 607–33); Renvoize, E., 'The Association of Medical Officers of Asylums and Hospitals for the Insane, the Medico-Psychological Association, and their Presidents', in G.E. Berrios and H. Freeman (eds), *150 years of British Psychiatry, 1841–1991* (London: Gaskell/Royal College of Psychiatrists, 1991) pp. 29–78

86 Spence, B., 'Presidential Address to the Medico-Psychological Association', *Journal of Mental Science* (1899; XLV: 635–42)

87 Turner, F.D., 'Mental Deficiency: Presidential Address at the 92nd Annual Meeting of the Royal Medico-Psychological Association, July, 1933', *Journal of Mental Science* (1933; 79: 563–77)

88 Masefield, W.G., 'Psychiatric Ruminations; The Presidential Address Delivered at the One Hundred and Sixth Annual Meeting of the Royal Medico-Psychological Association held at Eastbourne, 10 July 1947', *Journal of Mental Science* (1948; 94: 217–24)

89 The contents of earlier presidential addresses delivered by Irish presidents of the RMPA between 1860 and 1885 are explored in Healy, D., 'Irish Psychiatry. Part 2: Use of the Medico-Psychological Association by its Irish Members – Plus Ca Change!' in G.E. Berrios and H. Freeman H (eds), *150 Years of British Psychiatry, 1841–1991* (London: Gaskell/Royal College of Psychiatrists, 1991) pp. 314–20

90 This section of the book uses material drawn from: Kelly, B.D., 'Mental Health Law in Ireland, 1945 to 2001: Reformation and Renewal?' *Medico-Legal Journal* (2008; 76: 65–72)

91 Lyons, F.S.L., *Ireland Since the Famine* (London: Fontana, 1985)

92 Kelly, B.D., 'Penrose's Law in Ireland: An Ecological Analysis of Psychiatric Inpatients and Prisoners', *Irish Medical Journal* (2007; 100: 373–4)

93 Psychiatrist, 'Insanity in Ireland', *The Bell* (1944; 7: 303–10)

94 Dunne, J., 'Out-Patient Psychiatric Clinic – Report of Two Years' Work', *Journal of the Irish Medical Association* (1971; 64: 7–9)

95 Dunne, J., 'Survey of Modern Physical Methods of Treatment for Mental Illness Carried out in Grangegorman Mental Hospital', *Journal of the Medical Association of Eire* (1950; 27: 4–9)

96 Dunne, J., 'The Contribution of the Physical Sciences to Psychological Medicine', *Journal of Mental Science* (1956; 102: 209–20); Kelly, B.D., 'Physical Sciences and Psychological Medicine: The Legacy of Prof John Dunne', *Irish Journal of Psychological Medicine* (2005; 22: 67–72)

97 Shorter, E., *A History of Psychiatry: From the Era of the Asylum to the Age of Prozac* (New York: John Wiley & Sons, 1997)

98 Walsh, D. and A. Daly, *Mental Illness in Ireland 1750–2002: Reflections on the Rise and Fall of Institutional Care* (Dublin: Health Research Board, 2004)

99 Viney, M., 'Mental Illness: An Enquiry', *The Irish Times* (1968; October 23–30)

100 Department of Health, *Commission of Enquiry on Mental Illness 1966 Report* (Dublin: The Stationery Office, 1966); Healy, D., 'Irish Psychiatry in the Twentieth Century' in H. Freeman and G.E. Berrios (eds), *150 Years of British Psychiatry. Volume II: The Aftermath* (London: Athlone Press, 1996) pp. 268–91

101 Williamson, A., 'The Beginnings of State Care for the Mentally Ill in Ireland', *Economic and Social Review* (1970; 10: 281–90)

102 Walsh, D. and A. Daly, *Mental Illness in Ireland 1750–2002: Reflections on the Rise and Fall of Institutional Care* (Dublin: Health Research Board, 2004)

103 Department of Health, *The Psychiatric Services – Planning for the Future* (Dublin: The Stationery Office, 1984)

104 Kelly, B.D., 'Mental Health Policy in Ireland, 1984–2004: Theory, Overview and Future Directions', *Irish Journal of Psychological Medicine* (2004; 21: 61–8)

105 Expert Group on Mental Health Policy, *A Vision for Change* (Dublin: Stationery Office, 2006)

106 Guruswamy, S. and B.D. Kelly, 'A Change of Vision? Mental Health Policy', *Irish Medical Journal* (2006; 99: 164–5)

107 United Nations, *Principles for the Protection of Persons with Mental Illness and the Improvement of Mental Health Care* (New York: United Nations, Secretariat Centre For Human Rights, 1991)

108 O'Shea, B., 'The Mental Health Act, 2001: A Brief Summary', *Irish Medical Journal* (2002; 5: 153); Kelly, B.D., 'Ireland's Mental Health Act 2001', *Psychiatric Bulletin* (2007; 31: 21–4)

109 www.mhcirl.ie

110 Kelly, B.D., 'Viewpoint: The Mental Health Act 2001', *Irish Medical Journal* (2002; 95: 151–2); O'Shea, B., 'The Mental Health Act, 2001: A Brief

Summary', *Irish Medical Journal* (2002; 5: 153); Daly, I., 'Implementing the Mental Health Act 2001: What Should be done? What Can be Done?', *Irish Journal of Psychological Medicine* (2005; 22: 80–1); Ganter, K., 'Implementing the Mental Health Act 2001: What Should be Done? What Can be Done? *Irish Journal of Psychological Medicine* (2005; 22: 79–80); Lawlor, B., 'Implementing the Mental Health Act 2001: What Should be Done? What Can be Done? *Irish Journal of Psychological Medicine* (2005; 22: 79); Owens, J., 'Implementing the Mental Health Act 2001: What Should be Done? What Can be Done? *Irish Journal of Psychological Medicine* (2005; 22: 81–2)

111 Kelly, B.D., 'Ireland's Mental Health Act 2001', *Psychiatric Bulletin* (2007; 31: 21–4)

112 Ganter, K., 'Implementing the Mental Health Act 2001: What Should be Done? What Can be Done? *Irish Journal of Psychological Medicine* (2005; 22: 79–80)

113 Whelan, D., 'Mental Health Tribunals: A Significant Medico-Legal Change', *Medico-Legal Journal* of Ireland (2004; 10: 84–9); O'Neill, A-M., *Irish Mental Health Law* (Dublin: First Law, 2005)

114 O'Neill, A-M., *Irish Mental Health Law* (Dublin: First Law, 2005)

115 McGuinness, I., 'Tribunals Revoke 12 per cent of Detentions', *Irish Medical News* (2007; 26 October)

116 Department of Health and Children, *Review of the Operation of the Mental Health Act 2001: Findings and Conclusions* (Dublin: Department of Health and Children, 2007). See also: McGuinness, I., 'Report Addresses Serious Challenges', *Irish Medical News* (2007; 29 June); Ní Mhaoláin, Á. and B.D. Kelly, 'Ireland's Mental Health Act 2001: Where are we now?', *Psychiatric Bulletin* (2009; 33: 161–4)

117 Culliton, G., 'Review of Act is to be Built on "Human Rights"', *Irish Medical Times* (2011; 27 May)

118 Steering Group on the Review of the Mental Health Act 2001, *Interim Report of the Steering Group on the Review of the Mental Health Act 2001* (Dublin: Department of Health, 2012)

119 Quoted in: Macleod, S.M. and H.N. McCullough, 'Social Science Education as a Component of Medical Training', *Social Science and Medicine* (1994; 39: 1367–73)

120 Kennedy, H., *The Annotated Mental Health Acts* (Dublin: Blackhall Publishing, 2007)

121 Giblin, Y., A. Kelly, E. Kelly, H.G. Kennedy and D.J. Mohan, 'Reducing the Use of Seclusion for Mental Disorder in a Prison: Implementing a High Support Unit in a Prison Using Participant Action Research', *International Journal of Mental Health Systems* (2012; 6: 2); McInerney, C., M. Davoren, G. Flynn, D. Mullins, M. Fitzpatrick, M. Caddow, F. Caddow, S. Quigley, F. Black, H..G Kennedy and C. O'Neill, 'Implementing a Court Diversion and Liaison Scheme in a Remand

Prison by Systematic Screening of /New Receptions: A 6 Year Participatory Action Research Study of 20,084 Consecutive Male Remands', *International Journal of Mental Health Systems* (2013; 7: 18); Houston, M., 'Mountjoy Team Wins Top Psychiatric Care Award', *The Irish Times* (2011; 6 October)

122 See, for example: Davoren, M., S. O'Dwyer, Z. Abidin, L. Naughton, O. Gibbons, E. Doyle, K. McDonnell, S. Monks and H.G. Kennedy, 'Prospective In-Patient Cohort Study of Moves between Levels of Therapeutic Security; the DUNDRUM-1 Triage Security, DUNRDUM-3 Programme Completion and DUNDRUM-4 Recovery Scales and the HCR-20', *BMC Psychiatry* (2012; 12: 80)

123 Croudace, T.J., R. Kayne, P.B. Jones and G.L. Harrison, 'Non-Linear Relationship Between an Index of Social Deprivation, Psychiatric Admission, Prevalence and the Incidence of Psychosis', *Psychological Medicine* (2000; 30: 177–85)

124 Taylor, P.J. and J. Gunn, 'Violence and Psychosis, I: Risk of Violence among Psychotic Men,' *British Medical Journal (Clinical Research Edition)* (1984; 288: 1945–9); Teplin, L.A., 'Criminalizing Mental Disorder: The Comparative Arrest Rate of the Mentally Ill', *American Psychologist* (1984; 39: 794–803)

125 Fazel, S. and J. Danesh, 'Serious Mental Disorder in 23,000 Prisoners: A Systematic Review of 62 Surveys,' *The Lancet* (2002; 359: 545–50); Duffy, D., S. Linehan and H.G. Kennedy, 'Psychiatric Morbidity in the Male Sentenced Irish Prisons Population', *Irish Journal of Psychological Medicine* (2006; 23: 54–62.

126 O'Neill, C., H. Sinclair, A. Kelly and H. Kennedy, 'Interaction of Forensic and General Psychiatric Services in Ireland: Learning the Lessons or Repeating the Mistakes?', *Irish Journal of Psychological Medicine* (2002; 19: 48–54)

127 Psychiatrist, 'Insanity in Ireland', *The Bell* (1944; 7: 303–10)

Bibliography

PRIMARY SOURCES

Archival Sources

Central Mental Hospital (Central Criminal Lunatic Asylum), Dundrum, Dublin 14, Ireland
Male and Female Medical Case Records, 1868 to 1948 (except for female records for 1909)

Ballinrobe Parish, County Mayo, Ireland
Minutes from Ballinrobe Poor Law Union (Workhouse), County Mayo, 1845 to 1900

St Brendan's Hospital (Richmond Asylum), Rathdown Road, Phibsborough, Dublin 7, Ireland
Richmond Asylum Joint Committee Minutes, 1907

Legislation
Lunacy (Ireland) Act 1821 (1 & 2 Geo. 4, C. 33)
Criminal Lunatics (Ireland) Act 1838 (1 & 2 Vict. C. 27)
Central Criminal Lunatic Asylum (Ireland) Act 1845 (8 & 9 Vict. C. 107)
Lunacy Regulations (Ireland) Act 1871 (34 & 35 Vict. C. 22)
Local Government (Ireland) Act 1898 (61 & 62 Vict. C. 37)
Mental Deficiency Act 1913 (3 & 4, Geo. 5, C. 38)
Mental Treatment Act 1945 (No. 19 of 1945)
Infanticide Act 1949 (No. 16 of 1949)
Mental Health Act 2001 (No. 25 of 2001)

Court Cases

Blehein *v.* The Minister for Health and Children and Others (2008) IESC
40

Reports of the Inspectorates of Lunatics and Asylums

Inspector of Lunatic Asylums in Ireland, *Report of the District, Local, and Private
Lunatic Asylums in Ireland, 1846* (With Appendices (Dublin: Alexander Thom
for Her Majesty's Stationery Office, 1847)

Inspectors-General on District, Criminal and Private Lunatic Asylums in
Ireland, *Report of the Inspectors-General on District, Criminal and Private
Lunatic Asylums in Ireland* (Dublin: Her Majesty's Stationery Office, 1855)

Inspector of Lunatics (Ireland) *The Forty-Second Report (With Appendices) of
the Inspector of Lunatics (Ireland)* (Dublin: Thom and Co./Her Majesty's
Stationery Office, 1893)

Inspectors of Lunatics, *Special Report from the Inspectors of Lunatics to the Chief
Secretary: Alleged Increasing Prevalence of Insanity in Ireland* (Dublin: Her
Majesty's Stationery Office, 1894)

Inspector of Mental Health Services, *Report of the Inspector of Mental Health
Services 2004* (Dublin: Mental Health Commission, 2005)

Printed Works Published In or Before 1956

Anonymous, 'Increase in Insanity', *American Journal of Insanity* (1861; 18: 95)

Anonymous, 'Obituary: Daniel Hack Tuke', *The Lancet* (1895; 145: 718–9)

Beers, C.W., *A Mind That Found Itself: An Autobiography* (reprint) (Pittsburgh:
University of Pittsburgh Press, 1981) (originally published in 1908)

Boyd, Barrett E., 'Modern Psycho-Therapy and Our Asylums', *Studies*
(1924; 8: 29–43)

Bush, V., *Science: The Endless Frontier. A Report to the President* (Washington, DC:
US Government Printing Office, 1945)

Bynum, W.F., 'Rationales for Therapy in British Psychiatry: 1780–1835',
Medical History (1964; 18: 317–34)

Churchill, F., 'On the Mental Disorders of Pregnancy and Childbed', *Dublin
Quarterly Journal of Medical Science* (1850; 17: 39)

Cox, J.M., *Practical Observations on Insanity* (London: Baldwin and Murray,
1804)

Dillon, W., 'Law Adviser's Report on the Liability of the Joint Committee
of Management of the Richmond District Asylum to Maintain Lunatics
Sent From Workhouses and as to Their Powers to Erect and Maintain
Auxiliary Asylums for Harmless and Chronic Lunatics', *Richmond Asylum
Joint Committee Minutes* (Dublin: Richmond Asylum, 1907)

Drapes, T., 'On the Alleged Increase in Insanity in Ireland', *Journal of Mental
Science* (1894; 40: 519–43)

Dunne, J., 'Survey of Modern Physical Methods of Treatment for Mental Illness Carried Out in Grangegorman Mental Hospital', *Journal of the Medical Association of Éire* (1950; 27: 4–9)

Dunne, J., 'The Contribution of the Physical Sciences to Psychological Medicine', *Journal of Mental Science* (1956; 102: 209–20)

Esquirol, J-É., *Des Passions* (Paris: Didot Jeune, 1805)

Gralnick, A., 'Folie à Deux', *Psychiatric Quarterly* (1942; 16: 230–63)

Guthrie, D., *A History of Medicine* (London: Nelson, 1945)

Halberstadt, G., *La Folie par Contagion Mentale* (Paris: Baillière, 1906)

Hallaran, W.S., *An Enquiry into the Causes Producing the Extraordinary Addition to the Number of Insane Together with Extended Observations on the Cure of Insanity with Hints as to the Better Management of Public Asylums for Insane Persons* (Cork: Edwards and Savage, 1810)

Hallaran, W.S., *Practical Observations on the Causes and Cures of Insanity* (2nd edition) (Cork: Edwards and Savage, 1818)

Ireland, W.W., 'Folie à Deux – A Mad Family' in W.W. Ireland, *The Blot upon the Brain* (1st edition) (Edinburgh: Bell & Bradfute, 1885) pp. 201–208

Ireland, W.W., *The Blot upon the Brain* (1st edition) (Edinburgh: Bell & Bradfute, 1885)

Jones, K., *Lunacy, Law and Conscience* (London: Routledge and Kegan Paul, 1955)

Lasègue, C. and J. Falret, 'La Folie à Deux ou Folie Communiquée', *Annales Medico-Psychologiques* (1877; 18: 321–55)

Maudsley, H., 'Homicidal insanity', *Journal of Mental Science* (1863; 47: 327–43)

MacCabe, F., 'On the Alleged Increase in Lunacy', *Journal of Mental Science* (1869; 15: 363–6)

Menninger, W.C., 'Lessons from Military Psychiatry for Civilian Psychiatry', *Mental Hygiene* (1946; 30: 577–82)

Merrit, H.H., R. Adams and H.C. Solomon, *Neurosyphilis* (Oxford: Oxford University Press, 1946)

Mickaud, R., 'Translation of Lasègue and Farlet's Paper of 1877: Le Folie à ou Folie Communiquée', *American Journal of Psychiatry* (1964; 121 (suppl. 4))

M'Manus, L., 'Folk-Tales from Western Ireland', *Folklore* (1914; 25: 324–41)

Norman, C., 'Report of Dr Norman', *Richmond Asylum Joint Committee Minutes* (Dublin: Richmond Asylum, 1907)

Powell, R., 'Observations Upon the Comparative Prevalence of Insanity at Different Periods', *Medical Transactions* (1813; 4: 131–59)

Psychiatrist, 'Insanity in Ireland', *The Bell* (1944; 7: 303–10)

Ray, I., *A Treatise on the Medical Jurisprudence of Insanity* (3rd edition, with additions) (Cambridge, Massachusetts: Little, Brown and Company, 1853)

Ray, I., 'Confinement of the Insane', *American Law Review* (1869; 3: 193–221)

Ray, I. and W. Overholser (ed.), *A Treatise on the Medical Jurisprudence of Insanity* (reprint) (Cambridge, Massachusetts: Harvard University Press, 1962) (first published 1838)

Tuke, D.H., 'Folie à Deux', *Brain* (1888; 10: 408–21)

Tuke, D.H., 'Increase of Insanity in Ireland', *Journal of Mental Science* (1894; 40: 549–58)

Tuomy, M., *Treatise on the Principal Diseases of Dublin* (Dublin: William Folds, 1810)

Wilde, F.S., *Ancient Legends, Mystic Charms, and Superstitions of Ireland* (London: Ward and Downey, 1887)

Woods, O.T., 'Notes of a Case of Folie à Deux in Five Members of One Family', *Journal of Mental Science* (1889; 34: 535–39)

Yeats, W.B., *Irish Fairy Tales* (New York: Scott, 1907)

Secondary Sources

Allan, C., 'Blame Game Players are Thoughtless and Ill-Informed', *Guardian* (6 February 2008)

Amnesty International, *Amnesty International Report 2006: The State of the World's Human Rights* (London: Amnesty International UK, 2006)

Ances, B.M., R. Shelhaus, M.J. Brown, O.V. Rios, S.T. Herman and J.A. French, 'Neurosyphilis and Status Epilepticus: Case Report and Literature Review', *Epilepsy Research* (2004; 59: 67–70)

Andrews, J., 'The Boundaries of her Majesty's Pleasure: Discharging Child-Murderers from Broadmoor and Perth Criminal Lunatic Department, *c.*1860–1920' in M. Jackson (ed.), *Infanticide: Historical Perspectives on Child Murder and Concealment* (Aldershot: Ashgate, 2002) pp. 216–248

Andrews, J. and A. Digby, 'Introduction: Gender and Class in the Historiography of British and Irish Psychiatry', *Clio Medica* (2004; 73: 7–44)

Andrews, J. and A. Digby (eds), *Sex and Seclusion, Class and Custody: Perspectives on Gender and Class in the History of British and Irish Psychiatry* (Amsterdam: Rodopi, 2004)

Andrews, J. and A. Scull, *Customers and Patrons of the Mad-Trade: The Management of Lunacy in Eighteenth-Century London, with the Complete Text of John Munro's 1766 Case Book* (Berkeley CA: University of California Press, 2002)

Appleby, L., 'Suicide and Self-harm' in R. Murray, P. Hill, P. McGuffin (eds), *The Essentials of Postgraduate Psychiatry* (3rd edition) (Cambridge: Cambridge University Press, 1997) pp. 551–562

Aronson, J.K., *An Account of the Foxglove and Its Medical Uses, 1785–1985: Incorporating a Facsimile of William Withering's 'An Account of the Foxglove and Some of Its Uses' (1785)* (Oxford: Oxford University Press, 1985)

Ashton, M., W. Sopwith, P. Clark, D. McKelvey, L. Lighton and D. Mandal, 'An Outbreak No Longer: Factors Contributing to the Return of Syphilis in Greater Manchester', *Sexually Transmitted Infections* (2003; 79: 291–3)

Atkinson, D., M. Jackson and J. Walmsley, 'Introduction: Methods and Themes' in D. Atkinson, M. Jackson, J. Walmsley (eds), *Forgotten Lives: Exploring the History of Learning Disability* (Worcestershire, UK: British Institute of Learning Disabilities (BILD) 1997) pp. 1–20

Bardon, J., *A History of Ulster* (Belfast: Blackstaff Press, 1993)

Barrington, R., *Health, Medicine and Politics in Ireland 1900–1970*
(Dublin: Institute of Public Administration, 1987)

Bartlett, P., *The Poor Law of Lunacy* (London and Washington, DC: Leicester
University Press, 1999)

Benedek, E.P., 'Premenstrual Syndrome: A View from the Bench', *Journal of
Clinical Psychiatry* (1988; 49: 498–502)

Berrios, G.E., *The History of Mental Symptoms: Descriptive Psychopathology since the
19th Century* (Cambridge: Cambridge University Press, 1996)

Berrios, G.E., 'Introduction. Classic Text No. 35: Folie à Deux – A Mad
Family', *History of Psychiatry* (1998; 9: 383–95)

Bewley, T., *Madness to Mental Illness: A History of the Royal College of
Psychiatrists* (London: Royal College of Psychiatrists, 2008)

Bewley, T.H., 'The Health of Jonathan Swift', *Journal of the Royal Society of
Medicine* (1998; 91: 602–5)

Bewley, T.H., 'Swift's Pocky Queen', *Journal of the Royal Society of Medicine*
(1999; 92: 216)

Bourgeois, M.L., P. Duhamel and H. Verdoux, 'Delusional Parasitosis: Folie
à Deux and Attempted Murder of a Family Doctor', *British Journal of
Psychiatry* (1992; 161: 709–11)

Bourke, A., *The Burning of Bridget Cleary: A True Story* (London: Pimlico, 1999)

Brand, J.L., 'The National Mental Health Act of 1946: A Retrospect', *Bulletin
of the History of Medicine* (1965; 39: 231–45)

Breathnach, C.S. and J.B. Moynihan, 'An Irish Statistician's Analysis of the
National Tuberculosis Problem – Robert Charles Geary (1896–1983)',
Irish Journal of Medical Science (2003; 172: 149–53)

Breckenridge, A., 'William Withering's Legacy – For the Good of the Patient',
Clinical Medicine (2006; 6: 393–7)

Brown, E.M., 'Why Wagner-Jauregg Won the Nobel Prize for Discovering
Malaria Therapy for General Paralysis of the Insane', *History of Psychiatry*
(2000; 11: 371–382)

Buckingham, J., *Bitter Nemesis: The Intimate History of Strychnine* (Boca Raton,
Florida: CRC Press (Taylor and Francis Group), 2008)

Carlson, E.T. and N. Dain, 'The Psychotherapy that was Moral Treatment,'
American Journal of Psychiatry (1960; 117: 519–524)

Carter, R., 'James Joyce (1882–1941): Medical History, Final Illness and Death',
World Journal of Surgery (1996; 20: 720–724)

Cawte, J. and M. Tarrant, 'Capgras' Syndrome: Outmoded Term for
Changeling Delusions?' *Australian and New Zealand Journal of Psychiatry*
(1984; 18: 388–90)

Cherry, S. and R. Munting, '"Exercise is the Thing"? Sport and the Asylum
*c.*1850–1950', *International Journal of the History of Sport* (2005; 22: 42–58)

Claes, S.J., 'Corticotropin-Releasing Hormone (CRH) in Psychiatry: From
Stress to Psychopathology', *Annals of Medicine* (2004; 36: 50–61)

Clare, A.W., 'St Patrick's Hospital', *American Journal of Psychiatry* (1998; 155: 1599)

Clare, A.W., 'Swift, Mental Illness and St Patrick's Hospital', *Irish Journal of Psychological Medicine* (1998; 15: 100–104)

Clare, A., R.J. Daly, T.G. Dinan, D. King, B.E. Leonard, C. O'Boyle, J. O'Connor, J. Waddington, N. Walsh and M. Webb, 'Advancement of Psychiatric Research in Ireland: Proposal for a National Body', *Irish Journal of Psychological Medicine* (1990; 7: 93)

Clarke, C.R.A., 'Neurological Diseases and Diseases of Voluntary Muscle' in P. Kumar and M. Clark (eds), *Clinical Medicine* (3rd edition) (London: Baillière Tindall, 1994) pp. 871–955

Clark, M. and C. Crawford (eds), *Legal Medicine in History (Cambridge Studies in the History of Medicine)* (Cambridge: Cambridge University Press, 1994)

Coleborne, C., 'Passage to the Asylum: The Role of the Police in Committals of the Insane in Victoria, Australia, 1848–1900' in R. Porter and D. Wright (eds), *The Confinement of the Insane: International Perspectives, 1800–1965* (Cambridge: Cambridge University Press, 2003) pp. 129–148.

Collins, A., 'Eleonora Fleury Captured', *British Journal of Psychiatry* (2013; 203: 5)

Condrau, F., 'The Patient's View meets the Clinical Gaze', *Social History of Medicine* (2007; 20: 525–540)

Conley, C.A., 'No Pedestals: Women and Violence in Late Nineteenth Century Ireland', *Journal of Social History* (1995; 28: 801–808)

Connolly, M. and N. Jones, 'Constructing Management Practice in the New Public Management: The Case of Mental Health Managers', *Health Services Management Research* (2003; 16: 203–210)

Cooney, T. and O. O'Neill, *Psychiatric Detention: Civil Commitment in Ireland (Kritik 1)* (Wicklow, Ireland: Baikonur, 1996)

Crompton, F., 'Needs and Desires in the Care of Pauper Lunatics: Admissions to Worcester Asylum, 1852–72' in P. Dale and J. Melling (eds), *Mental Illness and Learning Disability: Finding a Place for Mental Disorder in the United Kingdom (Routledge Studies in the Social History of Medicine)* (London & New York: Routledge/Taylor & Francis Group, 2006) pp. 46–64

Cronin, M., L. Domegan, L. Thornton, M. Fitzgerald, P. O'Lorcain, E. Creamer and D. O'Flanagan, 'The Epidemiology of Infectious Syphilis in the Republic of Ireland', *Euro Surveillance: Bulletin Européensur les Maladies Transmissibles (European Communicable Disease Bulletin)* (2004; 9: 14–17)

Croudace, T.J., R. Kayne, P.B. Jones and G.L. Harrison, 'Non-Linear Relationship Between an Index of Social Deprivation, Psychiatric Admission, Prevalence and the Incidence of Psychosis', *Psychological Medicine* (2000; 30: 177–85)

Culliton, G., 'Review of Act is to be Built on "Human Rights"', *Irish Medical Times* (2011; 27 May)

Cunningham, M.D. and M.P.Vigen, 'Death Row Inmate Characteristics, Adjustment, and Confinement: A Critical Review of the Literature', *Behavioural Sciences and the Law* (2002; 20: 191–210)

Dale, P. and J. Melling, 'The Politics of Mental Welfare: Fresh Perspectives on the History of Institutional Care for the Mentally Ill and Disabled' in P. Dale and J. Melling (eds), *Mental Illness and Learning Disability: Finding a Place for Mental Disorder in the United Kingdom (Routledge Studies in the Social History of Medicine)* (London & New York: Routledge/Taylor & Francis Group, 2006) pp. 1–23

Daly, I., 'Implementing the Mental Health Act 2001: What Should Be Done? What Can Be Done?', *Irish Journal of Psychological Medicine* (2005; 22: 80–1)

Daly, R.J., 'Community Psychiatry and the National Institute of Mental Health', *Irish Journal of Psychological Medicine* (1990; 7: 5)

Damasio, A., *The Feeling of What Happens: Body, Emotion and the Making of Consciousness* (London: Vintage, 2000)

Davoren, M., S. O'Dwyer, Z. Abidin, L. Naughton, O. Gibbons, E. Doyle, K. McDonnell, S. Monks and H.G. Kennedy, 'Prospective In-Patient Cohort Study of Moves Between Levels of Therapeutic Security; the DUNDRUM-1 Triage Security, DUNRDUM-3 Programme Completion and DUNDRUM-4 Recovery Scales and the HCR-20', *BMC Psychiatry* (2012; 12: 80)

Dayan, L. and C. Ooi, 'Syphilis Treatment: Old and New', *Expert Opinion on Pharmacotherapy* (2005; 6: 2271–280)

Deacon, H., 'Insanity, Institutions and Society: The Case of the Robben Island Lunatic Asylum, 1846–1910' in R. Porter and D. Wright (eds), *The Confinement of the Insane: International Perspectives, 1800–1965* (Cambridge: Cambridge University Press, 2003) pp. 20–53

Deb, S., M. Thomas and C. Bright, 'Mental Disorder in Adults with Intellectual Disability. I: Prevalence of Functional Psychiatric Illness among a Community-Based Population Aged Between 16 and 64 years', *Journal of Intellectual Disability Research* (2001; 45: 495–505)

Dennett, D., *Consciousness Explained* (Boston: Little, Brown, 1991)

Department of Health, *Commission of Enquiry on Mental Illness 1966 Report* (Dublin: The Stationery Office, 1966)

Department of Health, *The Psychiatric Services – Planning for the Future* (Dublin: The Stationery Office, 1984)

Department of Health and Children, *Review of the Operation of the Mental Health Act 2001: Findings and Conclusions* (Dublin: Department of Health and Children, 2007)

Dewhurst, K. and J. Todd, 'The Psychosis of Association – Folie à Deux', *Journal of Nervous and Mental Disease* (1987; 74: 451–9)

Digby, A., 'Contexts and Perspectives' in D. Wright and A. Digby (eds), *From Idiocy to Mental Deficiency: Historical Perspectives on People with Learning Disabilities (Studies in the Social History of Medicine)* (London & New York: Routledge, 1996) pp. 1–21

Doherty, L., K.A. Fenton, J. Jones, T.C. Paine, S.P. Higgins, D. Williams and
    A. Palfreeman, 'Syphilis: Old Problem, New Strategy', *British Medical
    Journal* (2002; 325: 153–6)

D'Orban, P.T., 'Women Who Kill their Children', *British Journal of Psychiatry*
    (1979; 134: 560–71)

Dörries, A. and T. Beddies, 'The WittenauerHeilstätten in Berlin: A Case
    Record Study of Psychiatric Patients in Germany, 1919–1960' in R. Porter
    and D. Wright (eds), *The Confinement of the Insane: International Perspectives,
    1800–1965* (Cambridge: Cambridge University Press, 2003) pp. 149–172

Downs, L.L., 'PMS, Psychosis and Culpability: Sound or Misguided Defence?',
    Journal of Forensic Sciences (2002; 47: 1083–9)

Duffy D., S. Linehan and H.G. Kennedy, 'Psychiatric Morbidity in the Male
    Sentenced Irish Prisons Population' *Irish Journal of Psychological Medicine*
    (2006; 23: 54–62)

Dunne, J., 'Out-Patient Psychiatric Clinic – Report of Two Years' Work',
    Journal of the Irish Medical Association (1971; 64: 7–9)

Eberly, S.S., 'Fairies and the Folklore of Disability: Changelings, Hybrids and
    the Solitary Fairy', *Folklore* (1988; 99: 58–77)

Edelman, G., *The Remembered Present* (New York: Basic Books, 1989)

Edemariam, A., 'I'm Ready', *Guardian* (20 September 2006)

Egan, M., 'The "Manufacture" of Mental Defectives: Why the Number
    of Mental Defectives Increased in Scotland, 1857–1939' in P. Dale and
    J. Melling (eds), *Mental Illness and Learning Disability: Finding a Place for
    Mental Disorder in the United Kingdom (Routledge Studies in the Social History
    of Medicine)* (London & New York: Routledge/Taylor & Francis Group,
    2006) pp. 131–53

Eigen, J.P., 'Delusion in the Courtroom: The Role of Partial Insanity in Early
    Forensic Testimony', *Medical History* (1991; 35: 25–49)

Eigen, J.P., *Witnessing Insanity: Madness and Mad-Doctors in the English Court*
    (New Haven, CT: Yale University Press, 1995)

Eigen, J.P., 'Criminal Lunacy in Early Modern England: Did Gender Make
    a Difference?', *International Journal of Law and Psychiatry* (1998; 21:
    409–419)

Eigen, J.P., *Unconscious Crime: Mental Absence and Criminal Responsibility in
    Victorian London* (Baltimore, MD: Johns Hopkins University Press, 2003)

Eigen, J.P., 'Delusion's Odyssey: Charting the Course of Victorian Forensic
    Psychiatry', *International Journal of Law and Psychiatry* (2004; 27: 395–412)

Enoch, D. and H. Ball, *Uncommon Psychiatric Syndromes* (4th edition) (London:
    Hodder Arnold, 2001)

Expert Group on Mental Health Policy, *A Vision for Change*
    (Dublin: The Stationery Office, 2006)

Farmar, T., *Patients, Potions and Physicians: A Social History of Medicine in
    Ireland* (Dublin: A & A Farmar in association with the Royal College of
    Physicians of Ireland, 2004)

Farthing, M.J.G., D.J. Jeffries and J.M. Parkin, 'Infectious Diseases, Tropical
    Medicine and Sexually Transmitted Diseases', in P. Kumar and M. Clark (eds),
    Clinical Medicine (3rd edition) (London: BaillièreTindall, 1994) pp. 1–105

Fazel, S. and J. Danesh, 'Serious Mental Disorder in 23,000 Prisoners:
    A Systematic Review of 62 Surveys', *The Lancet* (2002; 359: 545–550)

Ferris, K., *James Joyce and the Burden of Disease* (Lexington: University Press of
    Kentucky, 1996)

Ferriter, D., *The Transformation of Ireland 1900–2000* (London: Profile
    Books, 2004)

Finkelhor, D., 'The Homicides of Children and Youth: A Developmental
    Perspective' in G.K. Kantor and J.L. Jasinski (eds), *Out of the Darkness:
    Contemporary Perspectives on Family Violence* (Thousand Oaks, CA: Sage
    Publications, 1997) pp. 17–34

Finnane, M., *Insanity and the Insane in Post-Famine Ireland* (London: Croon
    Helm, 1981)

Fleetwood, J.F., *The History of Medicine in Ireland* (2nd edition) (Dublin: Skellig
    Press, 1983)

Fleshner, M. and M.L. Laudenslager, 'Psychoneuroimmunology: Then and
    Now', *Behavioral and Cognitive Neuroscience Reviews* (2004; 3: 114–30)

Foley, S.R. and B.D. Kelly, 'Psychological Concomitants of Capital
    Punishment: Thematic Analysis of Last Statements from Death Row',
    American Journal of Forensic Psychiatry (2007; 28: 7–13)

Franzini, L.R. and J.M. Grossberg, *Eccentric and Bizarre Behaviours* (New York:
    John Wiley, 1995)

Fraser, W.I., 'Forensic Learning Disabilities: The Evidence Base: Executive
    Summary', *Journal of Intellectual Disability Research* (2002; 46 (Suppl. 1): 1–5)

Friedel, R.O., 'Dopamine Dysfunction in Borderline Personality Disorder:
    A Hypothesis', *Neuropsychopharmacology* (2004; 29: 1029–39)

Friedman, S.H, Horowitz, S.M. and P.J. Resnick, 'Child Murder by Mothers:
    A Critical Analysis of the Current State of Knowledge and a Research
    Agenda', *American Journal of Psychiatry* (2005; 162: 1578–87)

Gabbard, G.O. and J. Kay, 'The Fate of Integrated Treatment: Whatever
    Happened to the Biopsychosocial Psychiatrist?' *American Journal of
    Psychiatry* (2001; 158:1956–63)

Ganter, K., 'Implementing the Mental Health Act 2001: What Should be Done?
    What Can be Done?', *Irish Journal of Psychological Medicine* (2005; 22: 79–80)

Gasser, J. and G. Heller, 'The Confinement of the Insane in Switzerland,
    1900–1970: Cery (Vaud) and Bel-Air (Geneva) Asylums' in R. Porter and
    D. Wright (eds), *The Confinement of the Insane: International Perspectives,
    1800–1965* (Cambridge: Cambridge University Press, 2003) pp. 54–78

George, S.L., N.J. Shanks and L. Westlake, 'Census of Single Homeless People
    in Sheffield', *British Medical Journal* (1991; 302: 1387–9)

Gerbase, A.C., J.T. Rowley and T.E. Mertens, 'Global Epidemiology of
    Sexually Transmitted Diseases', *The Lancet* (1998; 351 (suppl. 3): 2–4)

Germine, M., 'Information and Psychopathology', *Journal of Nervous and Mental Disease* (1993; 181: 382–7)

Gibbons, P., N. Mulryan and A. O'Connor, 'Guilty but insane: The Insanity Defence in Ireland, 1850–1995', *British Journal of Psychiatry* (1997; 170: 467–72)

Giblin, Y., A. Kelly, E. Kelly, H.G. Kennedy and D.J. Mohan, 'Reducing the Use of Seclusion for Mental Disorder in a Prison: Implementing a High Support Unit in a Prison Using Participant Action Research', *International Journal of Mental Health Systems* (2012; 6: 2)

Gladstone, D., 'The Changing Dynamic of Institutional Care: The Western Counties Idiot Asylum, 1864–1914' in D. Wright and A. Digby (eds), *From Idiocy to Mental Deficiency: Historical Perspectives on People with Learning Disabilities (Studies in the Social History of Medicine)* (London & New York: Routledge, 1996) pp. 134–60

Glaser, W. and D. Flood, 'Beyond Specialist Programmes: A Study of the Needs of Offenders with Intellectual Disability Requiring Psychiatric Attention', *Journal of Intellectual Disability Research* (2004; 48: 591–602)

Goodey, C.F. and T. Stainton, 'Intellectual Disability and the Myth of the Changeling', *Journal of the History of the Behavioural Sciences* (2001; 37: 223–240)

Gordon, A.G., 'Swift's Pocky Queen', *Journal of the Royal Society of Medicine* (1998; 92: 102)

Grossberg, S. and J.W. Merrill, 'A Neural Network Model of Adaptively Timed Reinforcement Learning and Hippocampal Dynamics', *Brain Research. Cognitive Brain Research* (1992; 1: 3–38)

Guilbride, A., 'Infanticide: The Crime of Motherhood' in P. Kennedy (ed.), *Motherhood in Ireland* (Cork: Mercier Press, 2004) pp. 170–80

Gürses, C., M. Kürtüncü, J. Jirsch, N. Yeşilot, H. Hanağasi, N. Bebek, B. Baykan, M. Emr, A. Gökyiğit and F. Andermann, 'Neurosyphilis Presenting with Status Epilepticus', *Epileptic Disorders* (2007; 9: 51–6)

Guruswamy, S. and B.D. Kelly, 'A Change of Vision? Mental Health Policy', *Irish Medical Journal* (2006; 99: 164–5)

Gustafsson, L. and A.P. Paplinski, 'Self-Organization of an Artificial Neural Network Subjected to Attention Shift Impairments and Familiarity Preference, Characteristics Studied in Autism', *Journal of Autism and Developmental Disorders* (2004; 34: 189–98)

Harris, R., '"Risk", Law and Hygiene in late Nineteenth-Century France', *Society for the Social History of Medicine Bulletin* (1987; 40: 86–89)

Harris, R., *Murders and Madness: Medicine, Law and Society in the 'Fin de Siècle'*, (Oxford: Oxford University Press, 1989)

Healy, D., 'Irish Psychiatry. Part 2: Use of the Medico-Psychological Association by its Irish Members – Plus ca Change!' in G.E. Berrios and H. Freeman (eds), *150 Years of British Psychiatry, 1841–1991* (London: Gaskell/Royal College of Psychiatrists, 1991) pp. 314–20

Healy, D., 'Irish Psychiatry in the Twentieth Century' in H. Freeman and
    G.E. Berrios (eds), *150 Years of British Psychiatry: Volume II: The Aftermath*
    (London: Athlone Press, 1996) pp. 268–91

Hesketh, T. and W.X. Zhu, 'The One Child Family Policy: The Good,
    the Bad, and the Ugly', *British Medical Journal* (1997; 314: 1685–7)

Hesketh, T., L. Lu and Z.W. Xing, 'The Effect of China's One-Child Family
    Policy after 25 Years', *New England Journal of Medicine* (2005; 353: 1171–6)

Hodgson, B., *In the Arms of Morpheus: The Tragic History of Morphine, Laudanum
    and Patent Medicines* (Buffalo, New York: Firefly Books (US) Inc., 2001)

Hoff, J. and M. Yeates, *The Cooper's Wife is Missing: The Ritual Murder of Bridget
    Cleary* (New York: Basic Books, 2000)

Holland, T., I.C. Claire and T. Mukhopadhyay, 'Prevalence of Criminal
    Offending by men and Women With Intellectual Disability and the
    Characteristics of Offenders: Implications for Research and Service
    Development', *Journal of Intellectual Disability Research* (2002; 46 (Suppl. 1):
    6–20)

Holohan, T.W., 'Health and Homelessness in Dublin', *Irish Medical Journal*
    (2000; 93: 41–43)

Hook, E.W. and R.W. Peeling, 'Syphilis Control – A Continuing Challenge',
    New England Journal of Medicine (2004; 351: 122–124)

Hopkins, S., F. Lyons, F. Mulcahy and C. Bergin, The Great Pretender Returns
    to Dublin, Ireland', *Sexually Transmitted Infections* (2001; 77: 316–318)

Hopkins, S., F. Lyons, C. Coleman, G. Courtney, C. Bergin and F. Mulcahy,
    'Resurgence in Infectious Syphilis in Ireland: An Epidemiological Study',
    Sexually Transmitted Diseases (2004; 31: 317–321)

Horwitz, B. and A.R. Braun, 'Brain Network Interactions in Auditory, Visual
    and Linguistic Processing', *Brain and Language* (2004; 89: 377–84)

Houston, M., 'Mountjoy Team Wins Top Psychiatric Care Award', *The Irish
    Times* (2011; 6 October)

Hunter, R. and I. Macalpine, *Three Hundred Years of Psychiatry, 1535–1860: A History
    Presented in Selected English Texts* (London: Oxford University Press, 1963)

Hutto, B., 'Syphilis in Clinical Psychiatry: A Review', *Psychosomatics* (2001; 42:
    453–460)

Irish College of Psychiatrists, *People with a Learning Disability Who Offend:
    Forgiven but Forgotten? (Occasional Paper OP63)* (Dublin: Irish College of
    Psychiatrists, 2008)

Ishay, M.R., *The History of Human Rights* (Berkeley and Los Angeles:
    University of California Press, 2004)

Jackson, M., 'Institutional Provision for the Feeble-Minded in Edwardian
    England: Sandlebridge and the Scientific Morality of Permanent
    Care' in D. Wright and A. Digby (eds), *From Idiocy to Mental Deficiency:
    Historical Perspectives on People with Learning Disabilities (Studies in the
    Social History of Medicine)* (London & New York: Routledge, 1996)
    pp. 161–183

Jackson, M. (ed.), *Infanticide: Historical Perspectives on Child Murder and Concealment, 1550–2000* (Hampshire, England: Ashgate, 2002)

Jain, S., 'Psychiatry and Confinement in India' in R. Porter and D. Wright (eds), *The Confinement of the Insane: International Perspectives, 1800–1965* (Cambridge: Cambridge University Press, 2003) pp. 273–98

Jeffery, K.J. and I.C. Reid, 'Modifiable Neuronal Connections: An Overview For Psychiatrists', *American Journal of Psychiatry* (1997; 154: 156–64)

Johnston, S.J., 'Risk Assessment in Offenders with Intellectual Disability: The Evidence Base', *Journal of Intellectual Disability Research* (2002; 46 (Suppl. 1): 47–56)

Jones, G., 'The Campaign Against Tuberculosis in Ireland, 1899–1914' in E. Malcolm and G. Jones (eds), *Medicine, Disease and the State in Ireland, 1650–1940* (Cork: Cork University Press, 1999) pp. 158–176

Kaplan, H.I. and B.J. Saddock, *Concise Textbook of Clinical Psychiatry* (Baltimore: Williams and Wilkins, 1996)

Kelly, B.D., 'Mental Health and Human Rights: Challenges for a New Millennium', *Irish Journal of Psychological Medicine* (2001; 18: 114–5)

Kelly, B.D., 'Viewpoint: The Mental Health Act 2001', *Irish Medical Journal* (2002; 95: 151–152)

Kelly, B.D., 'Mental Health Policy in Ireland, 1984–2004: Theory, Overview and Future Directions', *Irish Journal of Psychological Medicine* (2004; 21: 61–8)

Kelly, B.D., 'Mental Illness in Nineteenth Century Ireland: A Qualitative Study of Workhouse Records', *Irish Journal of Medical Science* (2004; 173: 53–55)

Kelly, B.D., 'Physical Sciences and Psychological Medicine: The Legacy of Prof John Dunne', *Irish Journal of Psychological Medicine* (2005; 22: 67–72)

Kelly, B.D., 'Structural Violence and Schizophrenia', *Social Science and Medicine* (2005; 61: 721–30)

Kelly, B.D., 'The Power Gap: Freedom, Power and Mental Illness', *Social Science and Medicine* (2006; 63: 2118–28)

Kelly, B.D., 'Ireland's Mental Health Act 2001', *Psychiatric Bulletin* (2007; 31: 21–24)

Kelly, B.D., 'Murder, Mercury and Mental Illness: Infanticide in Nineteenth-Century Ireland', *Irish Journal of Medical Science* (2007; 176: 149–52)

Kelly, B.D., 'One Hundred Years Ago: The Richmond Asylum, Dublin in 1907', *Irish Journal of Psychological Medicine* (2007; 24: 108–14)

Kelly, B.D., 'Penrose's Law in Ireland: An Ecological Analysis of Psychiatric Inpatients and Prisoners', *Irish Medical Journal* (2007; 100: 373–4)

Kelly, B.D., 'Clinical and Social Characteristics of Women Committed to Inpatient Forensic Psychiatric Care in Ireland, 1868–1908', *Journal of Forensic Psychiatry and Psychology* (2008; 19: 261–73)

Kelly, B.D., 'Dr William Saunders Hallaran and Psychiatric Practice in Nineteenth-Century Ireland', *Irish Journal of Medical Science* (2008; 177: 79–84)

Kelly, B.D., 'Learning Disability and Forensic Mental Healthcare in Nineteenth-Century Ireland', *Irish Journal of Psychological Medicine* (2008; 25: 116–8)

Kelly, B.D., 'Mental Health Law in Ireland, 1821–1902: Building the Asylums', *Medico-Legal Journal* (2008; 76: 19–25)

Kelly, B.D., 'Mental Health Law in Ireland, 1821–1902: Dealing with the "Increase of Insanity in Ireland"', *Medico-Legal Journal* (2008; 76: 26–33)

Kelly, B.D., 'Mental Health Law in Ireland, 1945 to 2001: Reformation and Renewal?' *Medico-Legal Journal* (2008; 76: 65–72)

Kelly, B.D., 'The Mental Treatment Act 1945 in Ireland: An Historical Enquiry', *History of Psychiatry* (2008; 19: 47–67)

Kelly, B.D., 'Poverty, Crime and Mental Illness: Female Forensic Psychiatric Committal in Ireland, 1910–1948', *Social History of Medicine* (2008; 21: 311–28)

Kelly, B.D., 'Folie à Plusieurs: Forensic Cases from Nineteenth-Century Ireland', *History of Psychiatry* (2009; 20: 47–60)

Kelly, B.D., 'Syphilis, Psychiatry and Offending Behaviour: Clinical Cases from Nineteenth-Century Ireland', *Irish Journal of Medical Science* (2009; 178: 73–77)

Kelly, B.D., 'Criminal Insanity in Nineteenth-Century Ireland, Europe and the United States: Cases, Contexts and Controversies', *International Journal of Law and Psychiatry* (2009; 32: 362–8)

Kelly, B.D., 'Intellectual Disability, Mental Illness and Offending Behaviour: Forensic Cases from Early Twentieth-Century Ireland', *Irish Journal of Medical Science* (2010; 179: 409–16)

Kelly, B.D., 'Tuberculosis in the Nineteenth-Century Asylum: Clinical Cases from the Central Criminal Lunatic Asylum, Dundrum, Dublin' in P. Prior (ed.), *Asylums, Mental Health Care and the Irish, 1800–2010* (Dublin and Portland, Oregon: Irish Academic Press, 2012) pp. 205–20

Kelly, B.D., and S.R. Foley, 'The Price of Life', *British Medical Journal* (2007; 335: 938)

Kelly, B.D., 'Mental Health Need among the Intellectually Disabled', *Irish Journal of Medical Science* (2013; 182: 359)

Kelly, B.D. and S.R. Foley 'Love, Spirituality and Regret: Thematic Analysis of Last Statements from Death Row, Texas (2006–2011)', *Journal of the American Academy of Psychiatry and the Law* (2013; 41: 540–50)

Kennedy, H., *The Annotated Mental Health Acts* (Dublin: Blackhall Publishing, 2007)

Kennedy, L., 'Bastardy and the Great Famine: Ireland, 1845–1850', *Continuity and Change* (1999; 14: 429–52)

Kennedy, L., P.S. Ell, E.M. Crawford and L.A. Clarkson, *Mapping the Great Irish Famine* (Dublin: Four Courts Press Ltd, 1999)

Kerridge, I.H. and M. Lowe, 'Bloodletting: the Story of a Therapeutic Technique', *Medical Journal of Australia* (1995; 163: 631–3)

Kraya, N.A.F. and C. Patrick, 'Folie à Deux in Forensic Setting', *Australian and New Zealand Journal of Psychiatry* (1997; 31: 883–8)

Laffey, P., 'Two Registers of Madness in Enlightenment Britain. Part 2', *History of Psychiatry* (2003; 14: 63–81)

Langan-Egan, M., *Galway Women in the Nineteenth Century* (Dublin: Open Air (Four Courts Press), 1999)

Lawlor, B., 'Implementing the Mental Health Act 2001: What Should be Done? What Can be Done?', *Irish Journal of Psychological Medicine* (2005; 22: 79)

Leask J., A. Leask and N. Silove. 'Evidence for Autism in Folklore?', *Archives of Disease in Childhood* (2005; 90: 271)

Leonard, E.C. Jr., 'Did Some 18th and 19th Century Treatments for Mental Disorders Act on the Brain?', *Medical Hypotheses* (2004; 62: 219–221)

Lewis, D.O., J.H. Pincus, M. Feldman, L. Jackson and B. Bard, 'Psychiatric, Neurological, and Psychoeducational Characteristics of 15 Death Row Inmates in the United States', *American Journal of Psychiatry* (1986; 143: 838–45)

Lindsay, W.R., A.H. Smith, K. Quinn, A. Anderson, A. Smith, R. Allan and J. Law, 'Women with Intellectual Disability who have Offended: Characteristics and Outcome', *Journal of Intellectual Disability Research* (2004; 48: 580–90)

Lyons, F.S.L., *Ireland Since the Famine* (London: Fontana, 1985)

Lyons, J.B., 'James Joyce: Steps Towards a Diagnosis', *Journal of the History of the Neurosciences* (2000; 9: 294–306)

Macleod, S.M. and H.N. McCullough, 'Social Science Education as a Component of Medical Training', *Social Science and Medicine* (1994; 39: 1,367–73)

Madden, E., 'Section of Mental Health Act was Unconstitutional', *Irish Medical Times* (2009; 30: 15)

Malcolm, E., *Swift's Hospital: A History of St Patrick's Hospital, Dublin, 1746–1989* (Dublin: Gill and Macmillan, 1989)

Malcolm, E., '"Ireland's Crowded Madhouses": The Institutional Confinement of the Insane in Nineteenth- and Twentieth-Century Ireland' in R. Porter and D. Wright (eds), *The Confinement of the Insane: International Perspectives, 1800–1965* (Cambridge: Cambridge University Press, 2003) pp. 315–333

Marland, H., '"Destined to a Perfect Recovery": The Confinement of Puerperal Insanity in the Nineteenth Century' in J. Melling and B. Forsythe (eds), *Insanity Institutions and Society, 1800–1914: A Social History of Madness in Comparative Perspective* (London and New York: Routledge, 1999) pp. 137–156

Marland, H., *Dangerous Motherhood: Insanity and Childbirth in Victorian Britain* (Basingstoke: Palgrave MacMillan, 2004)

Masefield, W.G., 'Psychiatric Ruminations; The Presidential Address Delivered at the One Hundred and Sixth Annual Meeting of the Royal Medico-Psychological Association held at Eastbourne, 10 July 1947', *Journal of Mental Science* (1948; 94: 217–24)

McAuley, F., *Insanity, Psychiatry and Criminal Responsibility* (Dublin: Round Hall Press, 1993)

McCandless, P., 'Curative Asylum, Custodial Hospital: The South Carolina Lunatic Asylum and State Hospital, 1828–1920' in R. Porter and

D. Wright D (eds), *The Confinement of the Insane: International Perspectives, 1800–1965* (Cambridge: Cambridge University Press, 2003) pp. 173–92

McCarthy, A., 'Hearths, Bodies and Minds: Gender Ideology and Women's Committal to Enniscorthy Lunatic Asylum, 1916–1925' in A. Hayes and D. Urguhart (eds), *Irish Women's History* (Dublin and Portland: Irish Academic Press, 2004) pp. 115–136

McCauley, M., S. Rooney, C. Clarke, T. Carey and J. Owens, 'Home-Based Treatment in Monaghan: The First Two Years', *Irish Journal of Psychological Medicine* (2003; 20: 11–4)

McClelland, R.J., 'The Madhouses and Mad Doctors of Ulster', *Ulster Medical Journal* (1988; 57: 101–120)

McGarry, R.C. and P. McGarry, 'Please Pass the Strychnine: The Art of Victorian Pharmacy', *Canadian Medical Association Journal* (1999; 161: 1556–8)

McGuinness, I., 'Tribunals Revoke 12 per cent of Detentions', *Irish Medical News* (2007; 26 October)

McGuinness, I., 'Report Addresses Serious Challenges', *Irish Medical News* (2007; 29 June)

McInerney, C., M. Davoren, G. Flynn, D. Mullins, M. Fitzpatrick, M. Caddow, F. Caddow, S. Quigley, F. Black, H..G Kennedy and C. O'Neill, 'Implementing a Court Diversion and Liaison Scheme in a Remand Prison by Systematic Screening of New Receptions: A 6 Year Participatory Action Research Study of 20,084 Consecutive Male Remands', *International Journal of Mental Health Systems* (2013; 7: 18)

Meehan, E. and K. MacRae, 'Legal Implications of Premenstrual Syndrome: A Canadian Perspective', *Canadian Medical Association Journal* (1986; 135: 601–8)

Mela, M. 'Folie à Trios in a Multilevel Security Forensic Treatment Center: Forensic and Ethics-Related Implications', *Journal of the American Academy of Psychiatry and the Law* (2005; 33; 310–316)

Mentjox, R., van Houten C.A. and C.G. Kooiman, 'Induced Psychotic Disorder: Clinical Aspects, Theoretical Considerations, and some Guidelines for Treatment', *Comprehensive Psychiatry* (1993; 34: 120–126)

Michael, P., *Care and Treatment of the Mentally Ill in North Wales, 1800–2000* (Cardiff: University of Wales Press, 2003)

Michael, P., 'Class, Gender and Insanity in Nineteenth-Century Wales', *Clio Medica* (2004; 73: 95–122)

Michael, P., and D. Hirst 'Establishing the "Rule of Kindness": The Foundation of the North Wales Lunatic Asylum, Denbigh' in J. Melling and B. Forsythe (eds), *Insanity, Institutions and Society, 1800–1914: A Social History of Madness in Comparative Perspective (Studies in the Social History of Medicine)* (London & New York: Routledge/Taylor & Francis Group, 1999) pp. 159–79

Millon, T., *Masters of the Mind: Exploring the Story of Mental Illness from Ancient Times to the New Millennium* (Hoboken, New Jersey: John Wiley & Sons, 2004)

Mokyr, J., *Why Ireland Starved: A Quantitative and Analytical History of the Irish Economy, 1800–1850* (London: Unwin Hyman, 1985)

Moran, R., *Knowing Right from Wrong: The Insanity Defence of Daniel McNaughtan* (New York: Free Press, 1981)

Muir, R., 'The Changeling Myth and the Pre-Psychology of Parenting', *British Journal of Medical Psychology* (1982; 55: 97–104)

Mulholland, M., *To Comfort Always: A History of Holywell Hospital, 1898–1998* (Ballymena: Homefirst Community Trust, 1998)

Mulryan, N., P. Gibbons and A. O'Connor, 'Infanticide and Child Murder – Admissions to the Central Mental Hospital, 1850–2000', *Irish Journal of Psychological Medicine* (2002; 19: 8–12)

Munro, A., *Delusional Disorder: Paranoia and Related Illnesses* (Cambridge: Cambridge University Press, 1999)

Myers, F., *On the Borderline? People with Learning Disabilities and/or Autism Spectrum Disorders in Secure Forensic and Other Specialist Settings* (Edinburgh: The Stationery Office/Scottish Development Centre for Mental Health, 2004)

Ní Mhaoláin, Á. and B.D. Kelly, 'Ireland's Mental Health Act 2001: Where Are We Now?', *Psychiatric Bulletin* (2009; 33: 161–164)

O'Neill, A-M., *Irish Mental Health Law* (Dublin: First Law, 2005)

O'Neill, C., H., Sinclair, A. Kelly and H. Kennedy, 'Interaction of Forensic and General Psychiatric Services in Ireland: Learning the Lessons or Repeating the Mistakes?' *Irish Journal of Psychological Medicine* (2002; 19: 48–54)

O'Shea, B., 'The Mental Health Act, 2001: A Brief Summary', *Irish Medical Journal* (2002; 5: 153)

Oppenheim, J., *Shattered Nerves: Doctors, Patients and Depression in Victorian England* (New York and Oxford: Oxford University Press, 1991)

Owens, J., 'Implementing the Mental Health Act 2001: What Should be Done? What Can be Done?', *Irish Journal of Psychological Medicine* (2005; 22: 81–2)

Payne, H. and R. Luthe, 'Isaac Ray and Forensic Psychiatry in the United States', *Forensic Science International* (1980; 15: 115–127)

Pearsall, J. and B. Trumble, *The Oxford English Reference Dictionary* (2nd edition) (Oxford and New York: Oxford University Press, 1996)

Perr I.N., 'The Insanity Defence: A Tale of Two Cities', *American Journal of Psychiatry* (1983; 140: 873–4)

Porter, R., *A Social History of Madness: Stories of the Insane* (London: Phoenix, 1996)

Porter, R., *Madness: A Brief History* (Oxford: Oxford University Press, 2002)

Porter, R., *Madmen: A Social History of Madhouses, Mad-Doctors and Lunatics* (Gloucestershire, UK: Tempus Publishing, 2004)

Prestwich, P.E., 'Family Strategies and Medical Power: "Voluntary" Committal in a Parisian Asylum, 1876–1914' in R. Porter and D. Wright (eds), *The Confinement of the Insane: International Perspectives, 1800–1965* (Cambridge: Cambridge University Press, 2003) pp. 79–99

Prior, P., 'Dangerous Lunacy: The Misuse of Mental Health Law in

Nineteenth-Century Ireland', *Journal of Forensic Psychiatry and Psychology*
    (2003; 14: 525-41)

Prior, P., 'Prisoner or Lunatic? The Official Debate on the Criminal Lunatic in
    Nineteenth-Century Ireland', *History of Psychiatry* (2004; 15: 177–92)

Prior, P., 'Murder and Madness: Gender and the Insanity Defence in
    Nineteenth-Century Ireland', *New Hibernia Review* (2005; 9: 19–36)

Prior, P., 'Roasting a Man Alive: The Case of Mary Reilly, Criminal Lunatic',
    Éire-Ireland (2006; 41: 169–91)

Prior, P.M., *Madness and Gender: Gender, Crime and Mental Disorder in Nineteenth-
    Century Ireland* (Dublin and Portland, Oregon: Irish Academic Press, 2008)

Putkonen, H., J. Collander, M.L Honkaslo and J. Lonnqvist, 'Finnish Female
    Homicide Offenders, 1982–1992', *Journal of Forensic Psychiatry* (1998; 9:
    672–684)

Quen, J.M., 'Isaac Ray: Have We Learned His Lessons?' *Bulletin of the
    American Academy of Psychiatry and the Law* (1974; 2: 137–47)

Quen, J.M., 'Isaac Ray and the Development of American Psychiatry and the
    Law', *Psychiatric Clinics of North America* (1983; 6: 527–37)

Quen, J.M., 'Law and Psychiatry in America Over the Past 150 Years', *Hospital
    and Community Psychiatry* (1994; 45: 1005–10)

Quetel, C., *The History of Syphilis* (Oxford: Polity Press, 1990)

Quin, J.D., 'James Joyce: Seronegative Arthropathy or Syphilis?' *Journal of the
    History of Medicine and Allied Sciences* (1991; 46: 86–88)

Rehman, A.U., D. St Clair and C. Platz, 'Puerperal Insanity in the 19th and
    20th Centuries', *British Journal of Psychiatry* (1990; 156: 861–865)

Renvoize, E., 'The Association of Medical Officers of Asylums and Hospitals
    for the Insane, the Medico-Psychological Association, and their Presidents'
    in G.E. Berrios and H. Freeman (eds), *150 years of British Psychiatry,
    1841–1991* (London: Gaskell/Royal College of Psychiatrists, 1991) pp. 29–78

Resnick, P., 'Murder of the Newborn: A Psychiatric Review of Neonaticide',
    American Journal of Psychiatry (1970; 126: 1414–20)

Reuber, M., 'The Architecture of Psychological Management: The Irish
    Asylums (1801–1922)', *Psychological Medicine* (1996; 26: 1179–89)

Reuber, M., 'Moral Management and the "Unseen Eye": Public Lunatic Asylums
    in Ireland, 1800–1845' in E. Malcolm and G. Jones (eds), *Medicine, Disease and
    the State in Ireland, 1650–1940* (Cork: Cork University Press, 1999) pp. 208–33

Reynolds, J., *Grangegorman: Psychiatric Care in Dublin since 1815*
    (Dublin: Institute of Public Administration in association with Eastern
    Health Board, 1992)

Riches, V.C., T.R. Parmenter, M. Wiese and R.J. Stancliffe, 'Intellectual
    Disability and Mental Illness in the NSW Criminal Justice System',
    International Journal of Law and Psychiatry (2006; 29: 386–396)

Ritson, E.B., J.D. Chick and I. Strang, 'Dependence on Alcohol and Other
    Drugs' in R.E. Kendell and A.K. Zealley (eds), *Companion to Psychiatric
    Studies* (5th edition) (Edinburgh: Churchill Livingstone, 1996) pp. 359–96

Robins, J., *Fools and Mad: A History of the Insane in Ireland* (Dublin: Institute of Public Administration, 1986)

Robinson, D., *Wild Beasts and Idle Humors: The Insanity Defence from Antiquity to the Present* (Cambridge, Massachusetts: Harvard University Press, 1998)

Rothschild, B.M., 'History of Syphilis', *Clinical Infectious Diseases* (2005; 40: 1454–63)

Ryan, L., 'The Press, Police and Prosecution: Perspectives on Infanticide in the 1920s' in A. Hayes and D. Urquhart (eds), *Irish Women's History* (Dublin and Portland, OR: Irish Academic Press, 2004) pp. 137–51

Schwartz, L.L. and N.K. Isser, *Endangered Children: Neonaticide, Infanticide and Filicide (Pacific Institute Series on Forensic Psychology)* (Boca Raton, FL: CRC Press Inc., 2000)

Scull, A.T., *Museums of Madness: The Social Organization of Insanity in Nineteenth-Century England* (London: Allen Lane, 1979)

Scull, A., *The Most Solitary of Afflictions: Madness and Society in Britain, 1700–1900* (New Haven and London: Yale University Press, 1993)

Shorter, E., *A History of Psychiatry: From the Era of the Asylum to the Age of Prozac* (New York: John Wiley & Sons, 1997)

Simmons, H.G., 'Explaining Social Policy: The English Mental Deficiency Act of 1913', *Journal of Social History* (1978; 11: 387–403)

Singh, A.E., K. Sutherland, B. Lee, J.L. Robinson and T. Wong, 'Resurgence of Congenital Syphilis in Alberta', *Canadian Medical Association Journal* (2007; 177: 33–36)

Skalevag, S.A., 'The Matter of Forensic Psychiatry: A Historical Enquiry', *Medical History* (2006; 50: 49–68)

Slovenko, R., *Psychiatry in Law/Law in Psychiatry* (New York: Routledge, 2002)

Smith, C., 'The Central Mental Hospital, Dundrum, Dublin' in R. Bluglass and P. Bowden (eds), *Principles and Practice of Forensic Psychiatry* (Edinburgh: Churchill Livingstone, 1990) pp. 1351–3

Smith, R., 'Scientific Thought and the Boundary of Insanity and Criminal Responsibility', *Psychological Medicine* (1980; 10: 15–23)

Smith, R., 'The Victorian Controversy about the Insanity Defence', *Journal of the Royal Society of Medicine* (1988; 81: 70–73)

Smith, R.P., 'The Presidential Address, on Paranoia, Delivered at the Sixty-third Annual Meeting of the Medico-Psychological Association, Held in London on July 21 and 22, 1904', *Journal of Mental Science* (1904; L: 607–33)

Sneader, W., 'The Prehistory of Psychotherapeutic Agents', *Journal of Psychopharmacology* (1990; 4: 115–9)

Spence, B., 'Presidential Address to the Medico-Psychological Association', *Journal of Mental Science* (1899; XLV: 635–42)

Spiegel, A.D., 'Temporary Insanity and Premenstrual Syndrome: Medical Testimony in an 1865 Murder Trial', *New York State Journal of Medicine* (1988; 88: 482–92)

Spiegel, A.D., 'Abraham Lincoln and the Insanity Plea', *Journal of Community Health* (1994; 19: 201–20)

Spiegel, A.D. and F. Kavaler, 'A. Lincoln, Esquire Defends the Murderer of a Physician', *Journal of Community Health* (2005; 30: 309–24)

Spiegel, A.D. and F. Kavaler, 'The Differing Views on Insanity of Two Nineteenth-Century Forensic Psychiatrists', *Journal of Community Health* (2006; 31: 430–51)

Spiegel, A.D. and M.B. Spiegel, 'Was it Murder or Insanity? Reactions to a Successful Paroxysmal Insanity Plea in 1865', *Women and Health* (1992; 18: 69–86)

Spiegel, A.D. and M.B. Spiegel, 'The Insanity Plea in Early Nineteenth-Century America', *Journal of Community Health* (1998; 23: 227–47)

Stone, M.H., *Healing the Mind: A History of Psychiatry from Antiquity to the Present* (London: Pimlico, 1998)

Steering Group on the Review of the Mental Health Act 2001, *Interim Report of the Steering Group on the Review of the Mental Health Act 2001* (Dublin: Department of Health, 2012)

Stone, J., K. O'Shea, S. Roberts, J. O'Grady and A. Taylor (eds), *Faulk's Basic Forensic Psychiatry* (3rd edition) (Oxford: Blackwell Sciences, 2000)

Suzuki, A., 'The State, Family, and the Insane in Japan, 1900–1945' in R. Porter and D. Wright (eds), *The Confinement of the Insane: International Perspectives, 1800–1965* (Cambridge: Cambridge University Press, 2003) pp. 193–225

Taylor, P.J. and J. Gunn, 'Violence and Psychosis, I: Risk of Violence Among Psychotic Men', *British Medical Journal (Clinical Research Edition)* (1984; 288: 1945–9)

Teesson, M., T. Hodde and N. Buhrich, 'Psychiatric Disorders in Homeless Men and Women in Inner Sydney', *Australian and New Zealand Journal of Psychiatry* (2004; 38: 162–8)

Tempest, M., *The Future of the NHS* (Hertfordshire: XPL Publishing, 2006)

Teplin, L.A., 'Criminalizing Mental Disorder: The Comparative Arrest Rate of the Mentally Ill', *American Psychologist* (1984; 39: 794–803)

Thorne, M.L., 'Colonizing the New World of NHS Management: The Shifting Power of Professionals', *Health Services Management Research* (2002; 15, 14–26)

Tikhonova, L., E. Salakhov, K. Southwick, A. Shakarishvili, C. Ryan and S. Hillis for the Congenital Syphilis Investigation Team, 'Congenital Syphilis in the Russian Federation: Magnitude, Determinants, and Consequences', *Sexually Transmitted Infections* (2003; 79: 106–10)

Torrey, E.F. and J. Miller, *The Invisible Plague: The Rise of Mental Illness from 1750 to the Present* (New Brunswick, New Jersey: Rutgers University Press, 2001)

Tschinkel, S., M. Harris, J. Le Noury and D. Healy, 'Postpartum Psychosis: Two Cohorts Compared, 1875–1924 and 1994–2005', *Psychological Medicine* (2007; 37: 529–36)

Turner, F.D., 'Mental Deficiency: Presidential Address at the 92nd Annual
    Meeting of the Royal Medico-Psychological Association, July, 1933',
    Journal of Mental Science (1933; 79: 563–77)

United Nations, *Principles for the Protection of Persons with Mental Illness and the
    Improvement of Mental Health Care* (New York: United Nations, Secretariat
    Centre For Human Rights, 1991)

United States Bureau of the Census, *Historical Statistics of the United States, Colonial
    Times to 1970, Bicentennial Edition, Part 2* (Washington, DC: GPO, 1975)

Viney, M., 'Mental illness: An Enquiry', *The Irish Times* (1968; October 23–30)

Wade, N.J., 'The Original Spin Doctors – The Meeting of Perception and
    Insanity', *Perception* (2005; 34: 253–60)

Wade, N.J., U. Norrsell and A. Presly, 'Cox's Chair: "A Moral and a Medical
    Mean in the Treatment of Maniacs"', *History of Psychiatry* (2005; 16: 73–88)

Waisbren, B.A. and F.L. Walzl, 'Paresis and the Priest. James Joyce's Symbolic use
    of Syphilis in "The Sisters"', *Annals of Internal Medicine* (1974; 80: 758–62)

Walsh, D., 'The Ups and Downs of Schizophrenia in Ireland', *Irish Journal of
    Psychiatry* (1992; 13: 12–16)

Walsh, D., 'Mental Illness in Ireland and its Management' in D. McCluskey
    (ed.), *Health Policy and Practice in Ireland* (Dublin: University College
    Dublin Press, 2006) pp. 29–43

Walsh, D., 'The Ennis District Lunatic Asylum and the Clare Workhouse
    Lunatic Asylums in 1901', *Irish Journal of Psychological Medicine* (2010; 26:
    206–211)

Walsh, D. and A. Daly, *Mental Illness in Ireland 1750-2002: Reflections on the Rise
    and Fall of Institutional Care* (Dublin: Health Research Board, 2004)

Walsh, O., '"A Lightness of Mind": Gender and Insanity in Nineteenth-
    Century Ireland' in M. Kelleher and J.H. Murphy (eds), *Gender Perspectives
    in 19th Century Ireland: Public and Private Spheres* (Dublin: Irish Academic
    Press, 1997) pp. 159–67

Walsh, O., '"The Designs of Providence": Race, Religion and Irish Insanity'
    in J. Melling and B. Forsythe (eds), *Insanity Institutions and Society,
    1800–1914: A Social History of Madness in Comparative Perspective* (London
    and New York: Routledge, 1999) pp. 223–42

Walsh, O., 'Gender and Insanity in Nineteenth-Century Ireland', *Clio Medica*
    (2004; 73: 69–93)

Ward, N.S., 'Functional Reorganization of the Cerebral Motor System after
    Stroke', *Current Opinion in Neurology* (2004; 17: 725–30)

Watson, A.S., 'The Evolution of Legal Methods for Dealing with Mind-States
    in Crimes', *Bulletin of the American Academy of Psychiatry and the Law*
    (1992; 20: 211–20)

Waugh, M.A., 'Alfred Fournier, 1832–1914: His Influence on Venereology',
    British Journal of Venereal Disease (1974; 50: 232–6)

Weber, M.M. and H.M. Emrich, 'Current and Historical Concepts of
    Opiate Treatment in Psychiatric Disorders', *International Journal of Clinical*

Psychopharmacology (1988; 3: 255–66)

Whelan, D., 'Mental Health Tribunals: A Significant Medico-Legal Change', *Medico-Legal Journal of Ireland* (2004; 10: 84–89)

White, R., 'The Trial of Abner Baker, Jr., MD: Monomania and McNaughtan Rules in Antebellum America', *Bulletin of the American Academy of Psychiatry and the Law* (1990; 18: 223–34)

White P., D. Chant, N. Edwards, C. Townsend and G. Waghorn, 'Prevalence of Intellectual Disability and Comorbid Mental Illness in an Australian Community Sample', *Australian and New Zealand Journal of Psychiatry* (2005; 39: 395–400)

Wiglesworth, J., 'The Presidential Address, Delivered at the Sixty-first Annual Meeting of the Medico-Psychological Association, Held at Liverpool on July 24th, 1902', *Journal of Mental Science* (1902; XLVIII: 611–45)

Williamson, A., 'The Beginnings of State Care for the Mentally Ill in Ireland', *Economic and Social Review* (1970; 10: 281–90)

Williamson, A.P., 'Psychiatry, Moral Management and the Origins of Social Policy for Mentally Ill People in Ireland', *Irish Journal of Medical Science* (1992; 161: 556–58)

World Health Organisation, *The ICD-Classification of Mental and Behavioural Disorders* (Geneva: World Health Organisation, 1992)

World Health Organisation, *The World Health Report 2001. Mental Health: New Understanding, New Hope* (Geneva: World Health Organisation, 2001)

Wright, D., '"Childlike in his Innocence": Lay Attitudes to "Idiots" and "Imbeciles" in Victorian England' in D. Wright and A. Digby (eds), *From Idiocy to Mental Deficiency: Historical Perspectives on People with Learning Disabilities* (London and New York: Routledge, 1996) pp. 118–33

Wright, D., J.E. Moran and S. Gouglas, 'The Confinement of the Insane in Victorian Canada: The Hamilton and Toronto Asylums, *c.* 1861–1891' in R. Porter and D. Wright (eds), *The Confinement of the Insane: International Perspectives, 1800–1965* (Cambridge: Cambridge University Press, 2003) pp. 100–28

Wu, Z., K. Viisainen, Y. Wang and E. Hemminki, 'Perinatal Mortality in Rural China: A Retrospective Cohort Study', *British Medical Journal* (2003; 327: 1319)

Index